HISTOPATHOLOGY – REVIEWS AND RECENT ADVANCES

Edited by **Enrique Poblet Martínez**

Histopathology – Reviews and Recent Advances
http://dx.doi.org/10.5772/2991
Edited by Enrique Poblet Martínez

Contributors

Maria Isabel Tovar Martín, Miguel Juan Martínez Carrillo, Rosario Guerrero Tejada, Anca Maria Cimpean, Vitalie Mazuru, Lilian Şaptefraţi, Marius Raica, Abdolrasoul Talei, Majid Akrami, Maral Mokhtari, Sedigheh Tahmasebi, Alina Maria Sisu, Loredana Gabriela Stana, Codruta Ileana Petrescu, Romulus Fabian Tatu, Roxana Folescu, Andrei Motoc, Sharmila P. Patil, Nitin J. Nadkarni, Nidhi R. Sharma, Shivani Sangha, Amarjit Singh, Bruno Carvalho, Manuel Pontes, Helena Garcia, Paulo Linhares, Rui Vaz, Jesmine Khan, Mohammed Nasimul Islam, Watchariya Purivirojkul, Neiva Knaak, Diouneia Lisiane Berlitz, Lidia Mariana Fiuza, Mohammed M.A. Al Barbarawi, Mohammed Z. Allouh, Suhair M.A. Qudsieh, Wei-Wen Hung, Kun-Bow Tsai, Pi-Jung Hsiao, Hussein A. Kaoud

Published by InTech

Janeza Trdine 9, 51000 Rijeka, Croatia

Publishing Process Manager Dragana Manestar
Technical Editor InTech Prepress, Novi Sad
Cover InTech Design team

Additional hard copies can be obtained from orders@intechopen.com

Histopathology – Reviews and Recent Advances, Edited by Enrique Poblet Martínez
p. cm.
ISBN 978-953-51-0866-5

For EU product safety concerns:
IN TECH d.o.o., Prolaz Marije Krucifikse Kozulić 3, 51000 Rijeka, Croatia,
info@intechopen.com or visit our website at intechopen.com.

Meet the editor

Enrique Poblet Martínez is professor of pathology since the year 2002. He is currently affiliated with the Department of Anatomic Pathology at the School of Medicine and Dentistry of the Murcia University, Spain.

Contents

Preface

Histopathology, the discipline that studies the lesions that produce the pathological states in living organisms, is in expansion. It applies basic knowledge obtained from biological and anatomic science to make diagnosis, determine the severity and progress of a condition and to evaluate the possible response to certain therapies. Thus, it is not surprising that this discipline constantly expands with progress produced in biology. In addition, novel technologies that have been recently incorporated and the adoption of the histopathological methods by different areas contribute to enlarge the fields that may apply the histopathological methodology.

A major goal of the book is to bring together reputable researchers from different countries in order to provide a comprehensive coverage of advanced and modern topics in pathology.

The papers selected for this book comprise a cross-section of topics that reflect the variety of perspectives that histopathology contemplates. This book presents selected reviews of areas that cover topics that are considered relevant, and introduce novel concepts and descriptions of new entities.

The 13 chapters that have been selected for this book adequately review representative and diverse fields that are considered of special interest for their innovation or for their relevance in diagnostic pathology.

The 1st chapter, **"Human Papillomavirus Detection In Head And Neck Squamous Cell Carcinomas And Its Clinical Implications"**, deal with one of the hot topics of recent pathology. It has been shown that the presence of Human Papillomavirus (HPV) is a necessary event for development of cervical carcinoma. Although HPV has been detected in other genital tumours and in head and neck tumours, its presence is not constant, and it is controversial if detection of the virus may implicate it as an etiopathogenic factor. The chapter analyzes several methods for human papillomavirus detection, analyze the implications that this detection may represent, and review the biological and clinical aspects of human papillomavirus related with squamous cell carcinoma of the head and neck.

The 2nd chapter, **"Shadow Keyplayers of the Uterine Cervix Lesions Progression and Metastasis"**, is focused on early steps of angiogenesis and lymphangiogenesis in preneoplastic and neoplastic lesions of the uterine cervix.
Cervical neoplasia remains one of the most controversial issues for clinicians, pathologists, and researchers. Screening programs has been very important for reducing the incidence of invasive neoplastic lesions because these programs detect early, preneoplastic lesions that can bee properly treated. However, the rate of precursor lesions remains intact, and the study of some of the pathogenetic events that occur in these early stages of neoplasia are afforded in this chapter. Angiogenesis and lymphangiogenesis are accepted as important factors favouring tumor growth and metastases. But, questions about (i) startpoint of angiogenesis and lymphangiogenesis in cervical lesions, (ii) proliferative and/or activated status of cervical neovessels or (iii) the origin of lymph vessels and prognostic impact of lymphangiogenesis in precursor lesions of the uterine cervix still remain without a precise response. This interesting chapter afforded these important issues.

The 3rd chapter, **"Surgical and Clinical Pathology of Breast Diseases"**, describes in a precise manner pathological aspects of the most common breast diseases. In addition, some indications regarding the proper management that should be considered for the correct diagnosis of these lesions are included in the text. Selected illustrations that are present in the chapter emphasize the importance of histopathology in the diagnosis of breast lesions.

The 4th chapter, **"On the Bone Tumours: Overview, Classification, Incidence, Histopathological Issues, Behavior and Review Using Literature Data"**, reviews several aspects of bone tumours. Although metastatic bone tumours are frequent, primary bone tumours account for 0.2% of all malignant neoplasms in humans. The authors review their own case serie according to the World Health Organization classification. The most important thing in dealing with a bone tumour is a correct and full diagnosis as is shown in this chapter.

The 5th chapter, **"Nocardiosis: Clinical and Pathological Aspects"**, Nocardiosis is an opportunistic, localized or disseminated granulomatous infection caused by an aerobic actinomycete. The chapter represents a comprehensive review of this infection. Although nocardiosis infection most commonly occurs through the respiratory tract, manifestations of disease range from cutaneous infection caused by traumatic inoculation of the organism in a normal host, to severe hematogenous spread, or to pulmonary or central nervous system disease in an immunocompromised host. The chapter review several aspects of epidemiology, microbiology, pathogenesis, clinical features, and treatment related to nocardiosis.

The 6th chapter, **"Cytopathology of Canine Mammary Gland Affections"**, represent a structured description of a novel, useful, and affordable technique used for diagnosis of tumours. The chapter review fine needle aspiration cytology as a quick, inexpensive, and easily repeatable diagnostic technique for diagnosis of mammary gland affections in dogs. All technical aspects of the fine needle aspiration cytology technique are precisely described. The diagnostic value of cytology in mammary gland affections is emphasized showing that cytological interpretation is quiet helpful in rapid screening of the mammary gland affections, and in differentiating benign and malignant neoplastic lesions. The citological findings and the diagnostic interpretation of the fine needle aspirates complete this chapter, that is supported with very helpful illustrations.

The 7th chapter, **"Ossifying Fibromas of the Craniofacial Skeleton"**, afford a controversial issue because the accurate nature and classification of ossifying fibromas has undergone considerable debate among pathologists. This debate has produced a confusing evolution of competing nomenclatures. Authors of this chapter achieve to clarify this issue, and show that the definitive diagnosis can rarely be rendered on the basis of histopathologic features alone. Definitive diagnosis is usually dependent upon assessment of microscopic, clinical and imaging features together. Described subtypes vary with regard to behavior and propensity for recurrence after surgical excision. The chapter discusses the clinical, microscopic, radiological and therapeutic aspects of ossifying fibromas.

The 8th chapter, **"Morphology of the Intestinal Barrier in Different Physiological and Pathological Conditions"**, discuss the factors responsible for gut barrier dysfunction and possible morphological changes of the barrier during several conditions. Discussion is made in an attempt to provide a generalized idea of morphological changes during several conditions. Many harmful factors such malnutrition, chronic psychological stress, infections, or drugs are responsible for the damage of the gut barrier. Understanding the morphological changes of the gut barrier during various illnesses would enhance the knowledge of different preventive or therapeutic modulating agents of the gut barrier.

The 9th chapter, **"Histological Change of Aquatic Animals by Parasitic Infection"**, focuses on the category and diversity of the parasites that infect the aquatic animals. Histological methods are becoming quiet common in diagnostic methodology in aquatic animals. The author has collected more than 120 species of parasites from wild and cultured fish from freshwater and marine fish. The chapter discusses the port of entry and the site of localization into the host system. The degree of pathogenicity in relation to the histological observations detected is also analyzed.

The 10th chapter, **"Toxicology of the Bioinsecticides used in Agricultural Food Production "**, introduces a relatively new problem, that is the consequence of increases in the quantity of chemical pesticides required to control the losses in production caused by insect. The authors address the toxicological aspects of microbial and botanical biopesticides that act by ingestion with emphasis on histopathological analysis of tissues and cells in the alimentary channel of the Lepidoptera, as well as the specificity of the *Bacillus thuringiensis* bacteria, aqueous extracts and essential oil of medicinal and forest. For the application of plant and microbial toxins as biopesticides it is fundamental to evaluate the range of action and the specificity of the active ingredients.

The 11th chapter, **"Neuronal and Mixed Neuronal-glial Tumors of the Central Nervous System"**, proposes to review in an organized way, and according to the World Health Organization (WHO) Classification of Tumors, neoplasias of the central nervous system that show neuronal differentiation. The iconography used in this chapter is relevant, and emphasized the importance of the correct histopathological diagnosis for the proper management of these tumours.

The 12th chapter "**Calcitonin Expression in the Metastatic Tissue of Medullary Thyroid Carcinoma**" is a case report of a metastatic medullary carcinoma that fail to express the biomarker calcitonin. It includes the information about the calcitonin expression of medullary thyroid carcinoma and about thyroid carcinomas in general, which is interesting for this histopathology book.

The 13th Chapter "**Molecular Histopathology**" describes techniques of molecular pathology and their applications. It is well illustrated and useful source of information on this topic.

This book is the result of many collaborating parties. I gratefully acknowledge the assistance provided by all the authors that have contributed to the publication of this volume, and by the InTech editorial office that initiated this project and that has completed the book edition.

Enrique Poblet Martínez
Universidad de Murcia
Facultad de Medicina
Spain

Human Papillomavirus Detection in Head and Neck Squamous Cell Carcinomas and Its Clinical Implications

Maria Isabel Tovar Martín,
Miguel Juan Martínez Carrillo and Rosario Guerrero Tejada

Additional information is available at the end of the chapter

http://dx.doi.org/10.5772/50510

1. Introduction

Squamous cell carcinomas of the head and neck are a biologically heterogeneous group of cancers with a variable clinical course (Tran et al., 2007).

Human tumor viruses account for approximately one-fifth of all cancers worldwide (Psyrri & Tsiodoras, 2008). The first association between human papillomavirus and head and neck cancer was observed during the 1960s (Rabbett, 1965). A possible role for human papillomavirus in the etiology of cancers at other sites within the head and neck was first suggested by Löning et al., in 1985. Since then, mounting epidemiological, molecular, and clinical evidence indicates that high-risk human papillomavirus (especially human papillomavirus-16) account for the development of head and neck carcinoma in some individuals who do not have the classical risk factors for this disease (Psyrri & Dimaio, 2008).

Distinguishing human papillomavirus positive from human papillomavirus negative head and neck squamous cell carcinoma can provide prognostic information, because different studies have shown better clinical outcome among patients with human papillomavirus positive head and neck squamous cell carcinoma. Although there are innumerable options for human papillomavirus detection in head and neck squamous cell carcinoma, there isn´t any standardization of procedures to use in clinical practice. Several authors propose a testing algorithm of first screening for human papillomavirus using p16 immunohistochemistry, after positive p16 results confirmatory testing with polymerase chain reaction or similar technique is carried out (Pannone et al., 2012; Smeets et al., 2007).

The demonstration that human papillomavirus have a role in human carcinogenesis has allowed the development of preventive and therapeutic strategies aimed at reducing the incidence and mortality of human papillomavirus-associated cancers (Psyrri & Dimaio, 2008).

This chapter reviews the human papillomavirus detection in head and neck squamous cell carcinoma and its clinical implications. Our search strategy included an electronic search of MEDLINE (pubmed), to identify all published articles about this issue. We use the key words "Human papillomavirus", "head and neck neoplasm". We checked the titles and abstracs retrieved. Each author independently assessed the full text of studies relevant to this review.

2. Risk factors in head and neck cancer

The main risk factors for head and neck cancer globally are tobacco and alcohol (Dobrossy, 2005). These agents act by inducing mutations in key genetic pathways that govern normal cell turnover such as p53 and the product of the retinoblastoma gene (pRb) (Pfeifer et al., 2002)(figure1).

Approximately 20% of head and neck cancers occur in people lacking these established risk factors (Wiseman et al., 2003). There is strong epidemiologic and experimental evidence indicating that human papillomavirus accounts at least partly for this subset of cancers (Shanta et al., 2000), and it has suggested that human papillomavirus may be an independent risk factor for oropharyngeal carcinoma, as well as a modulator the malignancy process in some tobacco-and alcohol-induced oropharynx tumors (Turner et al., 2011).

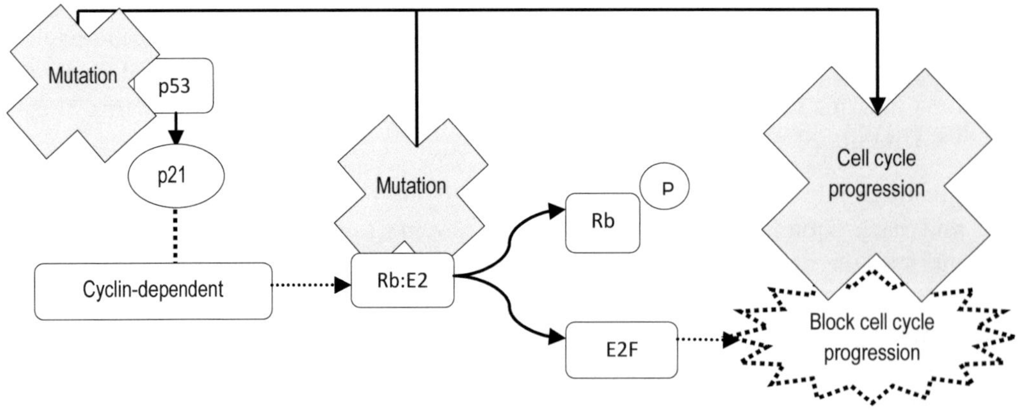

Figure 1. Inactivation of p53 and pRb by mutation by carcinogen agents. The p53 tetramers induce the expression of p21, which inhibits (dotted line) several cyclins. These cyclins induce the hyperphosphorylation of Rb, which normally binds to and inactives the E2F. The hyperphosphorylated form prevents the binding of E2F, which can then initiates uncontrolled cell division.

2.1. Human papillomavirus: Concept

Human papillomavirus is a member of the papillomaviridae family. They are small, non-enveloped, DNA viruses. They may be found integrated into the host genome, non-integrated or episomal, or as a combination or mixture of these types in infected tissue (Turner et al., 2011) [figure 2].

Mucosal human papillomavirus can be categorized in 2 major groups based on oncogenic potential: "low-risk" and "high-risk". Human papillomavirus 16 and 18 are the major "high-risk" types, which are associated with precancerous lesions (Tran et al., 2007; Psyrri & Tsiodoras, 2008; Psyrri & Dimaio, 2008; Snow & Laudadio, 2010).

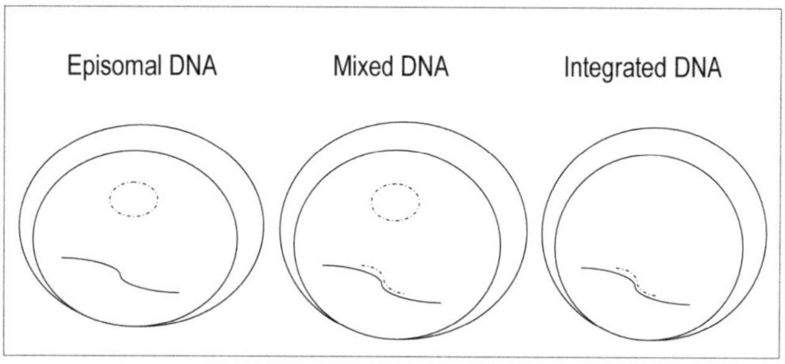

Figure 2. DNA viruses (dotted) and the host genome

2.2. Human papillomavirus life cycle and its role in the pathogenesis of head and neck squamous cell carcinoma (head and neck squamous cell carcinoma)

Through wounds or abrasions, the papillomaviruses infect basal epithelial cells. The viral DNA is maintained in the nuclei of infected epithelial cells (Stubenrauch & Laimins, 1999). human papillomavirus-DNA replicates to a high copy number only in terminally differentiated cells near the epithelial surface (Stubenrauch & Laimins, 1999). The late viral genes, which encode the L1 and L2 proteins that constitute the virus particle, are expressed only in the highly differentiated cells (Bedell et al., 1991).

Replication of the human papillomavirus genome is critically dependent on the host-cell DNA replication machinery (Cheng et al., 1995). The papillomavirus E1 and E2 proteins are required for viral DNA replication and papilloma formation (Wu et al., 1994). E1 is an ATP-dependent helicase that initiates viral replication in cooperation with the E2 protein. In addition, the E2 protein can function as a transcriptional repressor of E6 and E7 oncogene expression among other functions (Psyrri & Dimaio, 2008). E2 loss of function allows up-regulation of E6 and E7 oncoproteins (Pannone et al., 2012).

Transcription of human papillomavirus-16 E6/E7 mRNA in tonsillar carcinomas is not necessarily dependent on viral DNA integration, and the viral DNA is predominately in episomal form (Mellin et al., 2002). It has been also demonstrated that high risk human papillomavirus episomal DNAs up-regulate the activity of E6/E7 promoter, which in turn gives rise to elevated E6 and E7 protein expression in cancer cell (Pannone et al., 2012). Mellin et al (Mellin et al., 2002) concluding that in oropharyngeal carcinomas human papillomavirus is almost exclusively not integrates and its carcinogenic activity is due to E6/E7 oncoproteins expressed from episomal viral sequences. It is unknown whether the physical state of the virus influences tumor biology (Tran et al., 2007; Koskinen et al, 2003). However, the data suggested that a higher viral load cloud be a favourable prognostic indicator and that tumours with episomal DNA had larger tumours than patients with mixed or integrates forms of viral DNA. Higher copy number of episomal viral DNA was able to induce more rapid growth, perhaps by higher expression of the viral oncogenes (Pannone et al., 2011).

Human papillomavirus encode E6 and E7 proteins that create a state competent for DNA replication. The E6 protein of the high-risk human papillomavirus binds and induces the degradation of the p53 tumor suppressor protein via an ubiquitin-mediated process. E6 also activates telomerase allowing the regenesis of the ends of chromosomes after cell division. While, the human papillomavirus-E7 protein binds and destabilizes the retinoblastoma (Rb) tumor suppressor protein and related proteins. The molecular consequence of the expression of these viral oncoproteins is cell cycle entry and inhibition of p53-mediated apoptosis (figure 3). The E6 and E7 proteins also interact with other cellular targets. Together, these effects promote cell-cycle progression and viral DNA replication in differentiated keratinocytes (Tran et al., 2007; Leemans et al., 2011; Hobbs et al., 2006).

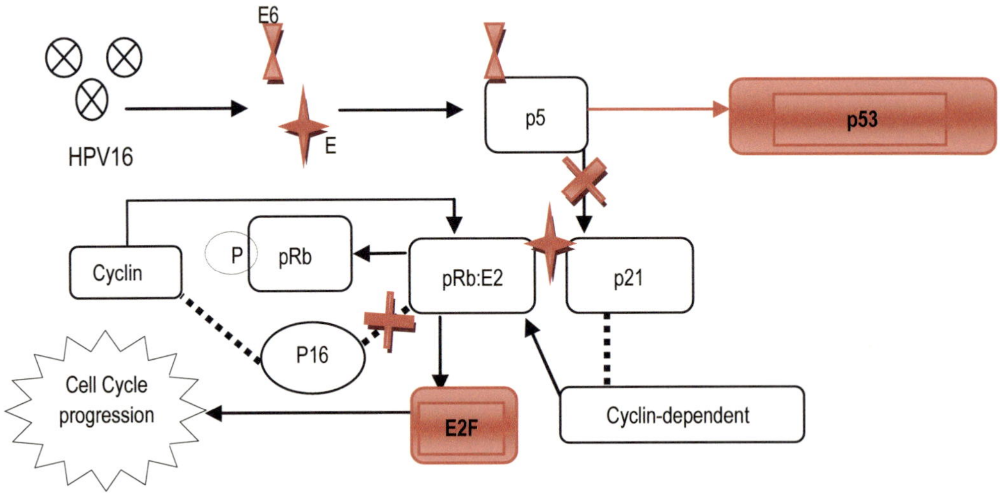

Figure 3. Inactivation of p53 by E6, inactivation of pRb by E7, and p16 over-expression. The E6 protein binds p53 and targets the protein for degradation, whereas the E7 protein binds and inactivates the Rb protein. pRB family proteins negatively regulate p16 gene expression. When E7 binds to pRB, this protein is inactivated, thus, p16 expression increase. Although p16 levels rise, normal feedback is by-passed, as human papillomavirus (HPV)-mediated cell proliferation is not dependent on cyclinD/Cdk4/6 (Dotted line = inhibition)

As a result, somatic mutation in TP53 (encoding p53), cyclin D1, and deletion or silencing CDKN2A (encoding p16) are established cancer genes in human papillomavirus-negative head and neck squamous cell carcinoma. In contrast, human papillomavirus-associated tumors are less likely to harbor TP53 mutation and the genes encoding the Rb family are established cancer genes in human papillomavirus-positive head and neck squamous cell carcinoma. In addition, human papillomavirus-positive head and neck squamous cell carcinoma has strong expression of p16 (as a component of the retinoblastoma tumor suppressor pathway) (Snow & Laudadio, 2010; Leemans et al., 2011). In the other hand, p16 expression loss defines a subgroup of head and neck squamous cell carcinoma patients with human papillomavirus-negative tumors.

So, the etiology of head and neck cancer is complex. Human papillomavirus, tobacco and alcohol represent three independent risk factors for head and neck carcinoma in the oral cavity and oropharynx.

The different risk factors can be combined. Smith et al (Smith et al., 2012) found that cancer in oral cavity or oropharyngeal risk was different among patients with several risk factors (Table 1). This investigation suggests that while risk of head and neck squamous cell carcinoma by tumor site is both different between oral cavity and oropharynx, both sites are nonetheless associated with independent effects for each of the three major head and neck squamous cell carcinoma risk factors.

The association between tobacco/alcohol, human papillomavirus, and tumor site is complex.

Oral Cavity/Oropharynx	*Human papillomavirus-positive*	*Human papillomavirus-negative*
Heavy alcohol user	**OR=3,5**/OR=4,7	**OR=1,4**/OR=11
Heavy tobacco user	**OR=9,8**/OR=8,5	**OR=3,1**/OR=24,3

Table 1. Risk of oral cavity and oropharyngeal carcinoma (Smith et al., 2012). OR=Odds Ratio

3. Epidemiologic and experimental evidence of an etiologic role for human papillomavirus in head and neck squamous cell carcinoma

Certain subsets of head and neck squamous cell carcinoma have fallen in parallel with the reduction in smoking, rates of oropharyngeal squamous cell carcinomas have risen by 2.1% and 3.9% among men and women respectively, from 1973 to 2001, particularly tongue and tonsillar cancers (Shiboski et al., 2005). Similarly, the incidence of tonsillar cancer increased by approximately 2–3% per year among men younger than 60 years from 1975 through 1998 (Canto & Devesa, 2002). In addition, the incidence of human papillomavirus-associated oropharyngeal cancer has increased between 1973 and 2004 (Chaturvedi et al., 2008).

These data suggest that human papillomavirus has emerged as an increasingly important cause of oropharyngeal cancer not only because tobacco-associated head and neck squamous cell carcinoma have decreased, but also because the incidence of human papillomavirus-associated oropharyngeal cancer is increasing (D'Souza & Dempsey, 2011).

This increase in the incidence of oropharyngeal cancer was paralleled by an increase in certain sexual behaviors. This change in the demographics of patients with head and neck squamous cell carcinoma is consistent with a role for genital human papillomavirus in the pathogenesis of oropharyngeal squamous cell carcinoma in individuals whose sexual practices are typically associated with sexual transmission of the virus (Psyrri & Dimaio, 2008). An elevated risk of oropharyngeal cancer has been associated with increasing number of sexual partners, younger age of first sexual intercourse, the practice of oral sex, and a history of genital warts (Trans et al., 2007).

One of the most important studies establishing the causal relationship between human papillomavirus and head and neck cancer was a multi-center case control study conduced by the International Agency for Research into Cancer (IARC) (Herrero et al., 2003). Findings confirmed that human papillomavirus-positive tumors cluster among non-smokers and nondrinkers.

There has been wide variation in human papillomavirus positivity rates in cancers at different sites within the head and neck. Approximately 25% of oropharyngeal cancers have tested human papillomavirus-positive, with rates in tonsillar cancer considerably higher (Trans et al., 2007). In fact, tonsillar crypts seem particularly susceptible to transformation by human papillomavirus, which is similar to the transformation zone of the uterine cervix, the location in which most cervical cancers originate (Psyrri & Dimaio, 2008).

4. Human papillomavirus detection

Since Syrjänen´s initial observations in 1983 (Syrjänen et al., 1983), there have been numerous reports on human papillomavirus-DNA detection in head and neck squamous cell carcinoma with rates varying from 0% to 100% of tumors studied (Clifford et al., 2003; Campisi et al., 2007). These differences in detection rate are due to at least two principal factors (Pannone et al., 2012):

1. Differences in the epidemiological distribution of oncogenic high risk human papillomavirus in the world
2. Different analytical methods utilized

So, there are nearly innumerable options for human papillomavirus detection in head and neck squamous cell carcinoma and no standardization of procedures to be used in clinical practice. The method choice depends greatly upon the desire information (test directed at identifying a broad group of high risk human papillomavirus or targeted at specific human papillomavirus genotypes), available tissue type (fresh tissue, fixed tissue, incision biopsy, brush cytology, saliva, serum, fine needle aspiration biopsy), the ubiquity and preservation of the candidate target molecule (DNA, RNA, and protein), and resources in (Snow & Laudadio, 2010; Robinson et al., 2010)

The **Southern blot** has long been considered the gold standard for detection of specific DNA sequence, however, with its technical demand, necessity for large quantities of DNA… Its use in clinical applications for human papillomavirus detection is rare (Snow & Laudadio, 2010).

Several **amplification techniques** (polymerase chain reaction [PCR]) have been developed for human papillomavirus type–specific using a specific primer set or for wide-spectrum human papillomavirus detection. Some of them adequately and equivalently amplify the target of interest, as L1 (late gene that encodes the viral capsid). However, multiple portions of the human papillomavirus genome, including L1, may be deleted in the process of integration to false negative results. For this reason, assays have been developed, which amplify portions of E6 and E7 (Snow & Laudadio, 2010). Many studies have shown reproductible results and high sensitivity with RNA-based assays (*reverse transcriptase polymerase chain reaction*) when using frozen tissue, but this material is not always available for testing. Multiple studies have compared RNA extraction from fresh or frozen tissue with that from formalin-fixed-paraffin-embedded tissue. The greatest decrease in RNA quality occurs immediately after fixation and processing (Snow & Laudadio, 2010).

Consensus polymerase chain reaction and genotyping is applicable to formalin-fixed-paraffin-embedded material and it has high sensitivity, however, it can detect of biologically irrelevant human papillomavirus, and the sample can be contaminated during biopsy acquisition. *Type specific polymerase chain reaction* has similar characteristics to consensus polymerase chain reaction. *Real time polymerase chain reaction* is applicable to formalin-fixed-paraffin-embedded material, it has high sensitivity and specificity, and it gives an estimate of the viral load, however, it requires tissue microdisecction and DNA extraction (Robinson et al., 2010).

The human papillomavirus-DNA test may be used in head and neck pathology departments with the following diagnostic and prognostic purposes (Reimers et al., 2007):

1. Distinguish human papillomavirus positive from human papillomavirus negative head and neck squamous cell carcinoma and providing prognostic information
2. Distinguish human papillomavirus positive metastases to the loco-regional lymph nodes derived from oropharyngeal cancers versus metastases of other origins
3. Furnish potentially useful indications for cancer treatment options
4. Contribute to the differential diagnosis of rhino-pharynx undifferentiated carcinoma (Worl Health Organization type I potentially related to human papillomavirus infection whereas Type II and III potentially related to Epstein Barr Virus)
5. Provide valuable information for head and neck cancer research

Table 2 shows the different types of primers (Hunsjak et al., 2000; Gravitt et al., 2003; Snow & Laudadio, 2010; Micalessi et al., 2012). Figure 4 shows the genomic structure of human papillomavirus.

Immunohistochemistry for the expression of viral human papillomavirus proteins as p16, E5, E6, E7 as surrogate markers of human papillomavirus infection. In the case of p16, human papillomavirus independent pathways of oncogenesis can lead to increased expression of p16 and the specificity is only 79% (Snow & Laudadio, 2010; Pannone et al., 2011). In fact, the immunohistochemistry detection of p16 protein has been proposed as surrogate marker of human papillomavirus infection in head and neck squamous cell carcinoma (Reimers et al., 2007).

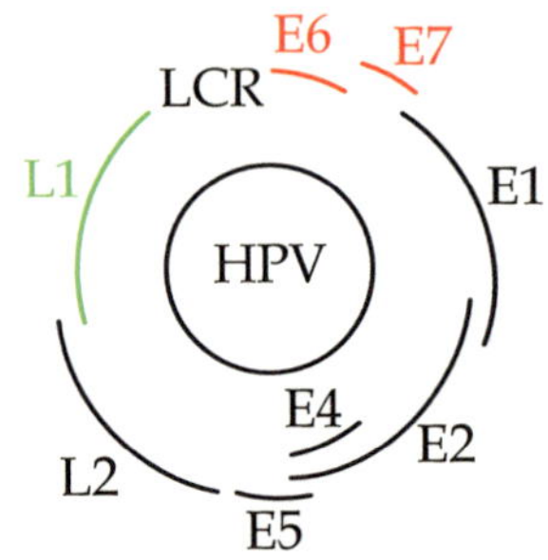

Figure 4. Genomic structure of human papillomavirus

Consensus Target: L1	*Degenerated* MY09, MY11 (450 base pairs) GP5+, GP6+ (140 base pairs)	*Not degenerated* SPF (65 base pairs)	***Advantages***: They have a larger spectrum of human papillomavirus detection. ***Disadvantages***: during the integration into the host DNA, parts of the L1 region may be deleted, contributing to false negative results. ***SPF:*** it has higher sensitivity compares to MY and GP because of its shorter amplification product (65 base pairs).
Specific Target: (for example: E6/E7)	Polymerase chain reaction directed at a single human papillomavirus The use of several specific primer pairs combined is called multiplex reaction		***Advantages***: they are available for target detection and type discrimination. ***Disadvantages:*** they require a polymerase chain reaction for each human papillomavirus type. ***Multiplex primer sets*** are directed at high or low-risk, but not specific human papillomavirus .

Table 2. Different types of primers.

In situ hybridization is a reproducible technique applicable to detection of a wide of human papillomavirus types particularly from formalin-fixed-paraffin-embedded tissues. However, in situ hybridization is considered method with a low sensitivity, because the low applicability in clinical routine for the long and hard technical word required in (Snow & Laudadio, 2010; Pannone et al., 2011).

A recent study (Pannone et al., 2012) has tested the reliability of a triple method which combines evaluation of p16 expression of viral human papillomavirus proteins by immunohistochemistry, human papillomavirus-DNA genotyping by polymerase chain reaction, and viral integration into the host by in situ hybridization. All the head and neck squamous cell carcinoma confirmed human papillomavirus positive by polymerase chain reaction and/or in situ hybridization were also p16 positive by immunohistochemistry. So immunohistochemistry showed a very high level of sensitivity as single test but lower specificity level. The double method, in situ hybridization and polymerase chain reaction increased significantly the specificity, but reduced the sensitivity. They observed different levels of p16-immunohistochemistry accuracy in the different cancer subpopulation studied. So, in a cohort of prevalently alcohol/tobacco associated cancers, p16-immunohistochemistry test showed a lower level of specificity in detecting human papillomavirus positive cases. In addition, a recent literature report demonstrates different p16 accuracy according to different anatomical sub-sites of head and neck region (Doxtader & Katzenstein, 2011). In this context, the p16-immunohistochemistry test alone could be used only as a screening method and need to be associated with molecular tests in order to detect human papillomavirus-DNA and to assess its integration status.

The hybrid capture technique is used extensively among pathology labs to detect 13 high-risk human papillomavirus genotypes in cervical cytology specimens. The use of this method is limited for head and neck squamous cell carcinoma human papillomavirus testing, but the technique has potential for screening oral brushings. However, at this time, oral brush cytology has not achieved a sensitivity or specificity sufficiently competitive with surgical biopsy for diagnosis and prospective studies are necessary to determine the clinical use of screening in (Snow & Laudadio, 2010; Pannone et al., 2011).

Luminex system combines PCR with hybridization to fluorescence-labeled polystyrene bead microarrays. This technology provides a new platform for high throughput nucleic acid detection and is being utilized with increasing frequency. It is a sensitive, reproducible technique for the simultaneous genotyping of all clinically relevant genital HPV types. However, these Luminex assays have shown low ability for type-specific genotyping and have missed variants with the type-specific probes. Multiple infections may occur in 20-40% of specimens. Luminex-based HPV genotyping can be used to differentiate between newly acquired HPV types and pre-existing infections when applied over time. Nevertheless, a limitation of the assay is the reduction of signal that occurs for a plasmid target in low abundance when it is amplified with another target that is 2 or 3 logs higher in abundance. This technology has been tested in cervical samples (Oh et al., 2007; Lowe B et al., 2010).

Human papillomavirus serology. The immune to human papillomavirus infection involves both the cell-mediated and humoral responses. Human papillomavirus seropositivity is potentially indicative not only of current oral infection but also of any past infection not limited to the oral cavity or oropharynx (Pannone et al., 2011). Antibodies to human papillomavirus E6 and E7 proteins are markers for an invasive human papillomavirus-associated cancer. The use of human papillomavirus viral load in conjunction with serological markers may serve to identify a subset of human papillomavirus-associated head and neck tumors in which human papillomavirus is biologically active (Ragin et al., 2007).

Table 3 resumes the characteristics of different methods for human papillomavirus detection (Dobrossy, 2005).

Method	Detect	Characteristics	Sample
Southern Blot	Specific DNA sequence	It needs large quantities of DNA. It don´t use in clinical practice. Low sensitivity	Frozen tissue
Polymerase chain reaction	Amplify particular DNA sequence	There are several sets. - *Consensus polymerase chain reaction*: high sensitivity, but it can detect biological irrelevant human papillomavirus. - *Type specific polymerase chain reaction*: as above - *Real time polymerase chain reaction*: high sensitivity and specificity, but it requires tissue microdissection and DNA extraction - *Reverse transcripase polymerase chain reaction*: high sensitivity and specificity, but adequate performance is limited to frozen tissue	Formalin-fixed-paraffin-embedded More accuracy in fresh frozen tissue for reverse trancriptase Polymerase chain reaction
Immuno-histochemistry	Viral human papillomavirus proteins	High sensitivity in screening. Specificity is low.	Formalin-fixed-paraffin-embedded
In situ hybridization	Specific DNA or RNA sequence	It has a low sensitivity	Formalin-fixed-paraffin-embedded
Hybrid Capture	High-risk human papillomavirus genotypes	It has potential for screening oral brushing. Lower sensitivity and specificity than surgical biopsy	Oral brush cytology
Serology	Cell-mediated and humoral responses	Minimally invasive test. It indicates human papillomavirus infection but not limited to the oral cavity or oropharynx. Low sensitivity and specificity.	Blood

Table 3. Characteristics of different methods for human papillomavirus detection

Establishing a diagnosis of head and neck cancer requires the acquisition of adequate biopsy material. Typically, tissue samples are fixed in formalin, processed in the laboratory and formalin-fixed-paraffin-embedded, whereas fine needle aspiration biopsy samples are usually treated with an alcohol-based fixative. So, for an human papillomavirus test to be useful it should be capable of reliably classifying 'human papillomavirus related' cancers in fixed cell and tissue samples. The techniques used should be reproducible, subject to standardization and quality assurance and be economically viable (Robinson et al., 2010).

The presence of the viral DNA does not establish causality, since the majority of human papillomavirus infections may be transient rather than persistent (Ragin et al., 2007). The important issue is that human papillomavirus is transcriptionally active (Trans et al., 2007; Hobbs et al., 2006). In fact, cases that are human papillomavirus positive but negative for p16 expression (or negative for E6/E7 mRNA) are molecularly more similar to human papillomavirus negative cases suggesting that in these instances human papillomavirus is not directly involved in carcinogenesis (Snow & Laudadio, 2010; Weinberger et al., 2006).

Detection of high-risk E6/E7 mRNA or protein would be the ideal test for classifying a tumor as truly human papillomavirus-associated, while it´s possible to perform quantitative polymerase chain reaction on formalin-fixed-paraffin-embedded samples the maximum accuracy is found using fresh frozen tissue (Pannone et al, 2012). Determination of p16 expression status by immunohistochemistry could serve as a reasonable surrogate marker for biologically relevant high-risk human papillomavirus infection (Psyrri & Dimaio, 2008).

Smeets et al (Smeets et al., 2007) propose a testing algorithm of first screening for human papillomavirus using p16 immunohistochemistry, after positive p16 resul'ts confirmatory testing with polymerase chain reaction is carried out. This approach had almost 100% sensitivity and specificity, with 2% risk of false positive. Others authors as Westra (Westra, 2009) propose confirmatory testing by in situ hybridization (Robinson et al., 2010). The majority of pathology laboratories have the capability of delivering the first algorithm.

Some authors are searching for other defining molecular characteristics. There is evidence that human papillomavirus positive head and neck squamous cell carcinoma tends to contain normal copies of the p53 gene (Braakhuis et al., 2004). However, p53 mutations have been described in these tumours (Westra et al., 2008). This presence of mutant p53 along with human papillomavirus infection in the same tumour raises the possibility that human papillomavirus infection is simultaneous and has no influence on pathogenesis (Robinson et al., 2010). Human papillomavirus viral oncoproteins are known to have epigenetic effects. They can silence the expression of key tumour suppressor genes by promoter methylation (Henken et al., 2007). The emergence of global genome methylation assays represents novel ways of refining the molecular classification of head and neck cancers in the future (Robinson et al., 2010).

5. Clinical implications

Several lines of clinical evidence also suggest that human papillomavirus-associated head and neck squamous cell carcinoma could be biologically distinct from classical head and neck squamous cell carcinoma (Table 4).

CHARACTERISTICS		HUMAN PAPILLOMAVIRUS +	HUMAN PAPILLOMAVIRUS -
MOLECULAR & HISTOPATHOLOGICAL	TP53 y RB1	Inactivation	Mutation
	p16	↑	↓
	Cyclin D1	↓	↑
	Histological grading	↑ Poorly differentiated tumours	Any
	Histotype	Often basaloid	Basaloid uncommon
CLINICAL	Sex	♂ y ♀ [or ♂ > ♀]	♂ >>♀
	Age	Younger [< 40 yrs]	Older
	Tobacco y alcohol	Generally NO	Generally YES
	Stage at diagnosis	Advanced and Later	Earlier
	Prognostic	Better	Worse

Table 4. Molecular & clinical characteristics in human papillomavirus + and human papillomavirus - head and neck squamous cell carcinoma

Several experiments delineated three biologically and clinically distinct types of oropharyngeal tumors (Weinberger et al., 2006) (Table 5):

		HUMAN PAPILLOMAVIRUS	
		Negative	Positive
P16 expressing	No	Class I	Class II
	Yes	Class IV	Class III

Table 5. Biologically and clinically distinct types of oropharyngeal tumors

- Class I, human papillomavirus-negative/p16 non expressing. Conventional head and neck squamous cell carcinoma with no evidence of human papillomavirus infection, typically exhibiting inactivation of p16, with p53 mutations and probably caused by tobacco and alcohol abuse.
- Class II, human papillomavirus-positive/p16 non expressing. Conventional head and neck squamous cell carcinoma that acquire simultaneous human papillomavirus infection late in its pathogenesis, with no consequences for p16 expression

- Class III, human papillomavirus-positive/ p16 expressing. "human papillomavirus related" head and neck squamous cell carcinoma that contains human papillomavirus DNA and shows evidence of oncogenic human papillomavirus protein expression, using p16 as a surrogate marker.
- Class IV, human papillomavirus-negative/p16 expressing. Small number of apparently human papillomavirus negative carcinomas that over express p16. There are two major reasons for this entity: a] misclassification as human papillomavirus negative, because the human papillomavirus test chosen lacks sensitivity, b] tumours where accumulation of p16 has been caused by perturbation of other cellular signaling pathways, or due to possible an as yet unidentified infectious agent.

Class III had the highest viral loads. The 5-year survival in class III was 79%, significantly higher than in the other two classes (20% and 18%, $P = 0.0095$). Disease free survival for class III was 75% compared with 15% and 13% for classes I and II, respectively ($P = 0.0025$). The 5-year local recurrence was 14% in class III compared with 45% and 74% ($P = 0.03$). Multivariate survival analysis confirmed the prognostic value of the three class model. It is clear that head and neck squamous cell carcinoma human papillomavirus-positive and p16 expressing is different from classic head and neck squamous cell carcinoma, but it is not clear whether head and neck squamous cell carcinoma human papillomavirus-positive and p16 non expressing (probably, tobacco/alcohol-related tumors that are infected by high-risk human papillomavirus) represents a group biologically distinct from human papillomavirus-negative tumors (Cheng et al., 1995). Other studies in (Smith et al., 2012; Harris et al., 2011) have confirmed better disease-specific and recurrence-free survival in human papillomavirus and/or p16 positive tumors.

About class IV, several studies (Reimers et al., 2007; Harris et al., 2011; Shah et al., 2009; Weinberger et al., 2004) have shown that patients with human papillomavirus negative and p16 positive tumors had better outcomes than patients with p16 negative tumors. So, p16 status could be the truly important prognostic marker in head and neck squamous cell carcinoma, independent of human papillomavirus infection.

For all this, p16 positivity has been proposed to be a more reliable and reproducible prognostic marker in head and neck squamous cell carcinoma (Harris et al., 2011).

On the basis of these results, we can refine a model for human papillomavirus-associated oropharyngeal cancer. The favorable outcome of human papillomavirus-induced oropharyngeal cancers might be attributable to the absence of field cancerization or enhanced radiation sensitivity (Lindel et al., 2001). In 1953, the term "field cancerization" was proposed to explain the high propensity to develop local recurrence after treatment of head and neck squamous cell carcinoma and the high likehood that multiple independent tumours will develop in the head and neck mucosa. This phenomenon is due to the presence of carcinogen induced early genetic changes in the epithelium from which multiple independent lesions arise (Slaughter et al., 1953).

Disrupting E6 and E7 in oropharyngeal cell lines results in increased levels of p53 and pRB and increased levels of p53-activated genes (Rampias et al., 2009). These findings indicate that in human papillomavirus-induced carcinoma the p53 and pRB pathways remain intact.

So, unlike tobacco associated oropharyngeal cancers that harbor mutant TP53, the apoptotic response of human papillomavirus-associated tumors to radiation and chemotherapy might be intact. Some authors have proposed that p16-expressing cells are less hypoxic and respond with less accelerated repopulation when irradiated (Lassen et al., 2009).

Given that the rate of p53 mutation is quite low in human papillomavirus-associated tumors, the addition of p53 mutation sequencing could have added valuable information had sufficient tissue been available (Harris et al., 2011). There have been conflicting data on p53 expression in human papillomavirus positive head and neck squamous cell carcinoma tumor cells. Some studies have observed high expression of nuclear p53 in some human papillomavirus-containing tumors with wild-type p53 (Hafkamp et al., 2003), and other studies demonstrating low p53 expression (Wilczynski et al., 1998). Mechanism of over-expression of wild-type p53 in the presence of the virus is known (Tang et al., 2011).

It has been suggested that less intensive treatment modalities should be examined in order to decrease treatment-toxicities. For that, the National Comprehensive Cancer Network Clinical Practice Guidelines in Oncology (USA) (Pfister et al., 2011) recommend that oropharyngeal squamous cell carcinoma is tested for high risk oncogenic human papillomavirus.

Furthermore, epidermal growth factor receptor expression has been suggested to be correlated with human papillomavirus status (Almadori et al., 2001). There are data suggesting a direct link between human papillomavirus-encoded proteins and epidermal growth factor receptor expression (Kim et al., 2006). Kumar et al (Kumar et al., 2008) reported the phenotype human papillomavirus positive and epidermal growth factor receptor high to be associated with poorer survival after chemotherapy and radiation than human papillomavirus positive and epidermal growth factor receptor low tumors.

Bonner et al (Bonner et al., 2010) tested the combination of cetuximab, a monoclonal antibody directed against epidermal growth factor receptor, and radiotherapy in head and neck squamous cell carcinoma. They demonstrated improved patient survival compared with radiation alone. The use of this combination increased skin irritation, but otherwise it had the same side effects as radiotherapy alone. An analysis of patients in this trial revealed that those with oropharyngeal squamous cell carcinoma who were male and younger, a group that mirrors the human papillomavirus-positive population, benefited most from the combination therapy. These results suggested that radiation plus cetuximab, instead of cisplatin-based chemotherapy, may reduce treatment toxicity without compromising cancer control for patients with human papillomavirus-positive oral squamous cell carcinoma. For this reason, Radiation Therapy Oncology Group (RTOG) has initiated a phase III randomized study of radiotherapy with cisplatin or cetuximab in patients with human papilloma virus-associated oropharyngeal cancer (RTOG-1016).

So, epidermal growth factor receptor, and p53 are also relevant markers that modify the prognostic effect of human papillomavirus and may help guide the development of targeted therapy in head and neck squamous cell carcinoma.

However, not all patients with human papillomavirus positive tumors respond well to therapy and the reasons for failure in some cases are not known (Maxwell et al., 2010). The variability of high risk human papillomavirus containing cell lines enhances our ability to study the role that human papillomavirus plays in head and neck squamous cell carcinoma development and response or resistance to therapy (Tang et al., 2011). Combination of several risk factors could explain this. A positive tobacco history in patients with human papillomavirus positive tumors may represent a distinct group of head and neck squamous cell carcinoma when all head and neck squamous cell carcinoma are divided by etiologic factors: human papillomavirus negative smokers, human papillomavirus positive never smokers, human papillomavirus positive ever smokers, etc… TPV status likely provided an additive and possibly synergistic effect with others risk factors (Tang et al., 2011).

In addition, in the patient with metastatic head and neck carcinoma of unknown origin, the presence of human papillomavirus in a fine needle aspiration biopsy sample can be used to direct the search to the oropharynx (Zhang et al., 2008).

All of this could lead to a new diagnosis and treatment algorithm (Figure 5).

Others implications are the preventions actions:

1. **Screening studies** have been performed in healthy adults using biopsy samples or less invasive saliva and oral lavage-based testing methods to identify human papillomavirus. These techniques revealed prevalence rate between 0-25% (Turner et al., 2011).

Detection of high risk human papillomavirus DNA may help identify individuals, including those with: a) any genetic predisposition to acquire high risk human papillomavirus infection and/or b) a limited immunologic ability to eliminate the virus. Whether oral exfoliated high risk human papillomavirus status is predictive of cancer before invasion or progression in patients with head and neck squamous cell carcinoma is unknown.

Quantitative measurement of salivary human papillomavirus16 DNA can be promise for surveillance and early detection of recurrence. Detection of high risk human papillomavirus in oral exfoliated cells may serve as clonal markers to monitor the presence of residual tumor after surgery or radiation, cancer recurrence, and progression (Pannone et al., 2011).

A recent study (Turner et al., 2011) recruited patients and screened saliva samples for high risk human papillomavirus using quantitative polymerase chain reaction. They confirmed human papillomavirus16, but not human papillomavirus18 in a small subset of the healthy adult patients. These patients were female and minority (2.6%).

2. **Prophylactic vaccines** that prevent persistent cervical human papillomavirus-16 infections might be effective in preventing these cases of head-and-neck cancer as well, either indirectly by eliminating an anogenital source of virus or directly by protecting the oropharyngeal epithelium itself from infection (Psyrri & dimaio, 2008).

In the U.S, two vaccines are currently available. The quadrivalent vaccine, Gardasil® (human papillomavirus4), protects against infection with human papillomavirus types -6, -11, -16, and 18. The second human papillomavirus vaccine, Cervarix® (human papillomavirus2), is a bivalent vaccine that provides protection against human papillomavirus types -16 and -18 in (D´Souza & Dempsey, 2011).

However, these vaccines do not alter the prognosis of established human papillomavirus infection. Therapeutic vaccines based on the viral oncogenes are still in the developmental stage, but they may eventually prove beneficial if used in association with conventional approaches for the management of advanced disease (Tran et al., 2007).

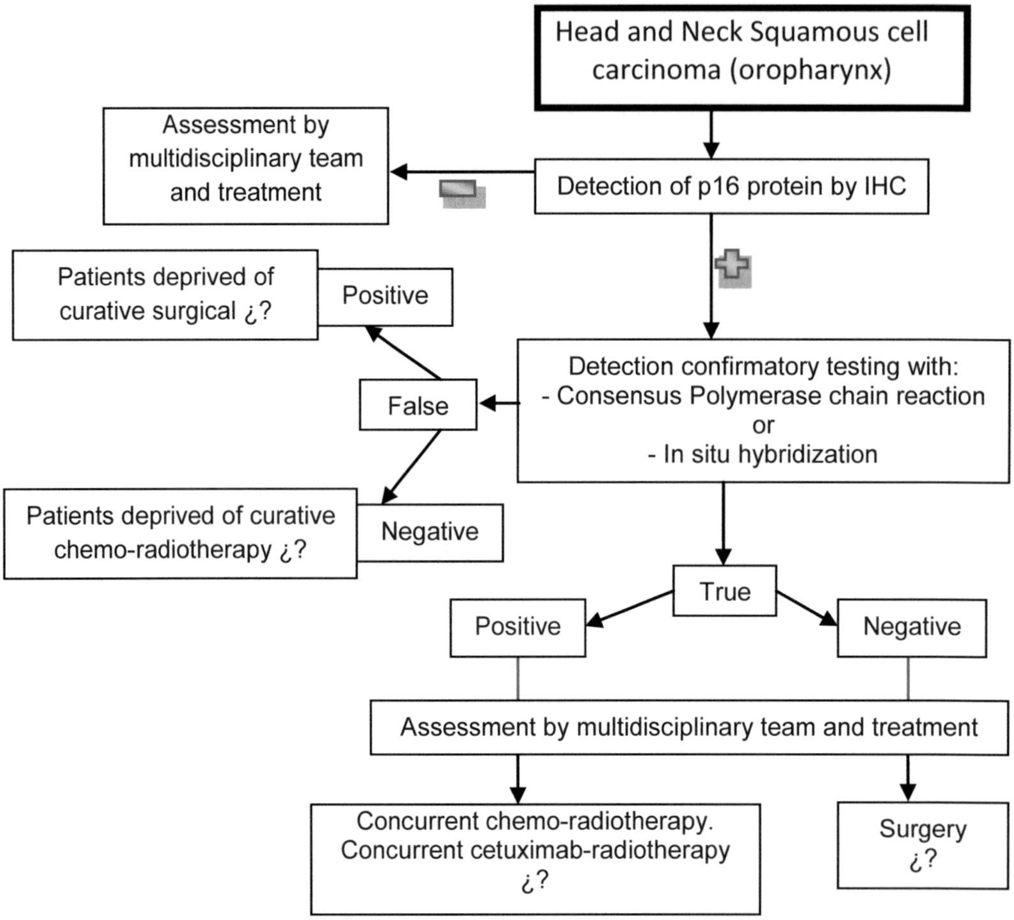

Figure 5. Diagnosis and treatment algorithm

6. Conclusion

Emerging evidences suggest that human papillomavirus-associated head and neck squamous cell carcinoma is a separate subgroup and biologically distinct from classical head and neck squamous cell carcinoma.

Human papillomavirus positive head and neck squamous cell carcinoma is typically found in the oropharynx and have been associated with younger patients who are less likely to be smokers or drinkers and with improved response to therapy and overall survival (Harris et al., 2011).

So, recognition that human papillomavirus has an etiologic role in head and neck squamous cell carcinoma has important implications for prognosis, treatment, disease prevention, and screening tests which are still being developed. Several authors have suggested that patients with human papillomavirus positive head and neck squamous cell carcinoma can be treated with chemo-radiotherapy or cetuximab-radiotherapy instead surgery.

Although high risk human papillomavirus detection is of utmost importance in clinical setting of head and neck squamous cell carcinoma, there is no agreement about the "golden standard" considering the number of molecular methods or combinations available.

There is evidence that detection of high risk human papillomavirus by consensus polymerase chain reaction alone is insufficient to accurately classify tumours, however, there is convincing evidence that the detection of p16 protein by immunohistochemistry can be used as a surrogate marker for the elaboration of oncogenic human papillomavirus proteins (Robinson et al., 2010). So, this is feasible as part of a routine diagnostic process using either a combination of p16 immunohistochemistry and in situ hybridization (Westra, 2009) or p16 detection and consensus polymerase chain reaction (Smeets et al., 2007).

Several studies have shown p16 expression status as a predictor of prognostic marker in head and neck squamous cell carcinoma, independent of human papillomavirus infection. In addition, epidermal growth factor receptor, and p53 are also relevant markers that modify the prognostic effect of human papillomavirus and may help guide the development of targeted therapy in head and neck squamous cell carcinoma.

Author details

Maria Isabel Tovar Martín, Miguel Juan Martínez Carrillo and Rosario Guerrero Tejada
Virgen de las Nieves University Hospital, Spain

7. References

Almadori, G; et al. (2001). Human papillomavirus infection and epidermal growth factor receptor expression in primary laryngeal squamous cell carcinoma. *Clinical Cancer Research*, Vol. 7, Nº.12, (December 2001), pp.3988-3993, ISSN 1078-0432 (Print) 1078-0432 (Linking)

Bedell, MA; et al. (1991). Amplification of human papillomavirus genomes in vitro is dependent on epithelial differentiation. *Journal Virology*, Vol.65, Nº.5, (May 1991), pp. 2254–2260, ISSN 0022-538X (Print) 1098-5514 (Electronic) 0022-538X (Linking)

Bonner, JA; et al. (2010). Radiotherapy plus cetuximab for locoregionally advanced head and neck cancer: 5-year survival data from a phase 3 randomised trial, and relation between cetuximab-induced rash and survival. *Lancet Oncology*, Vol.11, Nº.1, (January 2010),pp.21-8, ISSN 1470-2045 (Print) 1474-5488 (Electronic) 1470-2045 (Linking)

Braakhuis, BJ; et al. (2004). Genetic patterns in head and neck cancers that contain or lack transcriptionally active human papillomavirus. *Journal ot the National Cancer Institute*, Vol.96, Nº.13, (July 2004), pp.998–1006, ISSN 0027-8874 (Print) 1460-2105 (Electronic) 0027-8874 (Linking)

Campisi, G; et al. (2007). Human papillomavirus: its identity and controversial role in oral oncogenesis, premalignant and malignant lesions (review). *International Journal of Oncology*, Vol.30, Nº.4, (April 2007), pp.813– 823, ISSN 1019-6439 (Print) 1791-2423 (Electronic) 1019-6439 (Linking)

Canto, MT & Devesa, SS. (2002). Oral cavity and pharynx cancer incidence rates in the United States, 1975–1998. *Oral Oncology*, Vol.38, Nº.6, (September 2022), pp.610–617, ISSN 1368-8375 (Print) 1368-8375 (Linking)

Chaturvedi, AK; et al. (2008). Incidence trends for human papillomavirus-related and – unrelated oral squamous cell carcinomas in the USA. *Journal of Clinical Oncology: Official Journal of the American Society of Clinical Oncology*, vol.26, Nº.4, (February 2008), pp.612-619 ISSN 0732-183X (Print) 1527-7755 (Electronic) 0732-183X (Linking)

Cheng, S; et al. (1995). Differentiation-dependent up-regulation of the human papillomavirus E7 gene reactivates cellular DNA replication in suprabasal differentiated keratinocytes. *Genes & Development*, Vol.9, Nº.19, (October 1995), pp. 2335–2349, ISSN 0890-9369 (Print) 1549-5477 (Electronic) 0890-9369 (Linking)

Clifford, GM; et al. (2003.) Human papillomavirus types in invasive cervical cancer worldwide: a meta-analysis. *British Journal of Cancer*, Vol. 88, Nº1, (January 2003), pp.63–73, ISSN 0007-0920 (Print) 1532-1827 (Electronic) 0007-0920 (Linking)

Dobrossy, L. (2005). Epidemiology of head and neck cancer: magnitude of the problem. *Cancer Metastasis Reviews*. Vol.24, Nº.1, (January 2005), pp.9–17, ISSN 0167-7659 (Print) 1573-7233 (Electronic) 0167-7659 (Linking)

Doxtader, EE & Katzenstein, AL. (2011). The relationship between p16 expression and high-risk human papillomavirus infection in squamous cell carcinomas from sites other than – uterine cervix: a study of 137 cases. *Human Pathology*, Vol.43, Nº.3, (March 2012), pp.327–332 ISSN 0046-8177 (Print) 1532-8392 (Electronic) 0046-8177 (Linking)

D'Souza, G & Dempsey, A. (2011). The role of HPV in head and neck cancer and review of the HPV vaccine. *Preventive Medicine*, Vol.53, Nº1, (October 2011), pp.5-11, ISSN 0091-7435 (Print) 1096-0260 (Electronic) 0091-7435 (Linking)

Gravitt, PE; et al (2003). Reproducibility of HPV 16 and HPV 18 viral load quantitation using TaqMan real-time PCR assays. *Journal of virological methods*, Vol.112, Nº1-2 (September 2003), pp. 23-33, ISSN 0166-0934 (Print) 1879-0984 (Electronic) 0166-0934 (Linking)

Hafkamp, HC; et al. (2003). A subset of head and neck squamous cell carcinomas exhibits integration of HPV 16/18 DNA and overexpression of p16INK4A and p53 in the absence of mutations in p53 exons 5–8. *Internationl Journal of Cancer*, Vol.107, Nº.3 (November 2010), pp. 394–400, ISSN 0020-7136 (Print) 1097-0215 (Electronic) 0020-7136 (Linking)

Harris, SL; et al. (2011). Association of p16(INK4a) overexpression with improved outcomes in young patients with squamous cell cancers of the oral tongue. *Head & Neck*, Vol.33, Nº.11 (November 2011), pp.1622-7, ISSN 1043-3074 (Print) 1097-0347 (Electronic) 1043-3074 (Linking)

Henken, FE; et al. (2007). Sequential gene promoter methylation during HPV-induced cervical carcinogenesis. *British Journal of Cancer*, Vol.97, Nº. (10), (November 2007), pp.1457–64, ISSN 0007-0920 (Print) 1532-1827 (Electronic) 0007-0920 (Linking)

Herrero, R; et al. (2003). Human papillomavirus and oral cancer: the International Agency for Research on Cancer multicenter study. *Journal ot the National Cancer Institute*, Vol.95, Nº23, (December 2003), pp.1772-1783, ISSN, 0027-8874 (Print) 1460-2105 (Electronic) 0027-8874 (Linking)

Hobbs, CG; et al. (2006). Human papillomavirus and head and neck cancer: a systematic review and meta-analysis. *Clinical Otolaryngology: official journal of ENT-UK ; official journal of Netherlands Society for Oto-Rhino-Laryngology & Cervico-Facial Surgery*, Vol.31, Nº.4, (August 2006), pp.259-66, ISSSN 1749-4478 (Print) 1749-4486 (Electronic) 1749-4478 (Linking)

Hunsjak, H; et al. (2000). Comparison of five different polymerase chain reaction methods for detection of human papillomavirus in cervical call specimens. *Journal of virological Methods*, Vol.88, Nº2, (August 2000), pp.125-134, ISSN 0166-0934 (Print) 1879-0984 (Electronic) 0166-0934 (Linking)

Kim, SH; et al. (2006). Human papillomavirus 16 E5 up-regulates the expression of vascular endothelial growth factor through the activation of epidermal growth factor receptor, MEK/ ERK1,2 and PI3K/Akt. *Cellular and molecular life sciences : CMLS*, vol.63 Nº.7-8,(April 2006), pp.930–938, ISSN 1420-682X (Print) 1420-9071 (Electronic) 1420-682X (Linking)

Koskinen, WJ; et al. (2003). Prevalence and physical status of human papillomavirus in squamous cell carcinomas of the head and neck. *International journal of cancer. Journal international du cancer*, vol.107, Nº3., (November 2003), pp.401–406, ISSN 0020-7136 (Print) 1097-0215 (Electronic) 0020-7136 (Linking)

Kumar, B; et al. (2008). EGFR, p16, HPV titer, Bcl-xL and p53, sex, and smoking as indicators of response to therapy and survival in oropharyngeal cancer. *Journal of clinical oncology: official journal of the American Society of Clinical Oncology*, Vol.26, Nº.19, (July 2008), pp.3128–3137, ISSN 0732-183X (Print) 1527-7755 (Electronic) 0732-183X (Linking)

Lassen, P; et al. (2009). Effect of HPV-Associated p16INK4A Expression on Response to Radiotherapy and Survival in Squamous Cell Carcinoma of the Head and Neck. *Journal of clinical oncology: official journal of the American Society of Clinical Oncology*, Vol.27, Nº12., (April 2009), pp.1-7, ISSN 0732-183X (Print) 1527-7755 (Electronic) 0732-183X (Linking)

Leemans, CR; Braakhuis, BJ & Brakenhoff, RH. (2011). The molecular biology of head and neck cancer. *Nature reviews. Cancer*, Vol.11, Nº.1, (January 2011), pp.9-22, ISSN 1474 175X (Print) 1474-1768 (Electronic) 1474-175X (Linking)

Lindel, K; et al. (2001). Human papillomavirus positive squamous cell carcinoma of the oropharynx: a radiosensitive subgroup of head and neck carcinoma. *Cancer*, Vol.92, Nº4., (August 2001), pp.805–813, ISSN 0008-543X (Print) 1097-0142 (Electronic) 0008-543X (Linking)

Löning, T; et al. (1985). Analysis of oral papillomas, leukoplakias, and invasive carcinomas for human papillomavirus type related DNA. *The Journal of investigative dermatology*, Vol.84, Nº5., (May 1985), pp.417–420, ISSN 0022-202X (Print) 1523-1747 (Electronic) 0022-202X (Linking)

Lowe, B; et al. (2010). HPV genotype detection using hybrid capture sample preparation combined with whole genome amplification and multiplex detection with Luminex

XMAP. *The Journal of molecular diagnostics: JMD*, Vol.12, Nº6., (November 2010), pp.847-853, ISSN 1525-1578 (Print) 1943-7811 (Electronic) 1525-1578 (Linking)

Maxwell, JH; et al. (2010). Tobacco use in human papillomavirus-positive advanced oropharynx cancer patients related to increased risk of distant metastases and tumor recurrence. *Clin Cancer Res*, Vol.16, Nº4., (February 2010), pp.1226–1235, ISSN 1078-0432 (Print) 1078-0432 (Linking)

Mellin, H; et al. (2002). Human papillomavirus type 16 is episomal and a high viral load may be correlated to better prognosis in tonsillar cancer. *International journal of cancer*, Vol.102, Nº2., (November 2002), pp.152–158, ISSN 0020-7136 (Print) 1097-0215 (Electronic) 0020-7136 (Linking)

Micalessi, MI; et al. (2012). A real-time PCR approach based on SPF10 primers and the INNO-LiPA HPV genotyping extra assay for the detection and typing of human papillomavirus. *Journal of virological methods*,(May 2012) [Epub ahead of print. Article in press] ISSN 0166-0934 (Print) 1879-0984 (Electronic) 0166-0934 (Linking)

Oh, Y; et al. (2007). Polymerase chain reaction-based fluorescent Luminex assay to detect the presence of human papillomavirus types. *Cancer science*, Vol. 98, Nº4., (April 2007), pp.549-554. ISSN 1347-9032 (Print) 1349-7006 (Electronic) 1347-9032 (Linking)

Pfister, D; et al. (March 2011). Head and neck cancers V.2.2011, In: *National Comprehensive Cancer Network Clinical Practice Guidelines in Oncology*, April 2012, Available from: < http://www.nccn.org/professionals/physician_gls/pdf/head-and-neck.pdf>

Pannone, G; et al. (2011). The role of human papillomavirus in the pathogenesis of head & neck squamous cell carcinoma: an overview. *Infectious agents and cancer*, Vol.6, Nº4, (March 2011), pp.1-11, ISSN 1750-9378 (Electronic) 1750-9378 (Linking)

Pannone, G; et al. (2012). Evaluation of a combined triple method to detect causative HPV in oral and oropharyngeal squamous cell carcinomas: p16 Immunohistochemistry, Consensus polymerase chain reaction human papillomavirus-DNA, and In Situ Hybridization. *Infectious agents and cancer*, Vol.7, Nº4, (February 2012), pp.1-14. ISSN 1750-9378 (Electronic) 1750-9378 (Linking)

Pfeifer, GP; et al. (2002). Tobacco smoke carcinogens, DNA damage and p53 mutations in smokingassociated cancers. *Oncogene*, Vol.21, Nº.48, (October 2002), pp.7435–7451, ISSN 0950-9232 (Print) 1476-5594 (Electronic) 0950-9232 (Linking)

Psyrri, A & Dimaio, D. (2008). Human papillomavirus in cervical and head-and-neck cáncer. *Nature Clinical Practice. Oncology*, Vol.5, Nº.1, (January 2008), pp.24-31, ISSN 1743-4254 (Print) 1743-4262 (Electronic) 1743-4254 (Linking)

Psyrri, A & Tsiodoras, S. (2008) Optimizing approaches to head and neck cancers viruses in head and neck cancers: prevention and therapy. *Annals of Oncology: : official journal of the European Society for Medical Oncology / ESMO*, Vol.19, Nº. 7, (September 2008), pp.189–194, ISSN 0923-7534 (Print) 1569-8041 (Electronic) 0923-7534 (Linking)

Rabbett, WF. (1965). Juvenile laryngeal papillomatosis. The relation of irradiation to malignant degeneration in this disease. *The Annals of otology, rhinology, and laryngology*, Vol.74, Nº4., (December 1965), pp.1149–1163, ISSN 0003-4894 (Print) 0003-4894 (Linking)

Ragin, CC; Modugno, F & Gollin, SM. (2007). The epidemiology and risk factors of head and neck cancer: a focus on human papillomavirus. *Journal of dental research*, Vol.86, Nº.2,

(February 2007), pp.104-14, ISSN 0022-0345 (Print) 1544-0591 (Electronic) 0022-0345 (Linking)

Rampias, T; et al. (2009). E6 and E7 gene silencing and transformed phenotype of human papillomavirus 16-positive oropharyngeal cancer cells. *Journal of the National Cancer Institute*, Vol.101, Nº.6, (March 2009), pp.412–423, ISSN 0027-8874 (Print) 1460-2105 (Electronic) 0027-8874 (Linking)

Reimers, N; et al. (2007). Combined analysis of HPV-DNA, p16 and EGFR expression to predict prognosis in oropharyngeal cancer. *International journal of cancer. Journal international du cancer*, Vol.120, Nº.8, (April 2007), pp.1731–1738, ISSN 0020-7136 (Print) 1097-0215 (Electronic) 0020-7136 (Linking)

Robinson, M; Sloan, P & Shaw, R. (2010). Refining the diagnosis of oropharyngeal squamous cell carcinoma using human papillomavirus testing. *Oral Oncology*, Vol.46, Nº.7, (July 2010), pp.492-6, ISSN 1368-8375 (Print) 1368-8375 (Linking)

Shah, NG; et al. (2009). Prognostic significance of molecular markers in oral squamous cell carcinoma: a multivariate analysis. *Head & Neck*, Vol.31, Nº12., (December 2009), pp.1544–1556, ISSN 1043-3074 (Print) 1097-0347 (Electronic) 1043-3074 (Linking)

Shanta, V; et al. (2000). Epidemiology of cancer of the cervix: global and national perspective. *Journal of the Indian Medical Association*, Vol.98, Nº.2, (February 2000), pp.49–52, ISSN 0019-5847 (Print) 0019-5847 (Linking)

Shiboski, CH; et al. (2005). Tongue and tonsil carcinoma: increasing trends in the US population ages 20–44 years. *Cancer*, Vol.103, Nº.9, (May 2005), pp.1843–1849, ISSN 0008-543X (Print) 1097-0142 (Electronic) 0008-543X (Linking)

Slaughter, DP; et al. (1953). Field cancerization in oral stratified squamous epithelium; clinical implications of multicentric origin. *Cancer*, Vol.6, Nº.5, (September 1953), pp.963–968, ISSN 0008-543X (Print) 1097-0142 (Electronic) 0008-543X (Linking)

Smeets, SJ; et al. (2007). A novel algorithm for reliable detection of human papillomavirus in paraffin embedded head and neck cancer specimen. *International journal of cancer*, Vol.121, Nº.11, (December 2007), pp.2465-2472, ISSN 0020-7136 (Print) 1097-0215 (Electronic) 0020-7136 (Linking)

Smith, EM; et al. (January2012). Complex etiology underlies risk and survival in head and neck cancer human papillomavirus, tobacco, and alcohol: a case for multifactor disease. In: *Journal of oncology*, (March 2012), Available from: <http://www.ncbi.nlm.nih.gov/pmc/articles/PMC3270416/pdf/JO2012-571862.pdf>

Snow, AN & Laudadio, J. (2010). Human papillomavirus detection in head and neck squamous cell carcinomas. *Advances in anatomic pathology*, Vol.17, Nº.6, (November 2010), pp.394-403, ISSN 1072-4109 (Print) 1533-4031 (Electronic) 1072-4109 (Linking)

Stubenrauch, F & Laimins, LA. (1999). Human papillomavirus life cycle: active and latent phases. *Seminars in cancer biology*, Vol.9, Nº.6, (December 1999), pp.379–386, ISSN 1044-579X (Print) 1096-3650 (Electronic) 1044-579X (Linking)

Syrjänen, K; et al. (1983). Morphological and immunohistochemical evidence suggesting human papillomavirus (HPV) involvement in oral squamous cell carcinogenesis. *International journal of oral surgery*, Vol.12, Nº.6, (December 1983), pp.418–424, ISSN 0300-9785 (Print) 0300-9785 (Linking)

Tang, AL; et al. (December 2011). UM-SCC-104: A New human papillomavirus-16-positive cancer stem cell-containing head and neck squamous cell carcinoma cell line. In: *Head & Neck,* (March 2011), Available from:
<http://onlinelibrary.wiley.com/doi/10.1002/hed.21962/pdf>

Tran, N; et al. (2007). Role of human papillomavirus in the etiology of head and neck cancer. *Head & Neck,* Vol.29, Nº1., (January 2007) pp.64-70, ISSN 1043-3074 (Print) 1097-0347 (Electronic) 1043-3074 (Linking)

Turner, DO; et al. (October 2011). High-risk human papillomavirus (HPV) screening and detection in healthy patient saliva samples: a pilot study. In: *BMC oral health,* (March 2012), Available from:
<http://www.ncbi.nlm.nih.gov/pmc/articles/PMC3200164/pdf/1472-6831-11-28.pdf>

Weinberger, PM; et al. (2004). Prognostic significance of p16 protein levels in oropharyngeal squamous cell cancer. *Clinical cancer research : an official journal of the American Association for Cancer Research,* Vol.10, Nº.17, (September 2004), pp.5684–5691, ISSN 1078-0432 (Print) 1078-0432 (Linking)

Weinberger, PM; et al. (2006). Molecular classification identifies a subset of human papillomavirus–associated oropharyngeal cancers with favorable prognosis. *Journal of clinical oncology : official journal of the American Society of Clinical Oncology,* Vol.24, Nº.5, (February 2006), pp.736–747, ISSN 0732-183X (Print) 1527-7755 (Electronic) 0732-183X (Linking)

Westra, WH; et al. (2008). Inverse relationship between human papillomavirus-16 infection and disruptive p53 gene mutations in squamous cell carcinoma of the head and neck. *Clinical cancer research : an official journal of the American Association for Cancer Research,* Vol.14, Nº.2, (January 2008), pp.366–369, ISSN 1078-0432 (Print) 1078-0432 (Linking)

Westra, WH. (2009). The changing face of head and neck cancer in the 21st century: the impact of HPV on the epidemiology and pathology of oral cancer. *Head and neck pathology,* Vol.3, Nº.1, (March 2009), pp.78–81, ISSN 1936-055X (Print) 1936-0568 (Electronic)

Wilczynski, SP; Lin, BT; Xie, Y & Paz, IB. (1998). Detection of human papillomavirus DNA and oncoprotein overexpression are associated with distinct morphological patterns of tonsillar squamous cell carcinoma. *The American journal of pathology,* Vol.152, Nº.1, (January 1998), pp.145–156, ISSN 0002-9440 (Print) 1525-2191 (Electronic) 0002-9440 (Linking)

Wiseman, SM; et al. (2003). Squamous cell carcinoma of the head and neck in nonsmokers and nondrinkers: an analysis of clinicopathologic characteristics and treatment outcomes. *Annals of surgical oncology,* Vol.10, Nº.5, (January 2003), pp.551–557, ISSN 1068-9265 (Print) 1534-4681 (Electronic) 1068-9265 (Linking)

Wu, X; et al. (1994). Papilloma formation by cottontail rabbit papillomavirus requires E1 and E2 regulatory genes in addition to E6 and E7 transforming genes. *Journal of virology,* Vol.68, Nº.9, (September 1994), pp.6097–6102, ISSN 0022-538X (Print) 1098-5514 (Electronic) 0022-538X (Linking)

Zhang, MQ; El-Mofty, SK & Davila, RM. (2008). Detection of human papillomavirus-related squamous cell carcinoma cytologically and by in situ hybridisation in fine needle aspiration biopsies of cervical metastasis: a tool for identifying the site of an occult head and neck primary. *Cancer,* Vol.114, Nº.2, (April 2008), pp.118–123, ISSN 0008-543X (Print) 1097-0142 (Electronic) 0008-543X (Linking)

Chapter 2

Shadow Keyplayers of the Uterine Cervix Lesions Progression and Metastasis

Anca Maria Cimpean, Vitalie Mazuru,
Lilian Şaptefraţi and Marius Raica

Additional information is available at the end of the chapter

http://dx.doi.org/10.5772/51476

1. Introduction

Cervical neoplasia remains one of the most controversial issues for clinicians, pathologists and researchers. Screening programs have reduced the incidence of invasive neoplastic lesions but have not changed the rate of precursor lesions. Human papilloma virus (HPV) is confirmed to be involved in the etiology of uterine cervix lesions. Recently, Coutlée *et al.* reported that samples from women with low grade squamous intraepithelial lesions (LSIL) contained higher HPV-6 loads than women without this lesion.Despite the existence of an anti-HPV vaccine, HPV gene expression is dramatically altered during cervical carcinogenesis and novel biomarkers are needed for a better characterization of neoplastic cervical progression[2]. Incomplete characterization of the uterine cervix cancer from molecular point of view represents the main problem for the use of a proper therapy in this disease. Angiogenesis and lymphangiogenesis remain a paradigm of cervical lesions progression and metastasis. Most of the papers concerning angiogenesis were based on description of growth factors and/or microvessel density assessed in cervical lesions, especially in invasive carcinomas.The cellular and molecular mechanisms of the angiogenic switch in preneoplastic lesions of the uterine cervix are still less studied. The assessment of angiogenesis in uterine cervix lesions was performed using pan-endothelial markers such as CD31, CD34 and von Willebrand factor, which are not specific enough to differentiate between endothelial cells from normal, activated or tumor vessels[3-5]. All these antibodies stain both normal and tumor vessels. In 2008 Mazibrada *et al.* reported a correlation between CD105 microvascular density (MVD) and CD31 MVD and found an increase in both MVD as a continuum from benign lesions to invasive squamous cell carcinoma6. Endothelial cell activation and proliferation might be the clue for an early angiogenic switch and must be study more deeply.

Uterine cervical lesions and the involvement of LV in the tumor development, progression and metastasis still remains a field of debate. Few articles describe lymphatic vessel density and the potential role of lymphangiogenesis in the progression of cervical neoplasia[7-8]. The relationship between lymphangiogenesis and the invasion of cervical cancer was suggested by Hashimoto *et al.*, who considered that vascular endothelial growth factor C (VEGF)-C could be a promoter of pelvic lymph node metastasis in invasive cervical cancer [9]. Usually, malignant lesions of the uterine cervix are considered more important than precursor lesions. This fact may explain the lack of data about the promotion of lymphangiogenesis in pathological conditions of the uterine cervix. No data about the origin of lymph vessels, the prognostic impact of lymphangiogenesis in precursor lesions of the uterine cervix, or their involvement in nodal pelvic metastasis development have been confirmed. Available data about lymphatic vessels (LV) in tumors of the uterine cervix are scattered and controversial, and moreover, there are almost no references regarding lymphangiogenesis in precursor lesions and also for the normal cervix [10, 11].

Based on the controversial data concerning expression of CD105 and Ki-67 in endothelial cells from uterine cervix lesions, the aim of the present study was to investigate the distribution and co-localization of mentioned markers in benign and malignant conditions of the uterine cervix. Concerning early steps of lymphangiogenesis, the purpose was to evaluate morphology, distribution, lymphatic microvessel density and lymphatic proliferation in different stages of cervical lesions. Comparison of type-specific features of lymphangiogenesis in premalignant and malignant lesions, correlated with proliferative status of lymphatic endothelial cells, could help detect the early lymphangiogenesis in pathological conditions of the uterine cervix. A complete characterization of the morphological and immunohistochemical data of LV could have a prognostic and therapeutic impact and confirm diagnosis in cervical lesions.

2. Morphologic and immunohistochemical methods for blood and lymphatic vessels assessement in cervical neoplasia

One of our research included 128 retrospective targeted biopsies of the uterine cervix and specimens taken from conization in patients with macroscopically detectable lesions. Specimens were fixed in buffer formalin and embedded in paraffin, based on the conventional histological technique. Step sections, 5 mm thick, were prepared for each case. Initial sections were stained with HE, for the pathological diagnosis and grade of the tumor. Lesions were stratified as follows: squamous cell metaplasia (n = 27); cervical intraepithelial lesions (LSIL, n =25) and (high grade intraepithelial squamous lesions (HSIL),n = 23); carcinoma *in situ* (n = 10); microinvasive carcinoma (n = 15); and invasive carcinoma (n = 20). Normal uterine cervix specimens (biopsies collected from patients with inconclusive results of colposcopy when conization was recommended by gynecologist) were used as control (n=8). We applied a double stain method for colocalization of CD105 and Ki-67 markers on the same section. On dewaxed and rehydrated slides we performed endogenous peroxidase blocking with 3% hydrogen peroxide for 5 min followed by pretreatment with proteinase K for 15 min at room temperature. Incubation with primary CD105 antibody, clone SN6h from DakoCytomation (Glostrup, Denmark) for 1 h (dilution 1:10) preceeded the first application of avidin–biotin system LSAB+/HRP (Dako, Carpinteria, CA, USA), and visualization was performed with 3,3 diaminmobenzidine as chromogen. Automated method with PT Link module of heat-induced epitope retrieval in citrate buffer pH6 (DakoCytomation) was used for 30 min to unmask the Ki-67 epitope. After 30 min incubation with Ki-67 ready-to-use antibody (clone MIB1, Dako, Carpinteria, CA, USA), the LSAB+-HRP system was used, followed by visualization with amino-ethilcarbazol as chromogen for 10 min. Colocalization of the Ki67 proliferation marker (monoclonal antibody, clone MIB1 from Dako, (Carpinteria, CA, USA), with D2-40 in lymphatic endothelium was obtained by applying the double immunostainingmethod followed by the use of two different chromogens (3,3'diaminobenzidine for nuclear brown staining of Ki67 and amino ethyl carbazole for cytoplasmic red staining of D2-40 epitope). Basal cells of stratified squamous epithelium of the cervix and lymphatic endothelial cells were considered positive control. Also, PROX1, VEGF C and VEGFR3 were immunohistochemically assessed by using the same labeled streptavidin biotin methods. Counterstain was performed with Lillie's modified hematoxylin. The entire immunohistochemistry procedure was performed with DakoCytomation Autostainer.

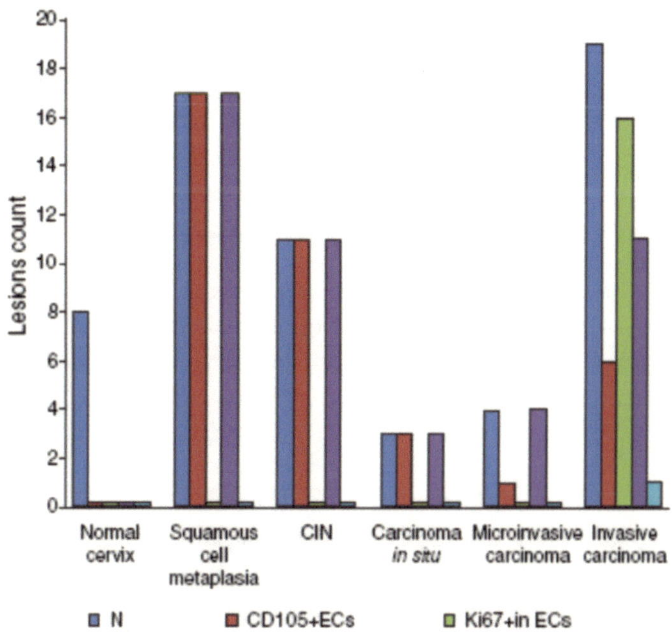

Figure 1. Statistic analysis of uterine cervix lesions based on CD105 and Ki-67 expression. Distribution of CD105-positive endothelial cells, Ki-67 immunoreactivity in endothelial cells and tumor cells according to histopathological type of uterine cervix lesions Note the presence of Ki-67+ endothelial cells only in invasive carcinoma. Coexpression of CD105 and Ki-67 was also restricted to the invasive type carcinoma. CIN, cervical intra-epithelial neoplasia; EC, endothelial cells.

3. Tumor blood vessels activation and proliferation is different for each histopathologic type of cervical neoplasia

CD105 expression was absent in all cases of normal cervix. CD105 imunoreaction was restricted to the vascular activated endothelium from dysplasia, carcinoma *in situ* and microinvasive carcinoma. Intense activation of blood vessels was observed in both squamous cell metaplasia and dysplasia, with a CD105-MVD that varied between 0 and 25 vessels/x400 field with a range of 6.5 vessels/x400 field. Also, *in situ* carcinoma had positive vessels for CD105 with no endothelial cell proliferation. The activated vessels were agglomerated close to the epithelial lesions and had a lower density far from them, similar to the dysplasia findings. In microinvasive carcinoma positive reaction for CD105 was found in only one case, and the other three cases were negative. Almost 68% of invasive carcinomas were negative for CD105 and most of them had a tumor cells proliferative index <5%. CD105-negative endothelial cells from invasive carcinoma had a higher proliferation rate compared with CD105-negative vascular endothelium from normal cervix blood vessels. We found a significant correlation between the lack of endoglin expression in proliferative endothelial cells and invasive type of cervix carcinoma (P = 0.004).Also, low proliferative index of tumor cells was correlated with lack of CD105 expression in tumor vessels (P = 0.003). Lack of coexpression for CD105 and Ki-67 in endothelial cells was a constant phenomenon. In only one case of invasive carcinoma with high CD105 MVD (13 vessels/x400 field) was a positive signal for Ki-67 observed in the nuclei of CD105-positive endothelial cells in the activated vessels located only in the tumor periphery.

4. Lymphangiogenesis and lympahtic vessels in cervical neoplasia- early development with a potential prognostic impact

Basal cells of the epithelium from normal exocervix and cervical squamous metaplasia were positive for D2-40 as a continuous layer over the lamina propria of the cervix. This distribution was also observed in LSIL. A lower intensity of immunostaining was detected for basal cells of HSIL. A discontinuous pattern of the basal layer or clusters of positive cells also characterized HSIL. There were differences concerning the distribution and density of LV between the histopathological types of cervical lesions included in our study. In the normal cervix we found large LV, round or oval in shape without branches, found deep in the lamina propria, far from the stratified squamous epithelium. In the normal cervix, D2-40-positive lymphatic vessels had no positive reaction for Ki67 in endothelial cells. The same pattern was found in squamous metaplasia of the uterine cervix. Lymphatic microvascular density (LMVD) ranged between 4.8 and 6.6 vessels/200 magnification, with an average of 5.8 in the normal cervix. In squamous cell metaplasia the number of LV was not significantly different from results found in the normal cervix. A significant increase in the number of LV was found in cases with HSIL and *in situ* carcinoma. All cases with LSIL, HSIL and carcinoma *in situ* showed D2/40+/Ki67+ proliferative lymphatic endothelial cells. Proliferative vessels were distributed close to the lesions. A significant correlation was found between the proliferative status of lymphatic endothelial cells in both cervical intraepithelial neoplasia types. In LSIL a higher correlation was found compared with HSIL (P = 0.009 in LSIL compared with P = 0.044 for HSIL). This finding supports early onset of lymphangiogenesis in cervical lesions. High proliferative activity of lymphatic endothelial cells found in LSIL, HSIL and *in situ* carcinoma was also present in microinvasive carcinoma A significant correlation of lymphatic proliferative activity and the microinvasive type of cervical cancer was also found (P = 0.002). In invasive carcinoma, LV were observed in the tumor and peritumoral areas. A few intratumoral LV were found as small D2-40-positive vessels with narrow or collapsed lumen, irregular walls and no tumor cells inside. Peritumoral LV were significantly more numerous, larger, sinuous, with a discontinuous wall and often containing proliferative lymphatic endothelial cells and tumor cells. Density of lymphatics varied between 1 and 15.2 with an average of 7.25. A significant correlation was also evident for invasive carcinoma (P = 0.002).

Expression of Prox1, VEGF-C and VEGFR3 was different concerning the histopathology of cervical lesions. Prox1 was restricted to the lymphatic and venous endothelial cell nuclei, whereas VEGF-C had a wide expression in the tumor, lymphatic endothelial and scaterred stromal cells. VEGFR3 had a strong expression in lymphatic endothelial cells from peritumoral or intratumoral lymphatic vessels, and also in the intravascular tumor emboli from invasive carcinoma cases.

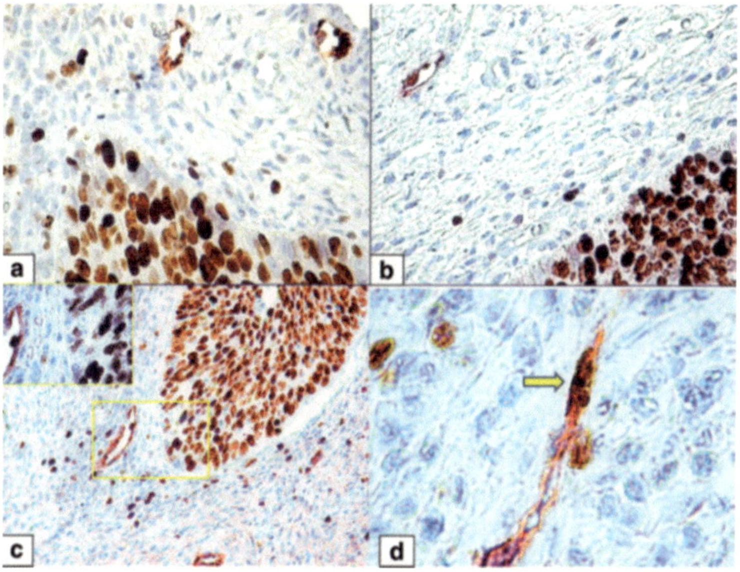

Figure 2. Proliferative status of lymphatic vessels in various cervical lesion types (D2-40 in red and Ki 67 brown immunostain). (**a**). High grade intraepithelial squamous lesions and (**b**) in situ carcinoma with a high number of Ki 67 proliferative endothelial cells (nuclear, brown) lining D2-40-positive lymphatic vessels (red). (**c**) Microinvasive carcinoma also presented proliferative lymphatic endothelial cells. (**d**) Intratumoral lymphatic vessel from invasive carcinoma with proliferating lymphatic endothelial cells at the tip of the lymphatic sprout (arrow) and collapsed lumen lined by D2-40-positive lymphatic endothelial cells.

Prox1 analysis showed the presence of positive reaction from CIN2 lesions (33,3% from total cases) to CIN3- 91,6% and microinvasive carcinoma – 14 cases (87,5%). Prox1 positive endothelial cells circumscribed the lumen of the lymphatic vessels in close vicinity with the epithelial proliferation of uterine cervix *"in situ"* preneoplastic lesions. The average number of Prox1 positive nuclei/x200 increased from CIN2 and CIN3 lesions to microinvasive carcinoma. All Prox1 positive lymphatic and venous blood vessels were also positive for VEGFR3. A significant correlation was found between density of Prox1 positive nuclei of lymphatic endothelial cells and LMVD assessed for VEGFR3 positive lymphatic vessels ($p=0.001$).

VEGF-C expression was found to be positive in all types of cervical lesions. Intensity of VEGF-C expression and number of positive cases increased from squamous metaplasia to invasive carcinoma. VEGF-C was highly expressed in tumor cells, less and inconstant in stromal cells and lymphatic vessel endothelial cells. , We obtained a significant correlation between intermediate grade of VEGF-C expression and Prox1 nuclear density ($p=0.044$). Tumor cells were negative for Prox-1 in 100% of cases. No positive reaction was found in normal specimens, squamous metaplasia, low grade intraepithelial neoplasia or invasive carcinoma.

5. Angiogenesis and lymphangiogenesis controversies in cervical neoplasia-review of the literature

Benign lesions has not been studied as much with regard to CD105 expression. We observed a high CD105 expression in vessels from cervical metaplasia and dysplasia, and absence of endothelial proliferation was quantified using Ki-67 marker. During the early stages of tumor development TGF-b acts as an inhibitor of neoplastic proliferation. When tumor cells escape from the anti-mitotic signal exerted by TGF-b, they secrete large amount of TGF-b, promote cell invasion and metastasis and create an optimal microenvironment for promoting neo-angiogenesis[2,13]. Also, it is known that as cells progress toward fully malignant tumor cells, they undergo changes that result in reduced expression of TGF-b receptors, increased expression of TGF-b ligands, and resistance to inhibition of growth by TGF-b. The present findings suggest the same changes in the endothelial cells of activated vessels from premalignant lesions and invasive carcinoma of the uterine cervix on expression of CD105 (co-receptor for TGF-receptors I and III) without Ki-67—in cervical metaplasia and dysplasia activated vessels— and lack of CD105 staining in Ki-67-positive endothelial cells from tumor vessels of cervical invasive carcinoma. This is sustained by significant correlation found by our team between low tumor cell proliferative index (<5%) and absence of CD105 expression in the vascular bed from cervical invasive carcinoma. Many studies associated CD105 immuno-expression with proliferating endothelial cells[14-16]. The present data showed that in CD105-positive endothelial cells from premalignant and malignant lesions of the uterine cervix, activation and proliferation are two distinct processes in most of the cases. In conclusion, activation of endothelial cells is an early event that predominates in benign and premalignant conditions of the uterine cervix, while endothelial cell proliferation is observed in tumor vessel endothelial cells from invasive carcinoma of the uterine cervix.

Using the method of step sections, Roche and Norris[17] and later Leman *et al.*[18] demonstrated lymphatic invasion in microinvasive carcinoma without association of lymph node metastasis. Later, Zivaljeviç *et al.* reported similar results and recommended a personalized treatment based on an exhaustive pathological evaluation of an adequate cone biopsy specimen[19]. These findings support the hypothesis that in microinvasive carcinoma the newly formed LV (based on a higher LMVD found in the present study compared with normal cervix) are already functional. The increase of LMVD in the early stages of LSIL and the similar LMVD value found in the present study in HSIL, LSIL, and carcinoma *in situ* could partially explain the early development of a lymphatic network and may promote early nodal metastases in cervical cancer. Scattered data characterizes lymphangiogenesis in cervical intraepithelial neoplasia lesions. Lymphangiogenic growth factors VEGF-C and VEGF-D, and their corresponding receptor VEGFR3 mRNA levels, significantly increase in HSIL lesions compared with LSIL. Correlation of these data with our findings concerning a doubled LMVD value in LSIL and HSIL compared to the normal cervix suggests an early lymphangiogenic switch in cervical carcinogenesis. Present findings concerning lymphangiogenesis correlated with our previous published data about proliferation of endothelial cells from blood vessels in cervical lesions[20] show an early lymphatic endothelial proliferation in preneoplastic stages of cervical lesions even before the development of the angiogenic response.

Prox1 has been extensively studied, mainly in the context of embryonic development of lymphatic vasculature, liver, pancreas, lens fibers cells and progenitor cells of retinal photoreceptor neurons.). In our study, no Prox1 positive immunostaining was found for normal cervix epithelium or dysplastic one. Up to now, there are no data about Prox1 expression in tumors derived from stratified squamous epithelia. Based on our results, we assume that Prox-1 is not involved in the uterine cervix epithelial carcinogenesis as previously described for other types of neoplasia. Committment of endothelial cells through a lymphatic phenotype by its Prox1 expression appear early in the development of cervical cancer. A high number of Prox1 positive cells was observed starting from the intraepithelial neoplastic stages (CIN2 and CIN3) to microinvasive carcinoma. These findings can be partially explained by previously published data concerning lymphangiogenesis. all Prox-1 positive lymphatic vessels were positive for VEGFR-3. Similar results were previously reported in lymphangiomas by Wilting et al. Furthermore, similar Prox1 and VEGFR-3 positivity of venous endothelial cells might be evidence for the origin of lymphatic endothelial cells from venous endothelium as a main lymphangiogenic mechanism during cervical neoplasia progression. No similar data has been previously reported in the uterine cervix cancer. Thus, we consider that in cervical neoplasia, venous endothelial cells could specify through a lymphatic phenotype, by activation of Prox1 expression during tumor progression, being able to give rise to lymphatic endothelial cells. The presence of stromal Prox1 positive cells found in the present study suggests the existence of a stromal pool of cells capable of acquiring the lymphatic phenotype.

In summary, the present findings suggests by microscopy, immunohistochemistry and statistical analysis that angiogenesis and lymphangiogenesis are early events in the lesions of the uterine cervix before an overt invasion certified by morphological and immunohistochemical tests. This explains the early development of metastasis from microinvasive carcinoma stage, aggressiveness and poor response to the therapy of cervical invasive carcinoma. Further studies are necessary to evaluate angiogenesis and lymphangiogenesis in preneoplastic lesions of the uterine cervix to show their value for prognosis and therapeutic management.

Author details

Anca Maria Cimpean and Marius Raica
Department of Histology, Angiogenesis Research Center,
"Victor Babeş" University of Medicine and Pharmacy Timişoara,
Romania

Vitalie Mazuru and Lilian Şaptefraţi
Department of Histology, „Nicolae Testemitanu"
University of Medicine and Pharmacy, Kisinev,
Moldavia

6. References

[1] Coutlée F, Trottier H, Gagnon S *et al*. Low-risk human papillomavirus type 6 DNA load and integration in cervical samples from women with squamous intraepithelial lesions. *J Clin Virol* 2009; 45: 96–9.

[2] Brandsma JL, Sun Y, Lizardi PM *et al*. Distinct human papillomavirus type 16 methylomes in cervical cells at different stages of premalignancy. *Virology* 2009; 389: 100–7

[3] Vieira SC, Zeferino LC, da Silva BB *et al*. Quantification of angiogenesis in cervical cancer: A comparison among three endothelial cell markers. *Gynecol Oncol* 2004; 93: 121–4.

[4] Vieira SC, Silva BB, Pinto GA *et al*. CD34 as a marker for evaluating angiogenesis in cervical cancer. *Pathol Res Pract* 2005; 201: 313–18.

[5] Lenczewski A, Terlikowski S, Famulski W, Sulkowska M, Kulikowski M. Angiogenesis as a prognostic factor in invasive carcinoma of the uterine cervix. *Folia Histochem Cytobiol* 2001; 39: 165–6.

[6] Mazibrada J, Rittà M, Mondini M *et al.* Interaction between inflammation and angiogenesis during different stages of cervical carcinogenesis. *Gynecol Oncol* 2008; 108: 112–20.

[7] Longatto-Filho A, Pinheiro C, Pereira SM *et al*. Lymphatic vessel density and epithelial D2-40 immunoreactivity in preinvasive and invasive lesions of the uterine cervix. *Gynecol Oncol* 2007; 107: 45–51.

[8] Van Trappen PO, Steele D, Lowe DG *et al*. Expression of vascular endothelial growth factor (VEGF)-C and VEGF-D, and their receptor VEGFR-3, during different stages of cervical carcinogenesis. *J Pathol* 2003; 201: 544–54.

[9] Hashimoto I, Kodama J, Seki N *et al*. Vascular endothelial growth factor-C expression and its relationship to pelvic lymph node status in invasive cervical cancer. *Br J Cancer* 2001; 85: 93–7.

[10] Urabe A, Matsumoto T, Kimura M *et al*. Grading system of lymphatic invasion according to D2-40 immunostaining is useful for prediction of nodal metastasis in squamous cell carcinoma of the uterine cervix. *Histopathology* 2006; 49: 493–97.

[11] Miyakuni Y, Matsumoto T, Arakawa A *et al*. Lymphatic invasion according to D2-40 immunostaining is a predictor of nodal metastasis in endometrioid adenocarcinoma of the uterine corpus. *Pathol Int* 2008; 58: 471–78.

[12] Derynck R, Akhurst RJ, Balmain A. TGF-b signaling in tumor suppression and cancer progression. *Nat Genet* 2001; 29: 117–29.

[13] Roberts AB, Wakefield LM. The two faces of transforming growth factor b in carcinogenesis. *Proc Natl Acad Sci USA* 2003; 100: 8621–3.

[14] Saad RS, Liu YL, Nathan G, Celebrezze J, Medich D, Silverman JF. Endoglin (CD105) and vascular endothelial growth factor as prognostic markers in colorectal cancer. *Mod Pathol* 2004; 17: 197–203.

[15] Wikström P, Lissbrant IF, Stattin P, Egevad L, Bergh A. Endoglin (CD105) is expressed on immature blood vessels and is a marker for survival in prostate cancer. *Prostate* 2002; 51: 268– 75.

[16] Dallas NA, Samuel S, Xia L *et al*. Endoglin (CD105): A marker of tumor vasculature and potential target for therapy. *Clin Cancer Res* 2008; 14: 1931–7.

[17] Roche WD, Norris HJ. Microinvasive carcinomaof the cervix: The significance of lymphatic invasion and confluent patterns of stromal growth. *Cancer* 1975; 36: 180–86.

[18] Leman MH, Benson WL, Kurman RJ *et al*. Microinvasive carcinoma of the cervix. *Obstet Gynecol* 1976; 48: 571–8.

[19] Zivaljeviç M, Vujkov T, Ninèiç D *et al*. Microinvasive carcinoma of the cervix. *Arch Oncol* 2004; 12: 142–44.

[20] Cimpean AM, Saptefrati L, Ceausu R, Raica M. Characterization of endoglin and Ki-67 expression in endothelial cells from benign and malignant lesions of the uterine cervix. *Pathol Int* 2009; 59: 695–700.

Chapter 3

Surgical and Clinical Pathology of Breast Diseases

Abdolrasoul Talei, Majid Akrami, Maral Mokhtari and Sedigheh Tahmasebi

Additional information is available at the end of the chapter

http://dx.doi.org/10.5772/52105

1. Introduction

Histopathology plays an important role in management of breast diseases. It is a necessary component of diagnosis, treatment and prognosis in most breast disorders. Also, when assessing the adequacy of treatment in breast cancer, pathologic assessment is the main criterion. The importance of the role of histopathology in treatment of breast cancer has encouraged the researchers to investigate the impact of pathology review on treatment of breast cancer. Kennecke HF and colleagues studied the impact of pathology review in treatment of 405 patients with breast cancer. A total of 102 pathology changes were documented among 81 patients (20%). These changes resulted in 27 treatment modifications among 25 patients (6%) (1). It seems that before decision making for treatment of breast disease, the pathology should review by an expert breast pathologist.

2. How to achieve tissue?

Fine needle aspiration or core needle biopsy versus surgical biopsy has remained a challenge in breast lesions suspicious to malignancy. An article published in December 2011 resulted from a report from the National Cancer Data Base concluded that tumor stage, hospital volume, and hospital location were the most statistically significant predictors of biopsy type (2). Rates of needle biopsy at high-volume hospitals suggest that appropriate utilization of this preferred diagnostic method should approach 90%. A meta-analysis has shown that FNA cytologic analysis of palpable breast masses is highly accurate in the diagnostic differentiation of benign from malignant tumors (3).

Sampling of nonpalpable or indistinct breast lesions can be done using stereotactic breast needle biopsy, a technique that enable the spatial localization of the lesion within the breast.

3. Estrogen receptor (ER) and progesterone receptor (PR) status

Receptors are proteins in or on certain cells that can attach to certain substances, such as hormones, that circulate in the blood. Normal breast cells and some breast cancer cells contain receptors that attach to estrogen and progesterone. These 2 hormones often fuel the growth of breast cancer cells.

An important step in evaluating a breast cancer is to test a portion of the cancer removed during the biopsy (or surgery) to see if they have estrogen and progesterone receptors. Cancer cells may contain neither, one, or both of these receptors. Breast cancers that have estrogen receptors are often referred to as *ER-positive* (or ER+) cancers, while those containing progesterone receptors are called *PR-positive* (or PR+) cancers. If either type of receptor is present, the cancer is said to be hormone receptor-postive.

Women with hormone receptor–positive cancers tend to live longer and are much more likely to respond to hormone therapy than women with cancers without these receptors.

All breast cancers, should be tested for these hormone receptors either on the the biopsy sample or when they are removed with surgery. About 2 of 3 breast cancers have at least one of these receptors. This percentage is higher in older women than in younger ones.

4. HER2/neu status

About 1 of 5 breast cancers have too much of a growth-promoting protein called *HER2/neu* (often just shortened to HER2). The HER2/neu gene instructs the cells to make this protein. Tumors with increased levels of HER2/neu are referred to as*HER2-positive.*

Women with HER2-positive breast cancers have too many copies of the HER2/neu gene, resulting in greater than normal amounts of the HER2/neu protein. These cancers tend to grow and spread more aggressively than other breast cancers.

All newly diagnosed breast cancers should be tested for HER2/neu because HER2-positive cancers are much more likely to benefit from treatment with drugs that target the HER2/neu protein, such as trastuzumab (Herceptin) and lapatinib (Tykerb).

Testing of the biopsy or surgery sample is usually done in 1 of 2 ways:

1. Immunohistochemistry (IHC): In this test, special antibodies that identify the HER2/neu protein are applied to the sample, which cause cells to change color if many copies are present. This color change can be seen under a microscope. The test results are reported as 0, 1+, 2+, or 3+.
2. Fluorescent in situ hybridization (FISH): This test uses fluorescent pieces of DNA that specifically stick to copies of the HER2/neu gene in cells, which can then be counted under a special microscope.

Many breast cancer specialists feel the FISH test is more accurate than IHC. However, it is more expensive and takes longer to get the results. Often the IHC test is used first. If the results are 1+ (or 0), the cancer is considered HER2-negative. People with HER2-negative tumors are not treated with drugs (like trastuzumab) that target HER2. If the test comes back 3+, the cancer is HER2-positive. Patients with HER2-positive tumors may be treated with drugs like trastuzumab. When the result is 2+, the HER2 status of the tumor is not clear. This often leads to testing the tumor with FISH.

A newer type of test, known as chromogenic in situ hybridization (CISH), works similarly to FISH, by using small DNA probes to count the number of HER2 genes in breast cancer cells. But this test looks for color changes (not fluorescence) and doesn't require a special microscope, which may make it less expensive. Right now, it is not being used as much as IHC or FISH.

5. Benign breast lesions

5.1. Fibrocystic disease

Fibrocystic disease is one of the most common benign breast lesions. The breast tissue in response of imbalanced estrogen and progesterone stimulation over time, undergoes a various morphologic changes of fibrocystic disease. The peak incidence is between 35 and 50 years of age. It is rare before 25 years. The term embraces a spectrum of histologic changes, and may encompass many patients who have cystic lesions detected clinically or sclerotic breast lesions detected on mammography as discussed elsewhere. Histologically it is characterized by overgrowth of both fibrous stroma, and of epithelial elements i.e. ducts and lobules, in differing proportions. These changes may be considered as aberrations of normal breast involution and not part of a disease process. The basic morphologic changes in the fibrocystic disease are cysts formation, apocrine metaplasia and fibrosis (4, 5, 6, 8,) Cysts may be grossly visible or evident in microscopic examination, usually contains yellow to clear fluid. The cyst lining may be flattened, or shows apocrine metaplasia and epithelial hyperplasia (5, 8). Apocrine metaplasia is characterized by abundant granular eosinophilic cytoplasm with apical snouts (5). Stromal fibrosis is also a common finding (5). Epithelial hyperplasia whether typical or atypical may be occurred in fibrocystic disease and put the patient in a higher risk of cancer development especially in patients accompanied by atypical ductal hyperplasia (Figure 1A &B) (4, 5, 6, 7).

Other rare morphologic variations include calcification and fibroadenoma-like picture, so called fibroadenomatoid mastopathy (9).

In most cases, symptoms of fibrocystic changes include breast pain and tender lumps or thickened areas in the breasts. These symptoms may change as the woman moves through different stages of the menstrual cycle. Sometimes, one of the lumps may feel firmer or have other features that lead to a concern about cancer. When this happens, a needle biopsy or a surgical biopsy may be needed to make sure that cancer is not present. Most women with fibrocystic changes and no bothersome symptoms do not need treatment, but closer follow-up may be advised. Women with mild discomfort may get relief from supportive bras or over-the-counter pain relievers. For a very small number of women with painful cysts,

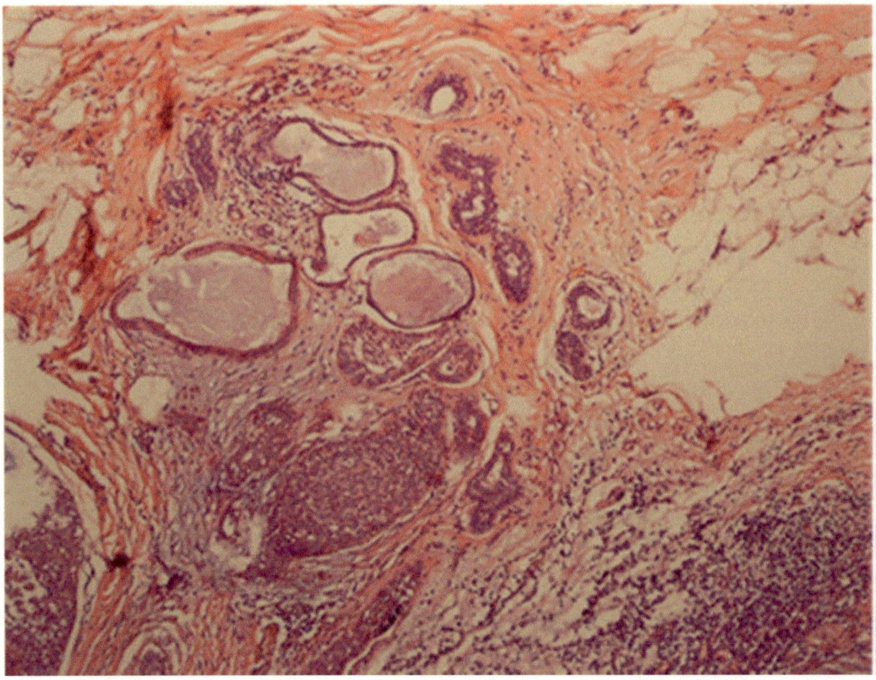

(a)

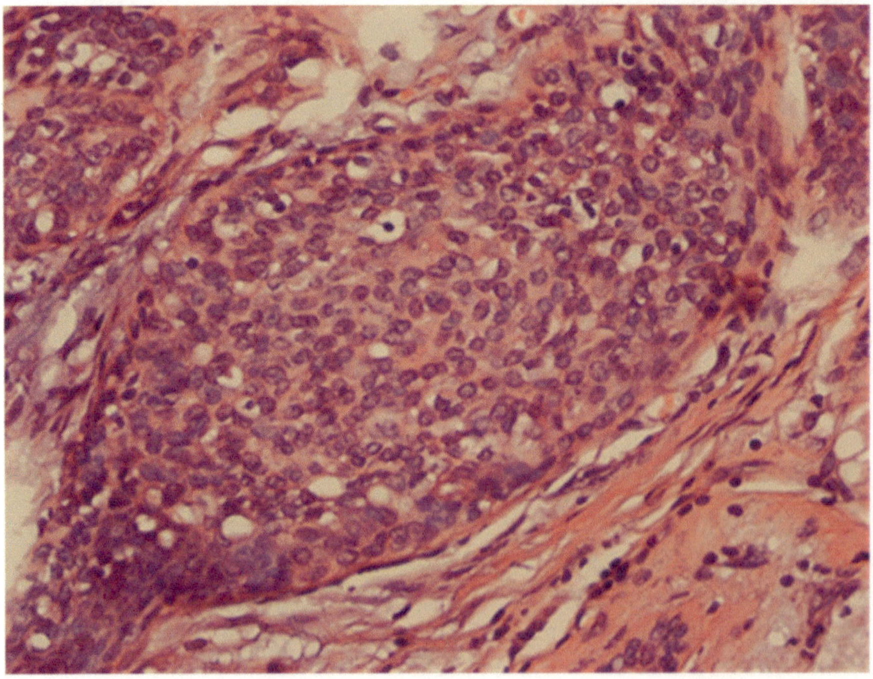

(b)

Figure 1. A: fibrocystic disease showing typical ductal hyperplasia, H & E, x100. B: typical ductal hyperplasia. The duct is obliterated by uniform cells with indistinc cytoplasmic border, H & E, x400.

draining the fluid with a needle can help relieve symptoms. Some women report that their breast symptoms improve if they avoid caffeine and other stimulants (called *methylxanthines*) found in coffee, tea, chocolate, and many soft drinks. Studies have not found those stimulants to have a significant impact on symptoms, but many women feel that avoiding these foods and drinks for a couple of months is worth trying. Because breast swelling toward the end of the menstrual cycle is painful for some women, some doctors recommend that women reduce salt in their diets or take diuretics. But studies have not found diuretics to be better than placebos. Many vitamin supplements have been suggested, but so far none are proven to be of any use, and some may have dangerous side effects if taken in large doses. Some doctors recommend hormones, such as oral contraceptives (birth control pills), tamoxifen, or androgens. But these are usually used only in women with severe symptoms because they can have serious side effects (10).

5.2. Breast cysts

Breast cysts are fluid filled, round or ovoid masses derived from the terminal duct lobular unit (TDLU). Cysts begin as fluid accumulation in the TDLU as a consequence of distension and obstruction of the efferent ductule (11). Breast cysts are influenced by hormonal function and therefore typically develop in premenopausal and perimenopausal women as a consequence of lobular development, cyclic changes, and lobular involution (12). Microscopically the cyst inner lining is flat or completely denuded and myopeithelial layer is recognizable.

Cysts are mostly occurs in women between 35-50 years old. It is uncommon for postmenopausal women to develop breast cysts, unless they are taking postmenopausal hormone replacement therapy. Breast cysts can present as gross palpable masses or as microcysts, usually found as an abnormality on an imaging examination. Acute enlargement of cysts may cause severe, localized pain of sudden onset. Cysts usually prompt women to seek medical attention because of a palpable mass or associated discomfort. FNA biopsy can confirm the diagnosis of a cyst and, at the same time, drain the cyst fluid. Removing the fluid may reduce pressure and pain for some time, but it is not necessary to remove the fluid unless it is causing discomfort. If removed, the fluid may come back later. Because needle biopsy of breast masses may produce artifacts that make mammography assessment more difficult, many radiologists prefer to image breast masses before performing needle biopsy (13, 14).

5.3. Intraductal papilloma

Papillomas are benign breast lesions usually affecting the lactiferous ducts, but smaller peripheral ducts may also be involved (4, 5, 6). The larger lesions may present with intramural fragile masses but smaller ones may be evident only on microscopic examination (4, 5). Microscopically, the papilloma consists of proliferation of ductal epithelium rested on fibrovascular stroma. Epithelial component consist of cuboidal to columnar cells without pleomorphism, nuclear atypia or mitotic figures (Figure 2A & B). Myoepithalial layer is also

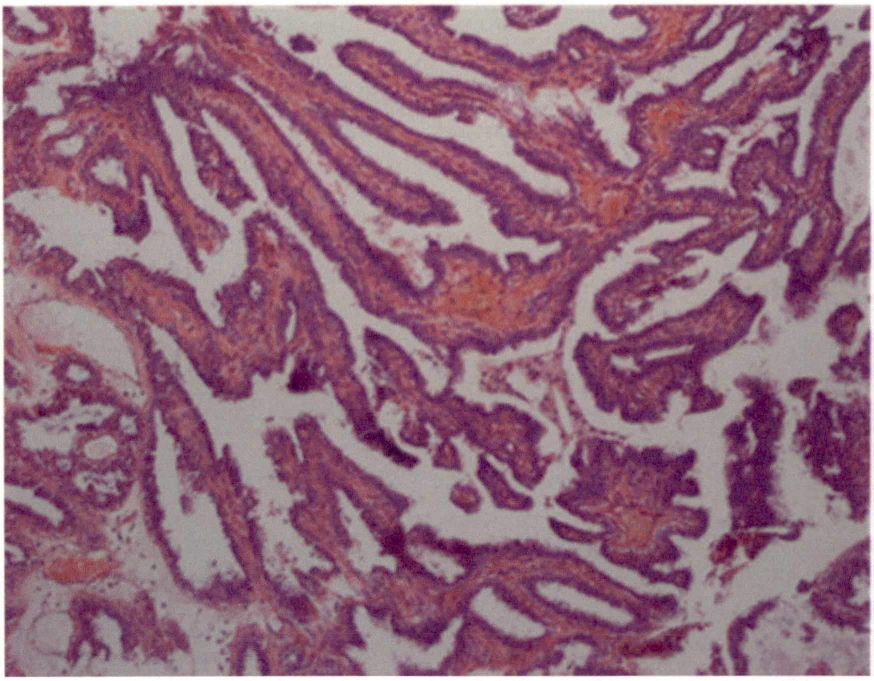

(a)

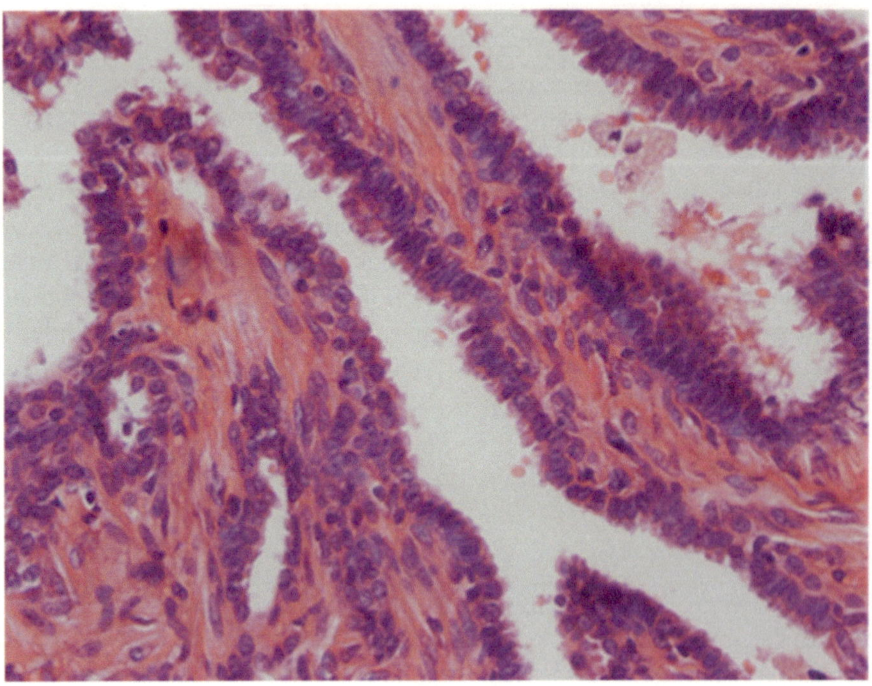

(b)

Figure 2. A & B: Papilloma. The epithelial cells are laying on fibrovascular core showing no atypia, H & E, x100 and x400

preserved (4, 5). Some papillomas have more complex structure accompanied by epithelial hyperplasia (4, 5, 6, 15). Atypical ductal hyperplasia and carcinoma in situ may occur in the setting of papillomas. Absence of myoepithelial layer is a useful marker for recognition of the malignant transformation (4, 5, 15). Papillomatosis (multiple papillomas) are usually bilateral with higher probability of association with carcinoma (6).

5.4. Sclerosing adenosis

Adenosis of breast is a proliferative lesion, characterized by increase number of glandular components. Various types of adenosis has been described: sclerosing, tubular, microglandular, and apocrine adenosis. Sclerosing adenosis is a kind of hyperplastic proliferation of glandular component of breast (5). It can occur as a focal or generalized proliferation of ducts and it may be accompanied by various forms of hyperplasia and even carcinoma (4, 6). Microscopically, the lesion has an oval to round configuration with central accentuation of cellularity. High power examination shows elongated and compressed glands formed by atrophied epithelial cells with preservation of myoepithelial layer, surrounded by sclerosed stroma (Figure 3A &B) (4, 5).

Some other morphologic variations include apocrine metaplasia and perineural invasion. Presence of myoepithelial layer distinguishes this lesion from an invasive carcinoma (4, 5, 16). The patients with sclerosing adenosis have a higher risk of subsequent development of malignancy, especially in patients that their lesion is accompanied by atypical lobular hyperplasia (4, 5). The clinical significance of sclerosing adenosis lies in its mimicry of cancer. It may be confused with cancer on physical examination, by mammography, and at gross pathologic examination. Excisional biopsy and histologic examination are frequently necessary to exclude the diagnosis of cancer. The diagnostic work-up for radial scars and complex sclerosing lesions frequently involves stereoscopic biopsy. It usually is not possible to differentiate these lesions with certainty from cancer by mammographic features, so biopsy is recommended. The mammographic appearance of a radial scar or sclerosing adenosis (mass density with spiculated margins) will usually lead to an assessment that the results of a core-needle biopsy showing benign disease are discordant with the radiographic findings. Breast radiologists will therefore often forego image-guided needle biopsy of a lesion suspicious for radial scar and refer the case directly to a surgeon for wire localized excisional biopsy.

5.5. Epithelial hyperplasia

Breast ducts are lined by two layers of epithelial cells, luminal and basal cells. Any increase in cell number within ductal space regarded as epithelial hyperplasia. Based on cytomorphology and presence of nuclear atypia, the lesion sub-classified as typical or atypical hyperplasia. The diagnosis of atypical epithelial hyperplasia (AEH) increases with breast cancer screening. AEH is divided in three groups: atypical ductal hyperplasia, columnar cell lesions with atypia, lobular neoplasia.

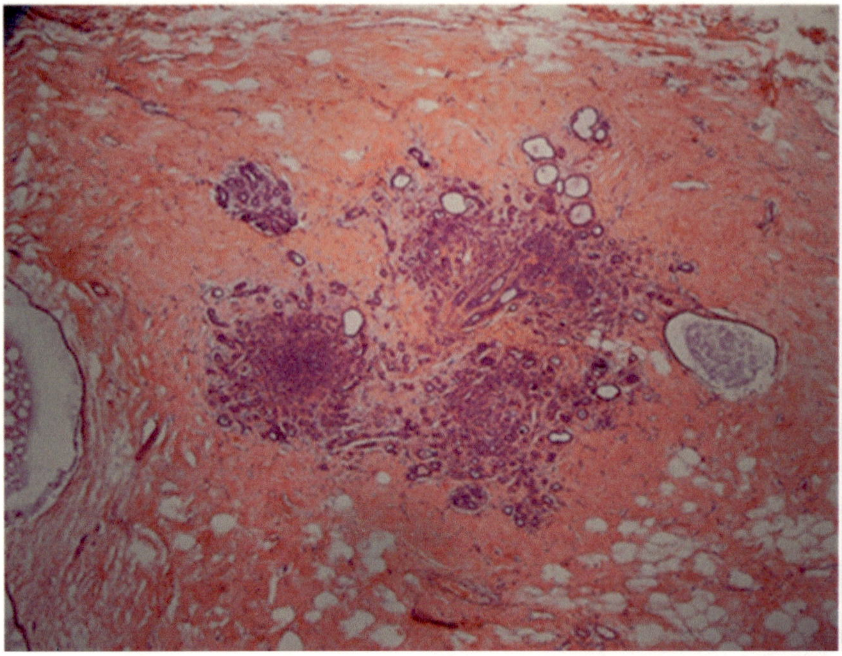

(a)

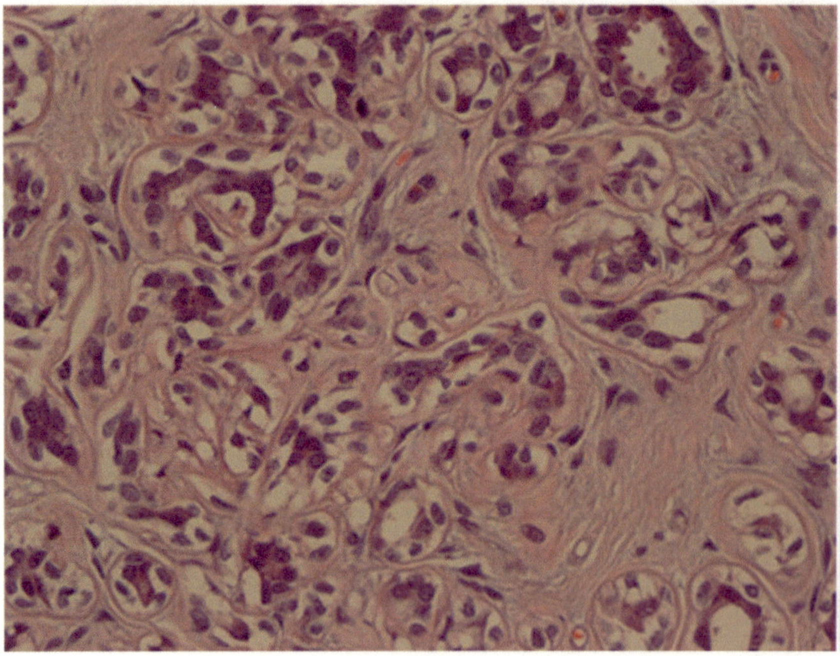

(b)

Figure 3. A & B: sclerosing adenosis. Glandular proliferation surrounded by sclerosed stroma. The glands are lined by two layer of epithelial and myoepithelial cells. The latter shows clear cell changes, H & E, X40 and X400

5.6. Ductal hyperplasia

Ductal hyperplasia is characterized by proliferation of ductal epithelium, resulting in increased cellularity and multi layering of ductal epithelium (4, 5). The pattern of growth varies greatly from case to case leading to different types of ductal hyperplasia (4, 5).

Features indicative of benign nature of the lesion includes oval nuclei with indistinct cytoplasmic border and eosinophilic rather than pale cytoplasm, arrangement of the cells in parallel bundles, presence of peripheral elongated clefts in ducts, presence of myoepithelial layer, apocrine metaplasia and absence of necrosis (4, 5). Ductal hyperplasia has been subdivided into mild, moderate and florid categories (4). In mild ductal hyperplasia, the epithelial thickness is 3 to 4 cell layer. In moderate hyperplasia, the thickness of epithelium is more than 4 layers and in florid hyperplasia, the gland lumen is often obliterated by proliferative epithelium and the affected duct is enlarged. Atypical ductal hyperplasia shares some features with intraductal carcinoma. The cells are monomorphic with round nuclei and distinct cytoplasmic border. Cytologic atypia is defined by high nuclear – to – cytoplasm ratio, hyperchromasia of nuclei and enlarged nucleoli. Mitotic activity is more seen in atypical ductal hyperplasia (Figure 4A & B). Presence of intermingled typical ductal hyperplasia or partial involvement of ducts aid in differentiating these lesions from ductal carcinoma insitu. (4, 5, 17). Patients with ductal hyperplasia especially with atypical ones have a higher risk for cancer development (4, 5, 6, 17, 18).

5.7. Columnar cell hyperplasia

The lesion is composed of ducts lined by tall columnar epithelial cells. Intraluminal secretion and calcification do occur. Atypical changes may be also encountered (4, 5, 6, 17).

5.8. Lobular hyperplasia

Lobular hyperplasia is a lesion in which lobules are larger and more cellular (4, 5). The lobular hyperplasia may occur in the setting of hormonal stimulation as in pregnancy (5). Atypical lobular hyperplasia characterized by proliferation of abnormal cells similar to the cell of lobular carcinoma in situ in one or more lobules. Atypical lobular hyperplasia increases the risk of cancer development (4, 5).

The management of women with AEH is not consensual because of uncertainty about their diagnosis related to the type of the biopsy sampling (core needle biopsy or surgical excision) and their controversial clinical signification between risk marker and true precursor of breast cancer. A systematic review performed by Lavoué V and colleagues showed that although according to immunohistochemistry and molecular studies, atypical epithelial hyperplasia (AEH) seems to be precursor of breast cancer; But, epidemiological studies show low rate of breast cancer in women with AEH. AEH were still classified as risk factor of breast cancer.

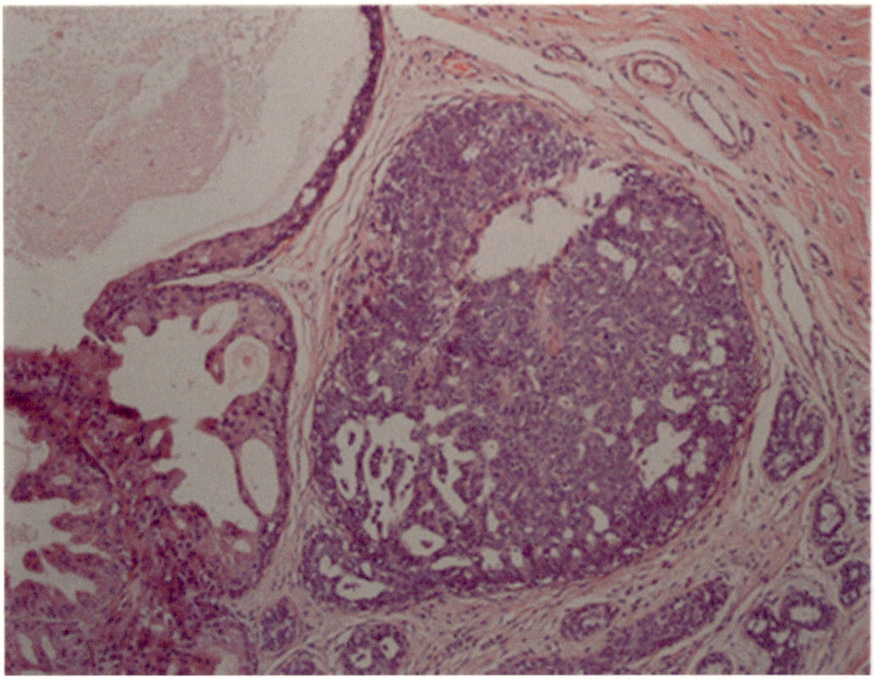

(a)

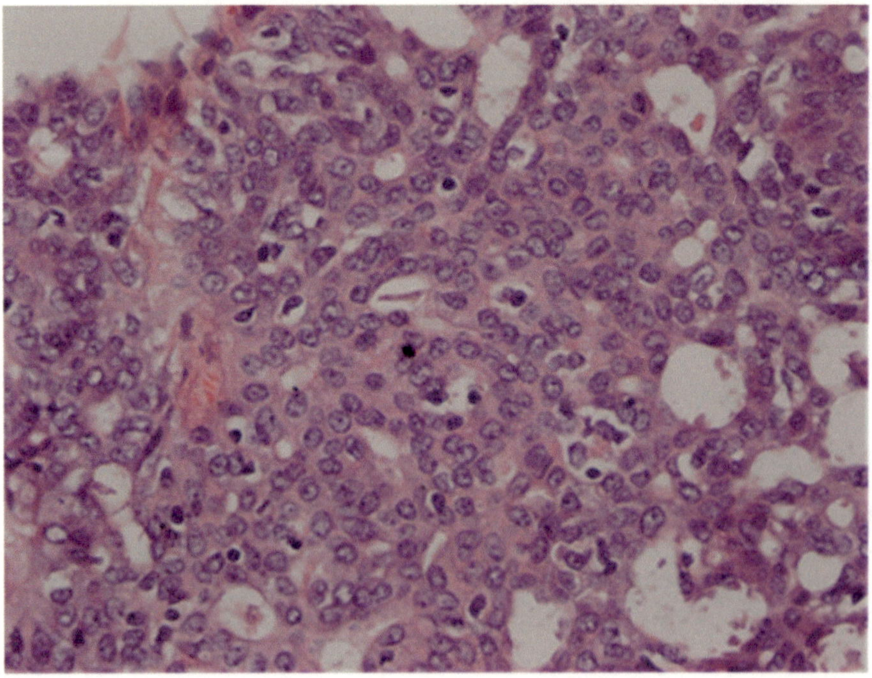

(b)

Figure 4. A & B: Atypical ductal hyperplasia. The duct is filled by atypical cells with pleomorphism and conspicuous nucleoli, H & E, x400.

5.9. Inflammatory lesions

Mastitis: inflammation of breast may caused by many etiologies, including infectious agents, local reaction to systemic disease, localized antigen-antibody reaction and idiopathic. Acute mastitis usually occurs in first 3 months of postpartum. The disorder is a cellulitis of the interlobular connective tissue within the mammary glands which can result in abscess formation. Granulomatous mastitis caused by infectious etiology, foreign material or systemic autoimmune disease. Idiopathic granulomatous mastitis can be diagnosed only when other causes were excluded. Histologically, chronic non-caseating granuloma confining to the lobule exist (Figure5A & B). Mammary duct ectasia or periductal mastitis characterized by dilatation of major ducts in the subareolar region. These ducts contain eosinophilic granular secretions within the duct epithelium or lumen.

Fat necrosis: is a benign non-suppurative inflammatory process secondary to trauma, surgery or radiation therapy. Microscopically, the lesion is characterized by infiltration of foamy histiocytes, lymphocytes, plasma cells and giant cells around anuclear fat cells (Figure 6) (4, 5, 6).

6. Neoplasms

Fibroadenoma is a common benign breast tumor, mostly occurs in second and third decade of life (4, 5). Grossly the tumor is circumscribed and firm. Microscopically, the fibroadenoma is a biphasic mass composing of epithelial and stromal components. The epithelial part is usually made up of tubules consisting of cuboidal to low columnar cells, resting on a myoepithelial cell layer. Stroma with varying degree of cellularity, contains loose connective tissue (Figure 7A & B) (4, 5, 6, 13).

Some morphologic variation exists in fibroadenoma including hyalinization, mixoid change, calcification, apocrine metaplasia and sclerosing adenosis. fibroadenoma showing cysts, sclerosing adenosis, apocrine neoplasia are called camplex fibroadenoma (4, 5).

Proliferative epithelial changes including ductal hyperplasia whether typical or atypical and lobular hyperplasia, are also noted in fibroadenoma (4, 5, 6, 13).

Malignant transformation in fibroadenoma do occur but it is rare, usually involving the epithelial component in the form of carcinoma in situ and invasive carcinoma (lobular and ductal) (4, 5, 13, 14).

The main differential diagnosis of fibroadenoma is phylloides tumor . The latter is usually occurring in older ages, has more cellular stroma with stromal overgrowth .

Mitotic figures may be seen in phylloides tumor, but they are usually absent in fibroadenoma (4, 13).

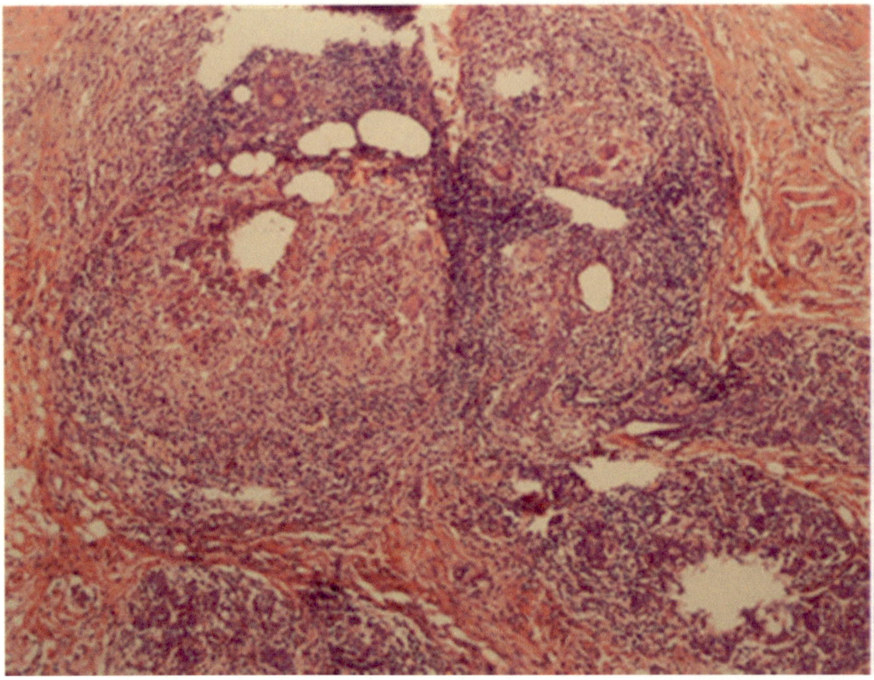

(a)

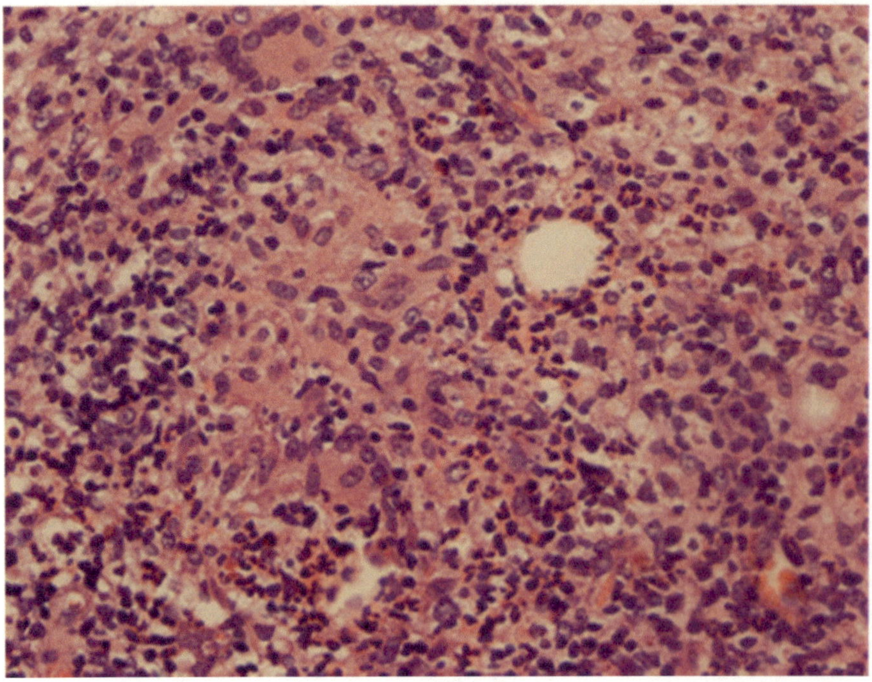

(b)

Figure 5. A & B: Granulomatous mastitis. The granulomatous reaction consistiong of epitheloid histiocytes, giant cells and inflammatory cells surrounds the breast lobules, H & E, x 100 and x400.

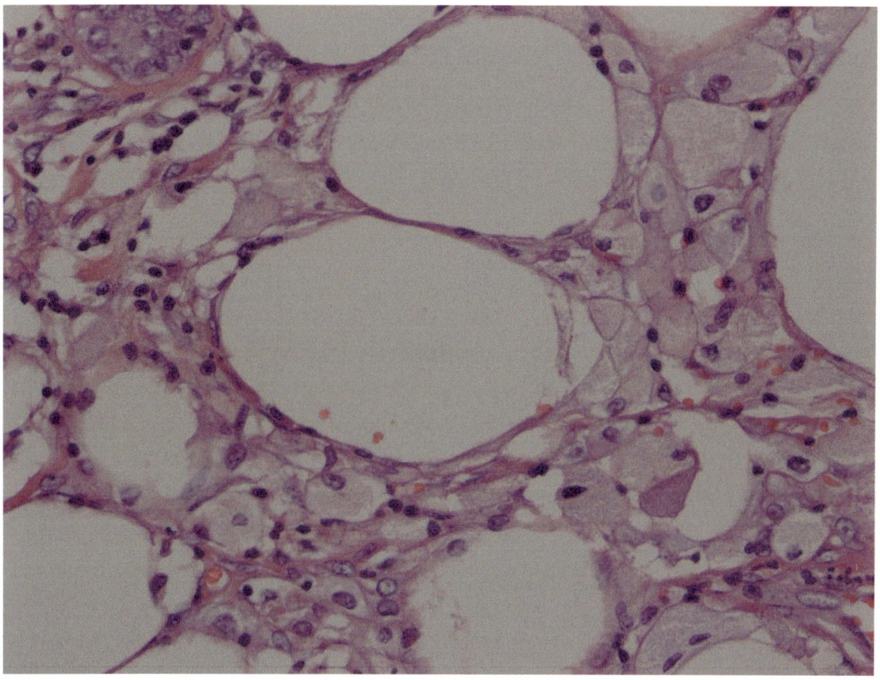

Figure 6. Fat necrosis. The breast parenchyma is infiltrated by foamy macrophages and inflammatory cells, H & E, X400.

7. Breast cancer

Breast cancer is the most common female cancer in the US, the second most common cause of cancer death in women, and the main cause of death in women ages 40 to 59. About 1 in 8 (12%) women in the US will develop invasive breast cancer during their lifetime (19). The American Cancer Society's most recent estimates for breast cancer in the United States are for 2012:

- About 226,870 new cases of invasive breast cancer will be diagnosed in women.
- About 63,300 new cases of carcinoma in situ (CIS) will be diagnosed (CIS is non-invasive and is the earliest form of breast cancer).
- About 39,510 women will die from breast cancer (20).

Many early breast cancers are asymptomatic. Among the symptomatic cases ,painless mass is the most common symptom. Pain or discomfort is not usually a symptom of breast cancer; only 5% of patients with a malignant mass present with breast pain. Diagnosis of the breast cancer is made based on history, physical examination, mammograms and/or ultrasound findings and the pathologic assessment of specimens. Once a diagnosis of breast cancer is made, the type of therapy offered to a breast cancer patient is determined by the stage of the disease. Laboratory tests and imaging studies are performed based on the initial stage.

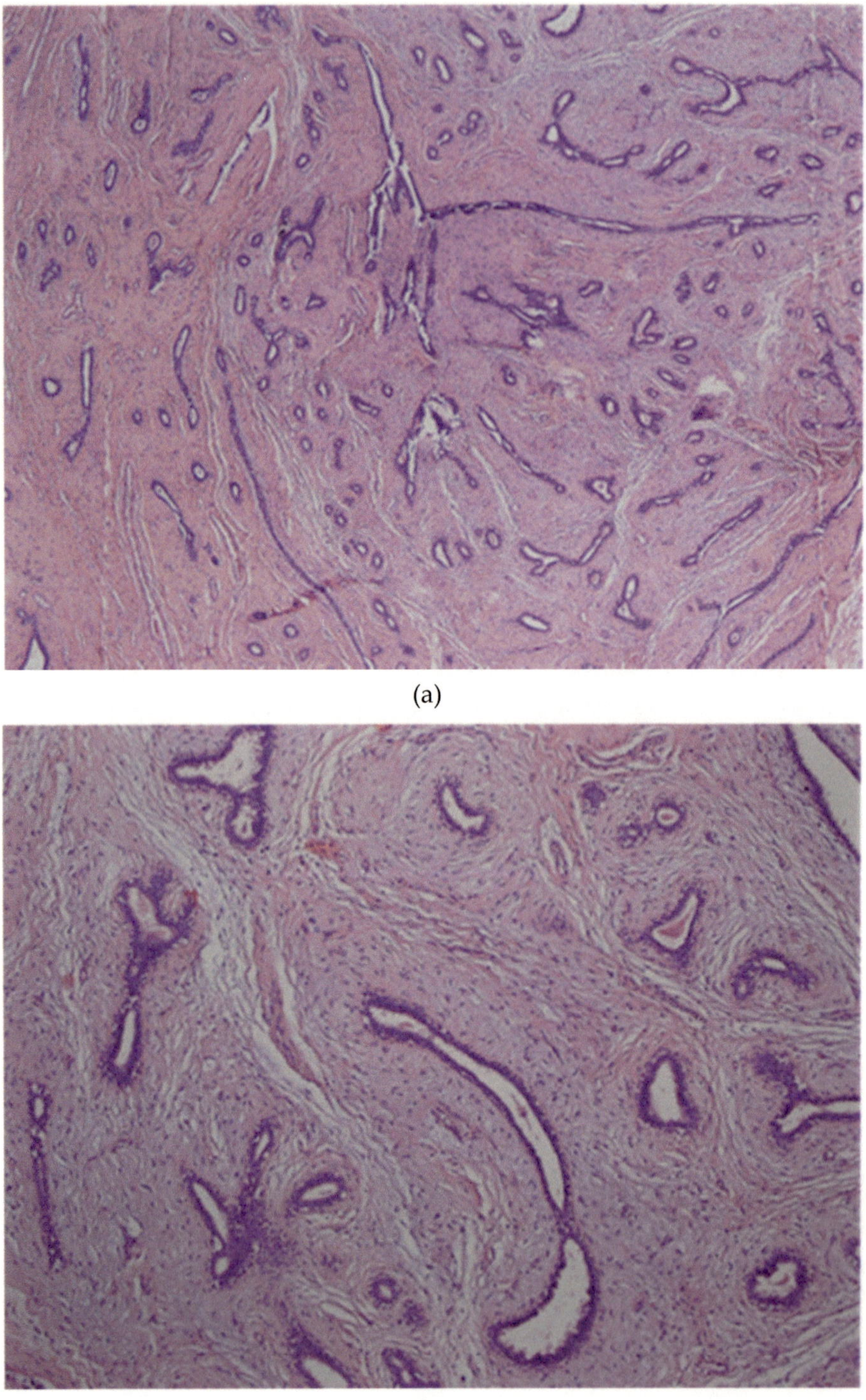

Figure 7. A & B: Fibroadenoma. The tumor is biphasic consisting of glanduar and stromal parts, H & E,x 40 and x100.

8. Pathology of the breast cancer

8.1. *In situ* carcinoma

8.1.1. Ductal carcinoma in situ (DCIS)

In situ ductal carcinoma is a malignant proliferation of epithelial cells, confined to the lumen of ducts, which was categorized into two grades: High grade comedocarcinoma, composed of pleomorphic cells showing central necrosis and low grade solid, cribriform and micropapillary group with uniform cells without area of necrosis. Clinging carcinoma, based on cytologic features was placed in either groups (4, 5, 21).

Recently, in situ carcinomas were divided into three grades, comedocarcinoma has been placed in grade 3, solid, cribriform and micropapillary carcinomas were designated as grade 1 if they and bland cytologic morphology and classified as grade 2 if they had intermediate cytomorphology (5).

8.2. Comedocarcinoma

Comedocarcinoma is characterized by solid growth of pleomorphic cells within the ducts with area of central necrosis and dystrophic calcification. Mitosis may be abundant. Grossly, thick walled ducts filled with creamy White necrotic material is a characteristic finding. Some comedocarcinoma may present with a palpable mass (4, 5, 22). Myoepithelial layer is usually present but it may have a discontinues fashions (Figure 8A & B) (4, 5).

8.3. *In situ* papillary carcinoma

In situ papillary carcinoma is defined by proliferations of epithelial cells resting on a fibrovascular core. The most important differential diagnosis of this lesion is papilloma. The proposed criteria in favor of in situ papillary carcinoma are older age, larger size, presence of uniform cells, lack of myoepithelial layer, presence of nuclear atypia (hyperchromasia and high nuclear-to-cytoplasmic ratio), high mitotic activity and absent intervening stroma (4, 5, 23, 24).

8.4. Solid *in situ* carcinoma

Solid In situ carcinoma is characterized by filling of the ducts lumen by malignant cells. These cells are uniform with distinct cytoplasmic border and pale cytoplasm (4, 5).

8.5. Cribriform *in situ* carcinoma

Cribriform in situ carcinoma is characterized by proliferation of uniform cells with distinct cytoplasmic border and pale cytoplasm forming round spaces. (Figure 9)(4, 5).

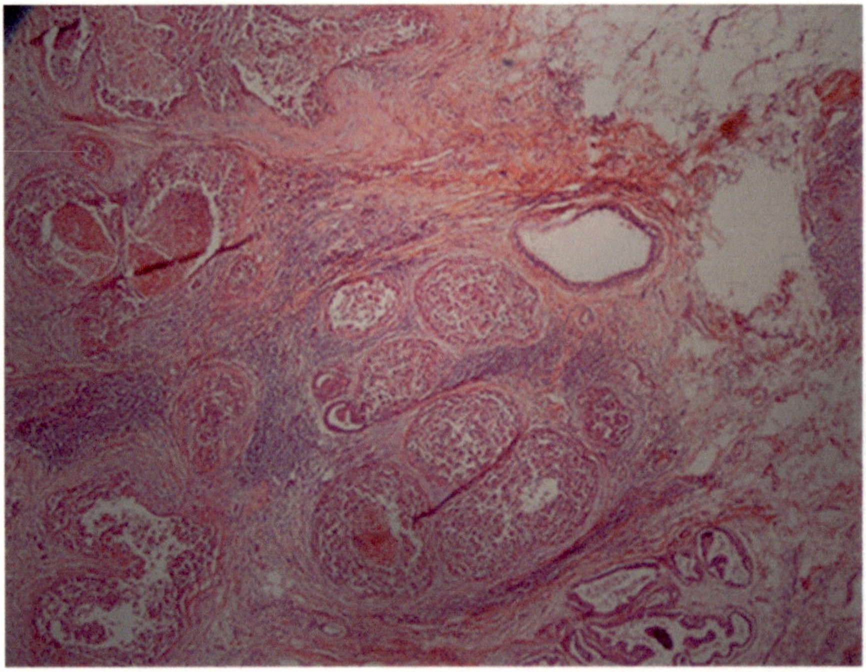

(a)

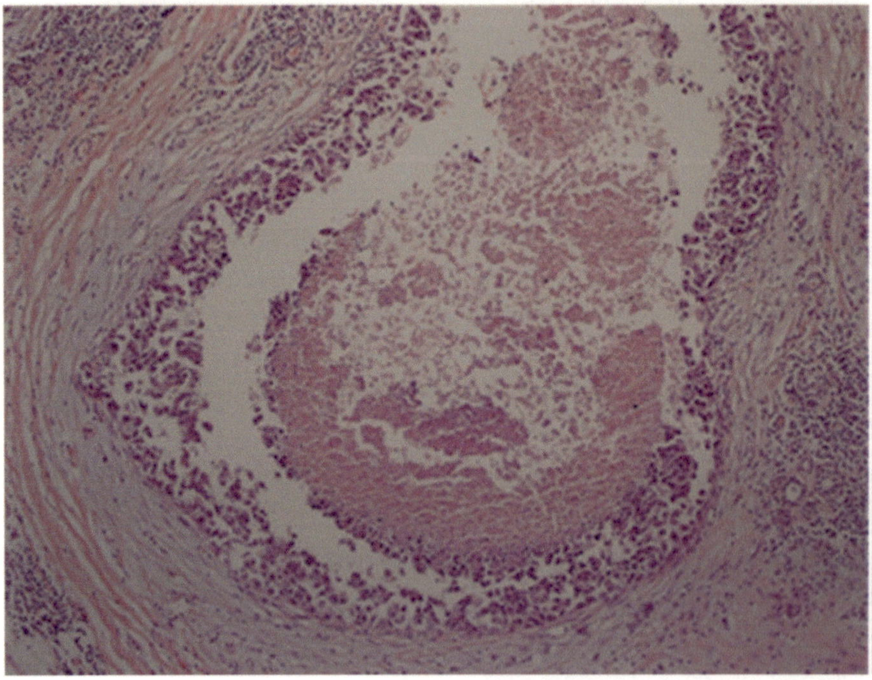

(b)

Figure 8. A & B: *In situ* comedo carcinoma. The dilated ducts are filled by atypical cells showing central necrosis, H & E, X40 and X100.

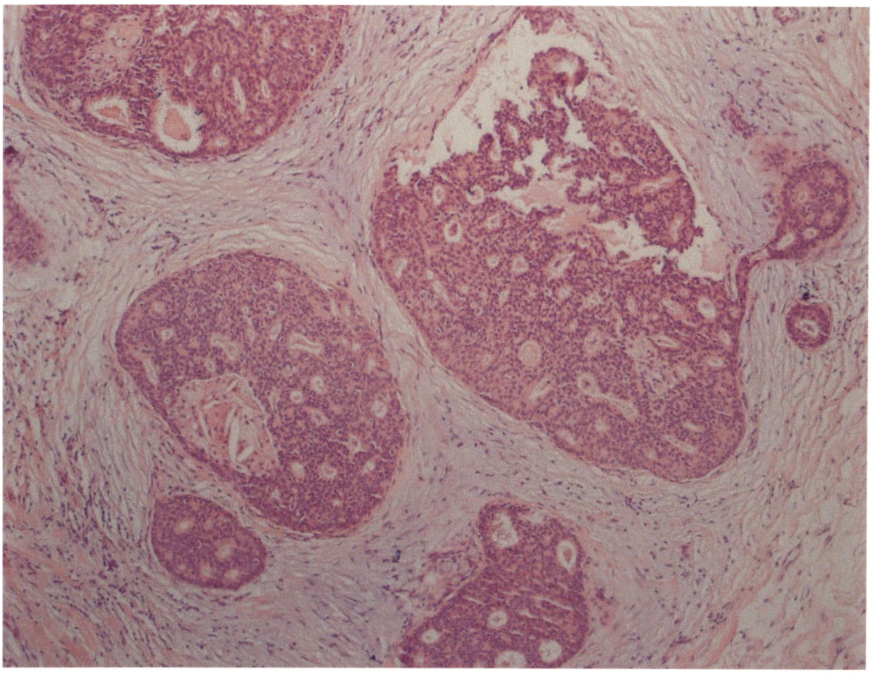

Figure 9. Ductal carcinoma in situ of cribriform type. The ducts are filled by cells forming round spaces, so called cribriform pattern, H & E, x100.

8.6. Micropapillary *in situ* carcinoma

Micropapillary in situ carcinoma is defined by intraluminal epithelial papillary projections. In contrast to papillary carcinoma, fibrovascular stroma is absent.

Pure micropapillary in situ carcinoma is significantly associated with foci of microinvasion and multicentricity (4, 5, 25).

8.7. Clinging *in situ* carcinoma

Clinging in situ carcinoma is a type of intraductal carcinoma in which one to two layer of malignant cells lined the ducts periphery (4, 5).

All types of in situ carcinomas have potential to transform into invasive carcinoma. It has been stated that the risk of subsequent invasive carcinoma development is related to cytologic grade of tumor (5, 21, 22).

8.8. Lobular carcinoma *in situ* (LCIS)

Lobular carcinoma in situ characterized by proliferations of neoplastic cells replacing the normal epithelial of breast lobules (4, 5, 26, 27, 28). Microscopically, the lobules are enlarged, filled with uniform, round, small to medium sized cells usually obliterating the lumen (Figure 10 A & B). The cells lost their cohesion. As a general rule the cells are more uniform

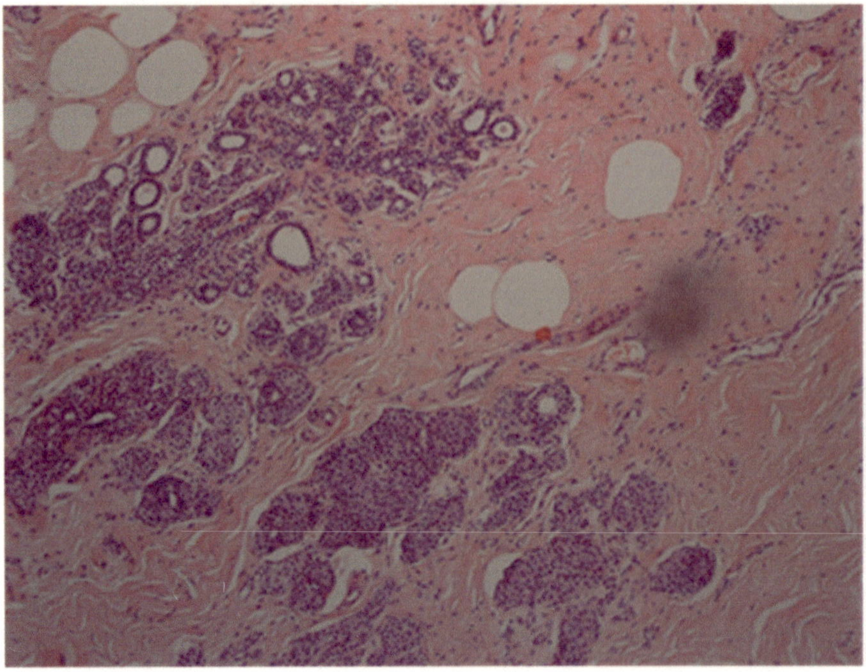

(a)

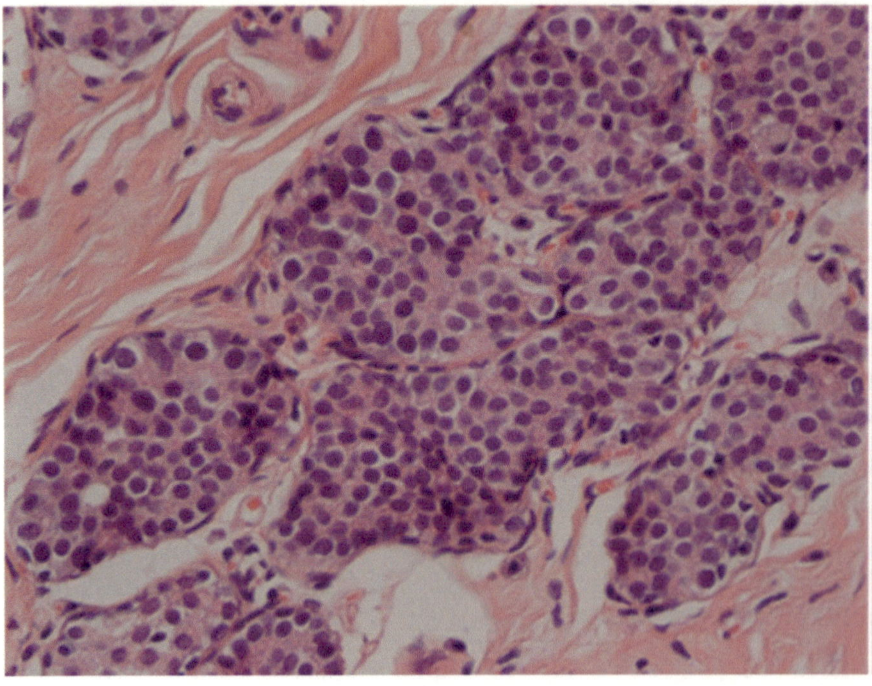

(b)

Figure 10. A & B: Lobular carcinoma *in situ*. The distended lobules obliterated by small and relatively uniform cells, H & E, X100 and X400.

and smaller than cells of DCIS, although cases with pleomorphic and large cells are present which are called " pleomorphic LCIS". So differentiation of this variant of LCIS from solid DCIS is an important task. Positive E-cadherin immune staining in DCIS distinguishes these two lesions (4, 5, 26, 27). Risk of invasive carcinoma development in breast harboring LCIS is significantly increased (4, 5).

8.9. Invasive carcinoma

Tumors, in which stromal invasions by malignant cells are evident, are called invasive carcinomas. Invasive tumors are categorized into two groups: ductal and lobular.

8.10. Invasive ductal carcinoma, Not-otherwise-specified (NOS)

This lesion is the most common malignant tumor of breast, consisting 75% to 80% of breast cancers. Grossly, the tumors are variable in size and consistency; in the prototype ones, the lesions are firm with ill-defined border and *"chalky streaks"* appearance on cut sections. Some tumors may have softer consistency with a better-defined border. Microscopically, the tumor cells may grow in sheets, nests, cords or single cell. Glandular formation varies between cases. The cells also show considerable variation, ranging from small cells with relatively uniform nuclei to markedly pleomorphic cells. Mitotic figures are evident and necrosis may occur (Figure 11). Myoepithelial cells are absent. Based on morphology some other subtypes of invasive ductal carcinoma are present (4, 5).

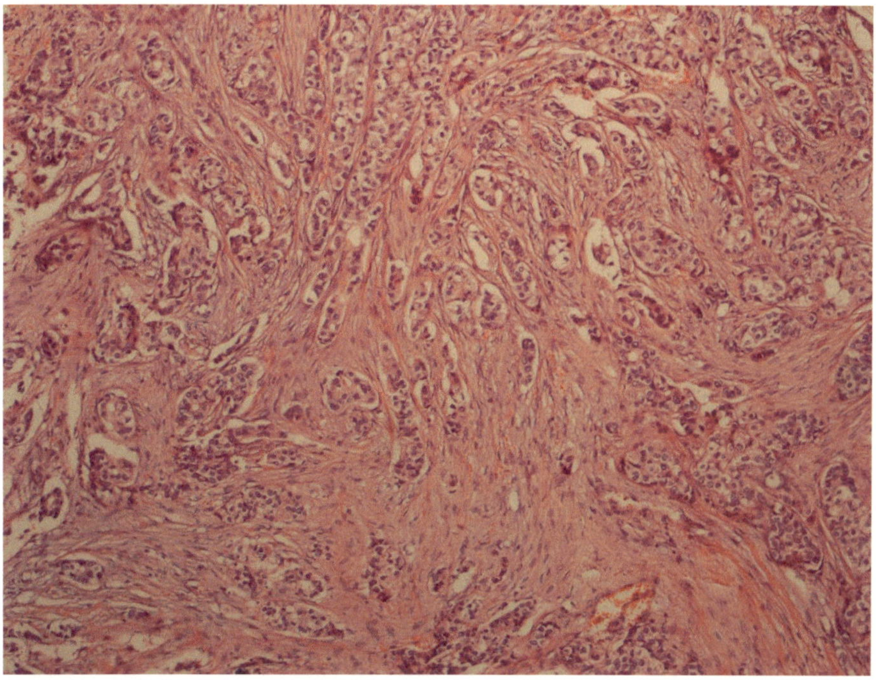

Figure 11. Invasive ductal carcinoma NOS. small nests of tumarl tissue infiltrating the breast stroma, H & E, X100.

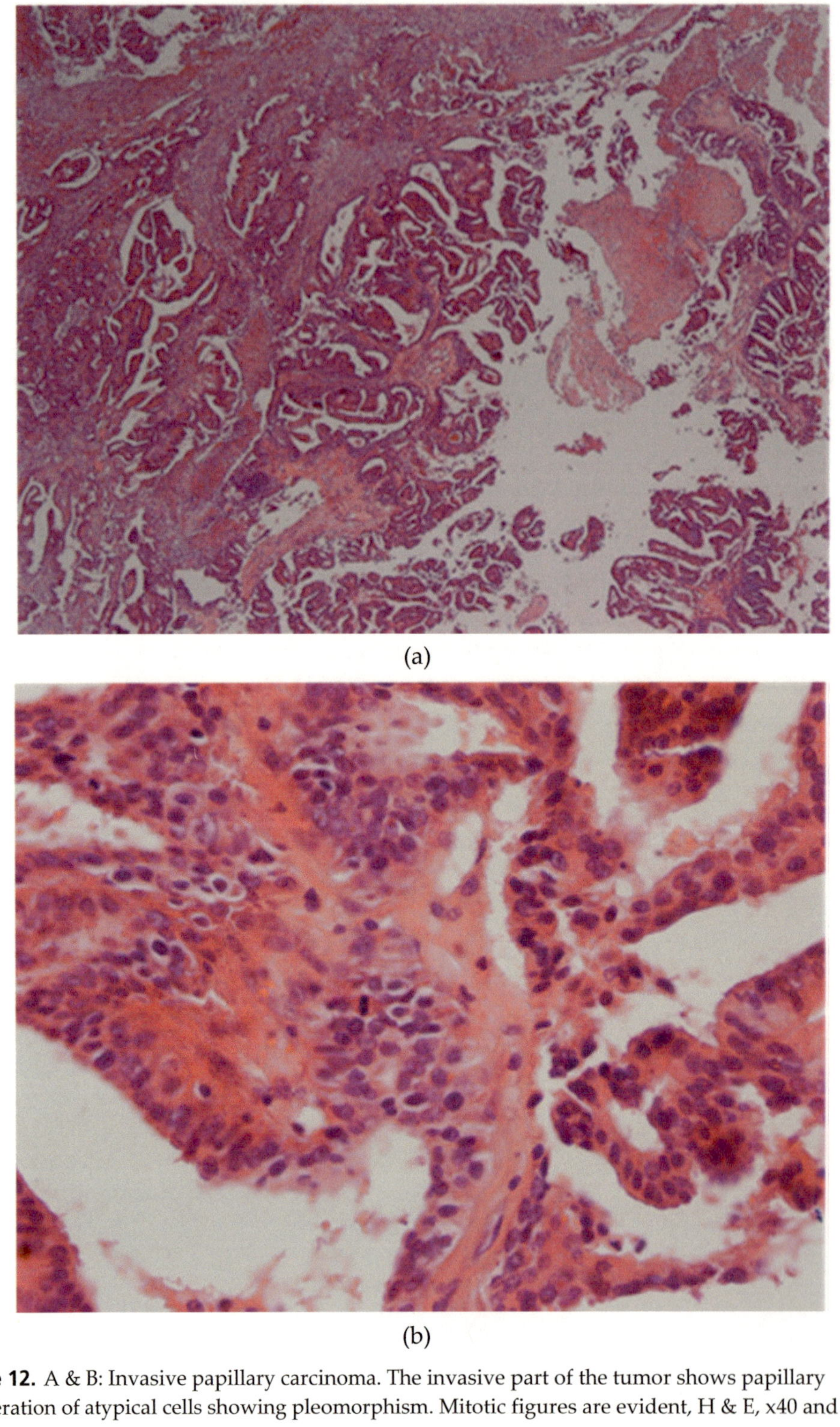

(a)

(b)

Figure 12. A & B: Invasive papillary carcinoma. The invasive part of the tumor shows papillary proliferation of atypical cells showing pleomorphism. Mitotic figures are evident, H & E, x40 and x400.

8.11. Tubular carcinoma

The lesion is a distinctive type of breast cancer. Grossly, the lesion is firm with ill-defined border. Microscopically, the tumor composed of small glands or tubules with irregular contours, lacking myoepithelial layer. Basement membrane is also absent (4, 5, 29). This lesion has a better prognosis than invasive ductal carcinoma with lower risk of lymph mode metastasis (4, 5, 30).

8.12. Papillary carcinoma

Papillary carcinoma usually occurs in the central part of breast. Microscopically, the invasive component shows papilla formation, although in some area solid sheet proliferation of tumor cells is seen (Figure 12A & B). Myoepithelial cells are consistently absent (4, 5, 22, 24).

8.13. Medullary carcinoma

Medullary carcinomas are usually occur in young patients and are commonly associated with BRCA-1 mutation. Grossly, the tumor is relatively well circumscribed. Microscopically, the sheets of syncyial poorly differentiated large pleomorphic cells with prominent nucleoli are seen. Mitotic figures are numerous and the tumor border is of pushing type. Infiltration of lympho-plasma cells of the periphery of the tumor is a constant histologic picture (Figure 13). As a general rule gland formation is absent or minimal (4, 5, 31, 32). Prognosis of medullary carcinoma is too better than invasive ductal carcinoma (4).

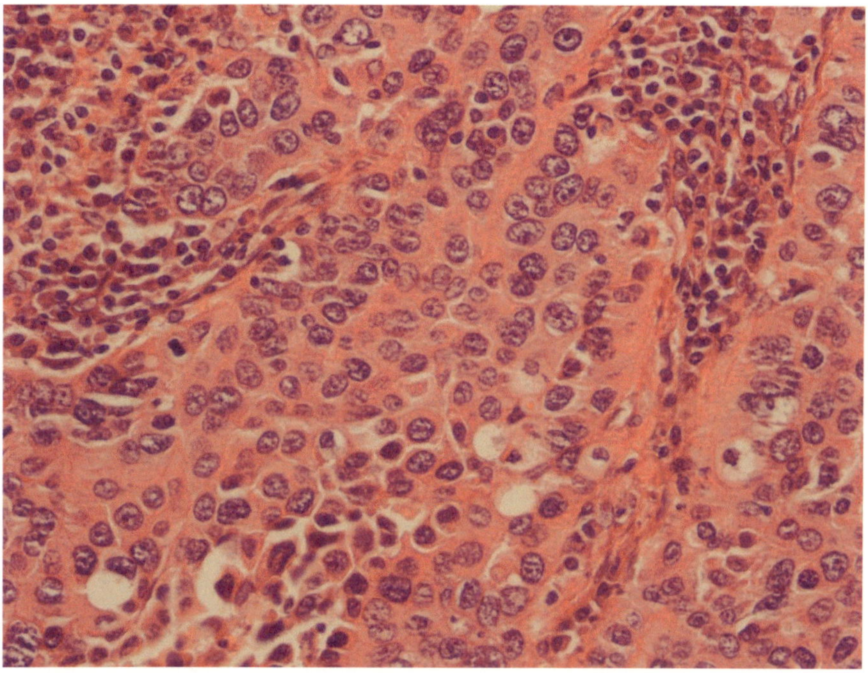

Figure 13. Medullary carcinoma. Sheet of atypical tumor cells infiltrated by lymphoplasma cells, H & E, X400.

8.14. Metaplastic carcinoma

Metaplastic carcinoma is a distinct type of ductal carcinoma in which the predominant growth pattern is nonglandular. The metaplastic change may be squamous or pseudosarcomatous (Figure 14A & B). Heterogeneous element such as bone or cartilage may also be found (4, 5, 33, 34). Metaplastic carcinoma is considered in differential diagnosis of any spindle cell lesions of the breast including primary breast sarcomas and phyllodes tumor. The behavior of metaplastic carcinoma is more aggressive than invasive ductal carcinoma (4).

Squamous cell carcinoma is a form of metaplastic carcinoma. Before establishing the diagnosis of primary squamous cell carcinoma, metastasis from extra mammary sites must be ruled out. Microscopically, this tumor is similar to squamous cell carcinoma of the other body organs in which keratinization may be evident (4, 5, 35).

8.15. Mucinous carcinoma:

Mucinous carcinoma also known as colloid carcinoma is a form of invasive ductal carcinoma, in which clusters of tumor cells floating in extracellular mucin lakes (Figure 15A & B). Grossly, the tumor is well circumscribed with a gelatinous cut surface. Some mucinous carcinomas may show neuroendocrine differentiation. Based on this observation mucinous carcinomas were categorized into type A and B with or without neuroendocrine differentiation, respectively (4, 5, 36, 37). Mucinous carcinoma has a better prognosis than invasive ductal carcinoma, NOS (4, 5, 36).

8.16. Secretory carcinoma

Secretory carcinoma was thought to occur in pediatric age groups but reported cases of this lesion in adults exist. Grossly, the tumor is well circumscribed and firm. Microscopically, the tumor shows glandular, cystic or papillary pattern. Individual tumor cells may be granular or vacuolated tend to form spaces containing a periodic acid-schiff (PAS) positive secretion. Atypia is minimal and mitotic activity is low (4, 5, 38, 39, 40). The prognosis is good and rate of lymph node metastasis is low (4, 5).

8.17. Inflammatory carcinoma

Inflammatory carcinoma is clinically present with edema and redness of the breast skin, resembling mastitis. Microscopically, inflammatory carcinoma is a type of ordinary breast cancer in which dermal lymphatic invasions by tumor is evident (4).

8.18. Paget's disease

Paget is an erythematous, eczema-like lesion of nipple and areola, accompanied by underlying breast carcinoma, which may be in situ or invasive. Microscopically, large cells with clear cytoplasm and atypical nuclei are seen in epidermis (Figure 16A & B). These cells

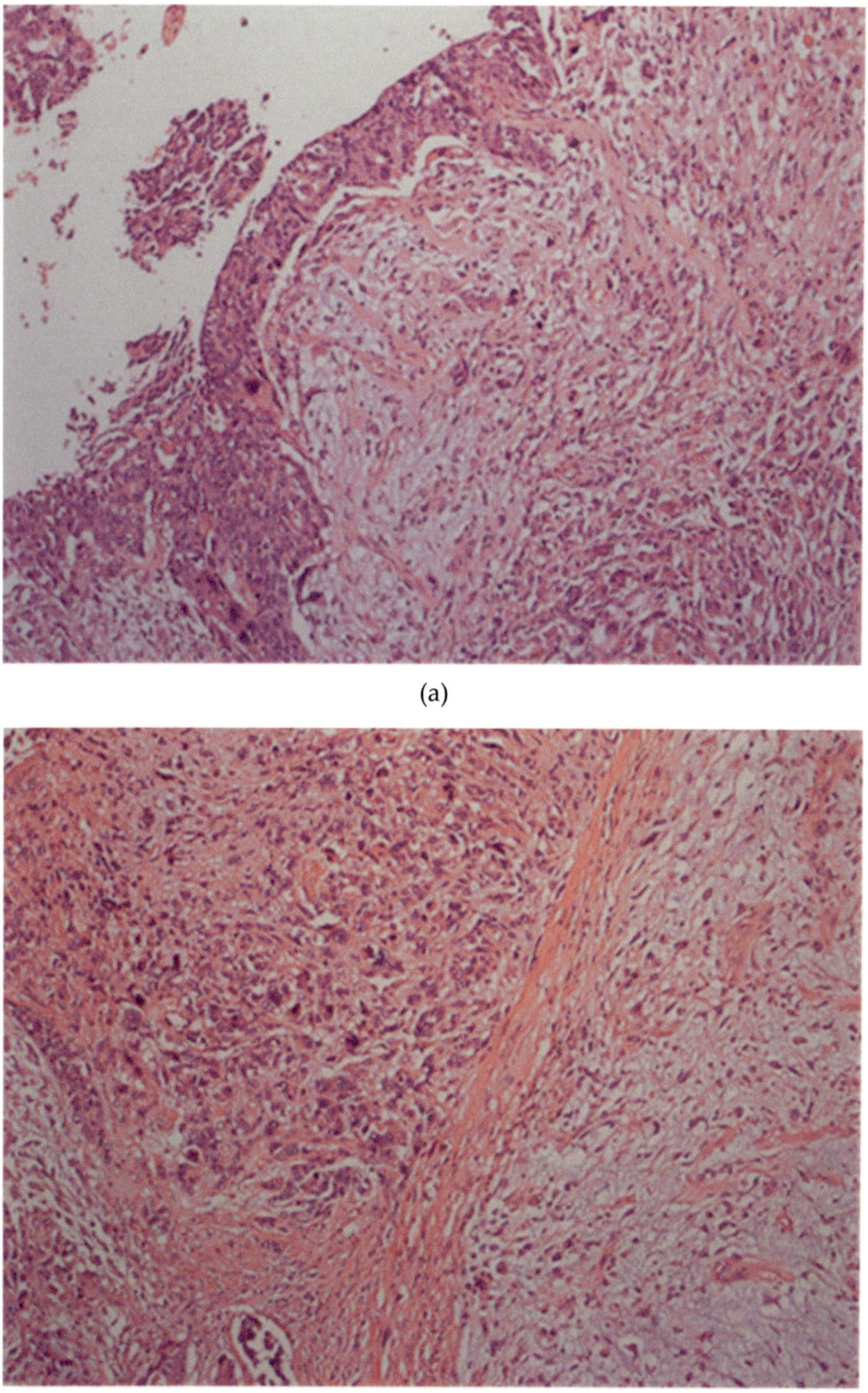

(a)

(b)

Figure 14. A & B: metaplastic carcinoma. The tumor composed of sarcomatous component (right side) and carcinomatous compnent (left side), so called carcinosarcoma, H & E, X100.

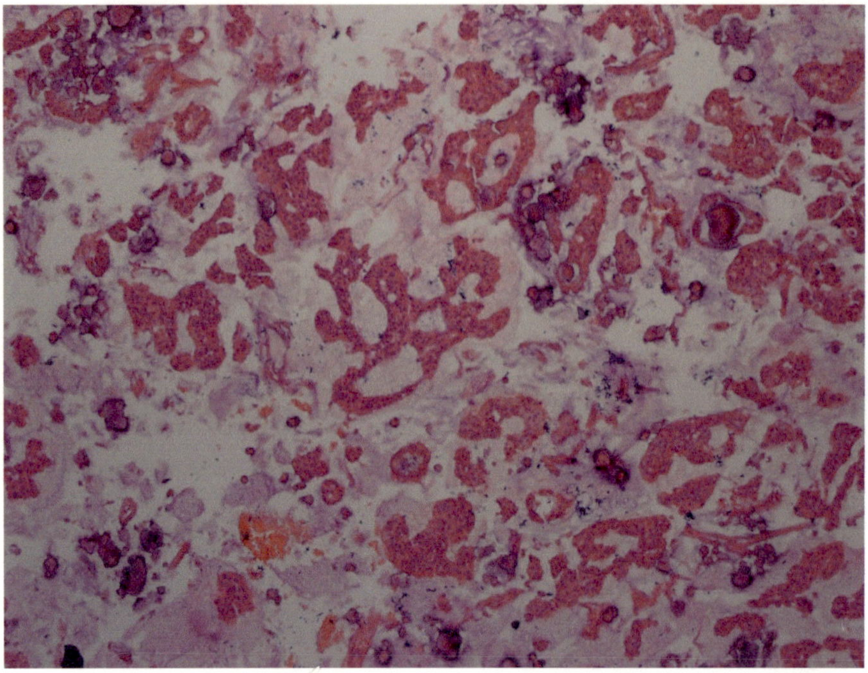

(a)

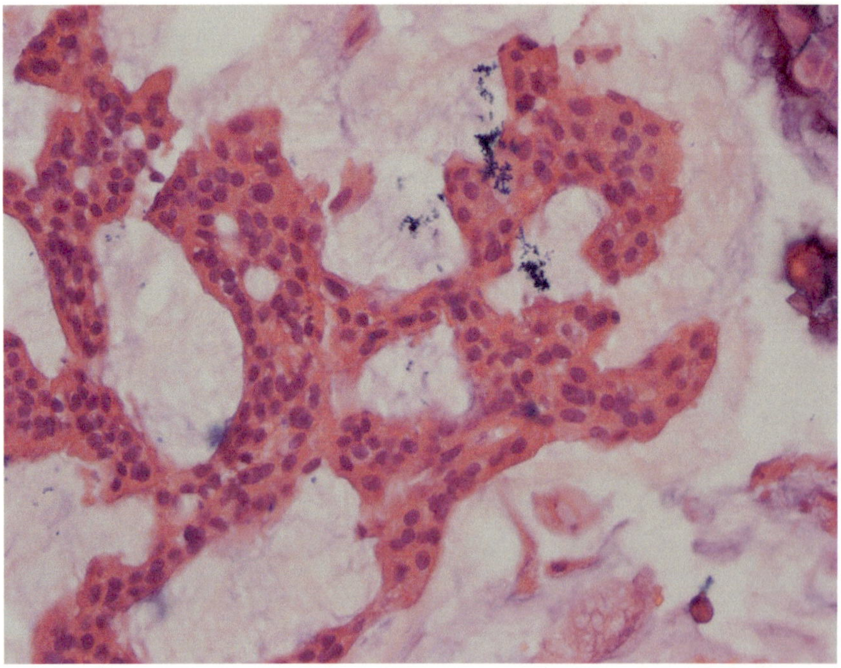

(b)

Figure 15. A & B: mucinous carcinoma. The tumor nests are floating in mucin lakes, H & E, X40 and X400.

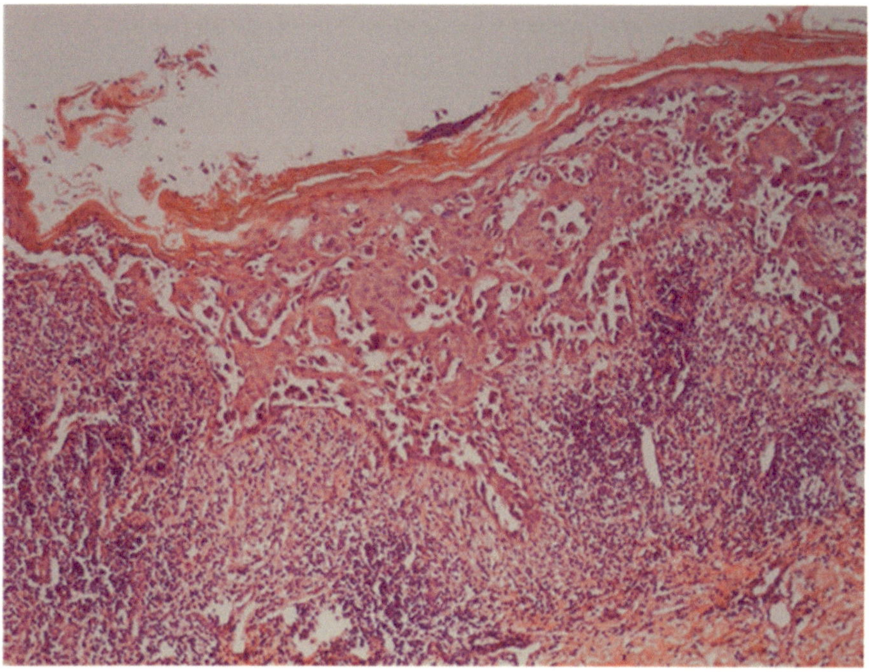

(a)

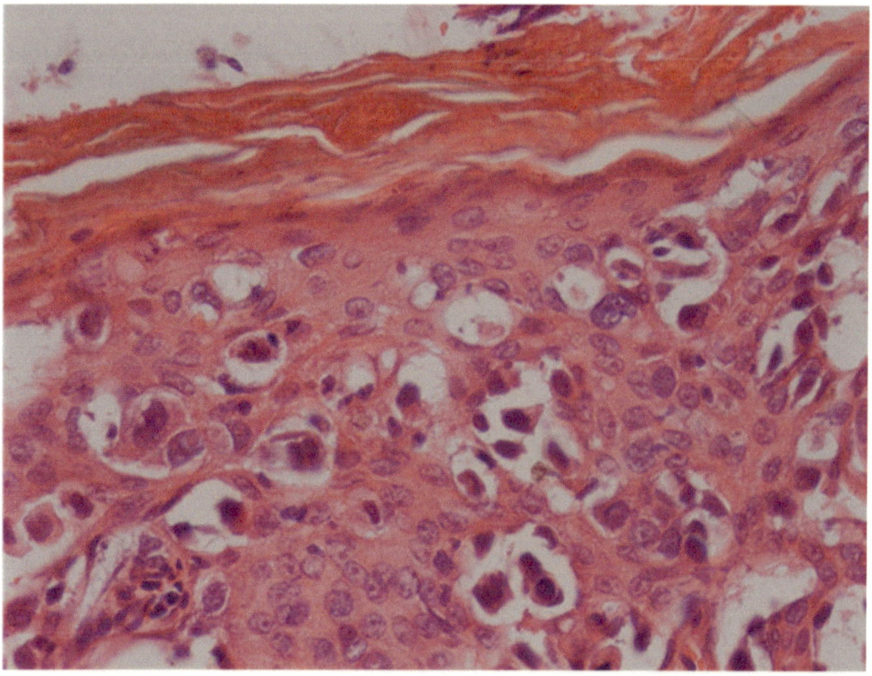

(b)

Figure 16. A & B: Paget's disease. The atypical cells with clear cytoplasm are infiltrating the epidermis, H & E, X100 and X400.

may be isolated or appeared in clusters especially in basal layer of epidermis (4, 5, 41, 42). Important differential diagnosis is malignant melanoma. Immunohistochemistry is of great help to reach a correct diagnosis. Paget's cells are immune reactive for EMA, CEA, CK-7, HER-2/neu and GCPFP-15 but S100 is negative (4).

The other rare types of invasive ductal carcinoma are apocrine carcinoma, carcinoma with neuroendocrine differentiation and cribriform carcinoma.

8.19. Invasive lobular carcinoma

Invasive lobular carcinoma is characterized by infiltration of discohesive small, monotonous tumor cells grow in Indian file or singly (Figure 17). Concentric arrangement of tumor cells around lobules is seen (4, 5, 28, 43). Discohesion of cells is due to loss of E-cadherin. For purpose of differentiating these tumors from invasive ductal carcinoma, an attention to cytomorphology and immunohistochemistry is helpful. In general, cells of lobular carcinomas are smaller, more uniform and discohesive. Other morphologic variants of invasive lobular carcinoma exist (4, 5). Pleomorphic lobular carcinoma shows larger tumor cells with nuclear pleomorphism. Pattern of growth and loss of E-cadherin points to lobular nature of the lesion (4, 5).

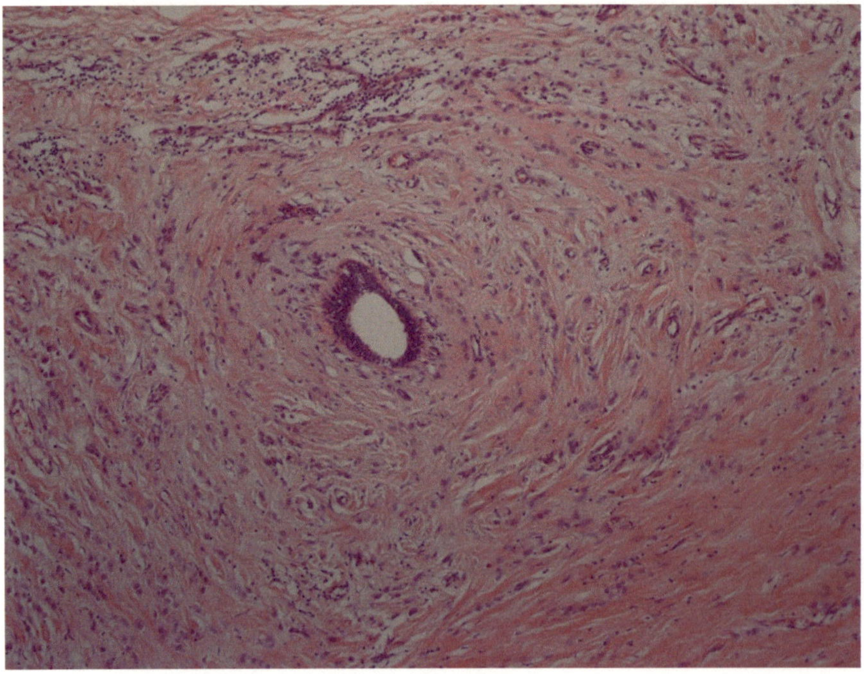

Figure 17. Invasive lobular carcinoama. The small tumoral cells infiltrating the stroma in indian file fashion concentrating around uninvolved duct, H & E, X100.

Other types of lobular carcinoma exist.

Histiocytic carcinoma is a type of lobular carcinoma in which tumor cells showing abundant foamy cytoplasm and apocrine differentiations. In signet ring carcinoma, accumulation of intracytoplasmic mucin pushes the nuclei to the periphery of cells (4, 5).

Tubulolobular carcinoma is characterized by small tubular formation in a tumor with typical appearance of lobular carcinoma. Immunohistochemical profile is intermediate between ductal and lobular carcinoma (4, 5).

8.20. Phylloides tumor

Phylloides tumor or cystosarcoma phylloides is a biphasic neoplasm usually affecting middle age woman. Grossly the tumor is firm, round and well circumscribed. Some cleft-like spaces may be evident on cut sections (4, 5).

Microscopically, the tumor is composed of epithelial and stromal components. Epithelial part is made of slit-like double layered ducts, surrounded by hypercellular stroma. The stromal hypercellularity and overgrowth distinguishes the phylloides tumor from fibroadenoma (Figure 18) (4, 5, 44, 45, 46, 47). Based on cytomorphology of stroma, mitotic count and status of margins, phyllodes tumor has been divided into three grades: benign, borderline and malignant.

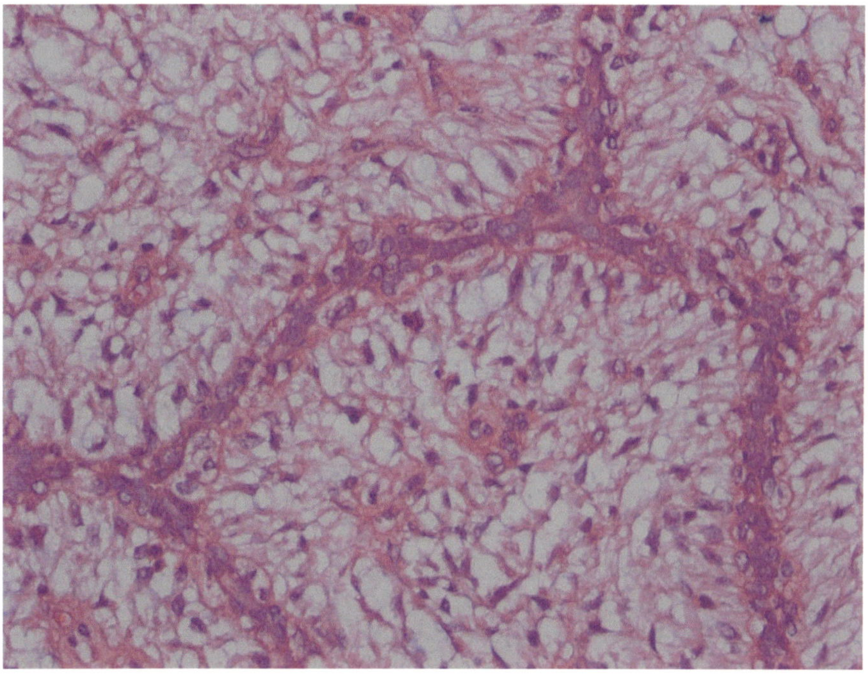

Figure 18. Phyllodes tumor. The biphasic tumor shows stromal hypercellularity surrounding the slit-like epithelial component, H & E, X400.

Benign phylloides tumor is characterized by less than two mitosis per ten high power field (HPF). The stroma is cellular with mild to moderate degree of cytologic atypia. The tumor border tends to be well defined.

Borderline lesions may have circumscribed or infiltrative margin. The stroma is hypercellular containing two to five mitosis per ten HPF (4).

Malignant phylloides shows marked degree of stromal hypercellularity and overgrowth. The border is usually invasive and mitotic count is more than five per ten HPF (4). Mitotic figure cut offs are different in various studies (44, 45, 46, 47).

Epithelial abnormalities ranging from hyperplasia to in situ carcinoma or rarely invasive carcinoma has been reported in phylloides tumor (4, 5).

Benign phylloides tumor has the potential for local recurrence but distant metastasis is a rare event in contrast to malignant phylloides tumor in which has the capacity for distant metastasis (5).

9. Conclusion

Histopathology plays an important role in management of breast diseases. It is a necessary component of diagnosis, treatment and prognosis in most breast disorders. When evaluating a breast lesion suspicious to malignancy pathologic assessment is a major consideration, because it not only differentiates the in situ lesions from invasive ones, but determines the grade and type of disease. An important step in evaluating a breast cancer is to test a portion of the cancer removed during the biopsy (or surgery) to see if they have estrogen and progesterone receptors; also All newly diagnosed breast cancers should be tested for HER2/neu because HER2-positive cancers are much more likely to benefit from treatment with drugs that target the HER2/neu protein, such as trastuzumab (Herceptin) and lapatinib (Tykerb). Fine needle aspiration or core needle biopsy versus surgical biopsy has remained a challenge in breast lesions suspicious to malignancy. Sampling of nonpalpable or indistinct breast lesions can be done using stereotactic breast needle biopsy, a technique that enable the spatial localization of the lesion within the breast.

Author details

Majid Akrami, Maral Mokhtari,
Sedigheh Tahmasebi and Abdolrasoul Talei
Shiraz University of Medical Sciences, Shiraz, Iran

10. References

[1] Kennecke HF, Speers CH, Ennis CA, Gelmon K, Olivotto IA, Hayes M. Impact of Routine Pathology Review on Treatment for Node-Negative Breast Cancer. J Clin Oncol. 2012 May 7. PMID: 22564990

[2] Williams RT, Yao K, Stewart AK, Winchester DJ, Turk M, Gorchow A, Jaskowiak N, Winchester DP. Needle versus excisional biopsy for noninvasive and invasive breast cancer: report from the National Cancer Data Base, 2003-2008. Ann Surg Oncol. 2011 Dec;18(13):3802-10. Epub 2011 Jun 1.

[3] Akçil M, Karaağaoğlu E, Demirhan B. Diagnostic accuracy of fine-needle aspiration cytology of palpable breast masses: an SROC curve with fixed and random effects linear meta-regression models. Diagn Cytopathol. 2008 May;36(5):303-10.

[4] Rosen PP. Rosen's breast pathology: Lippincott Williams; 2009

[5] Rosai J. Rosai and Ackerman's surgical pathdogy : Elsevier ; 2011

[6] Guray M , Sahin AA . Benign breast disease; classification, diagnosis and management. 7he oncologist 2006;11:435-449

[7] Hartman LC, Sellers TA , Frost MH, Lingle WL, Degnim AC, Ghosh K, et al . Benign breast disease and the risk of breast cancer. N Engl J Med 2005;352:229-237

[8] Batemam AC. Pathology of benign breast disease. wohm 2006;Doi:10.1383

[9] Hanson CA, Snover DC, Dehner LP. Fibroadenomatosis (fibroadenomatiid mastopathy): a benign breast lesion with composite pathologic features. Pathology 1987;19:393-6.

[10] American cancer society. http://www.cancer.org/Healthy/FindCancerEarly/WomensHealth/Non-CancerousBreastConditions/non-cancerous-breast-conditions-fibrocystic-changes

[11] Courtillot C, Plu-Bureau G, Binart N, et al. Benign breast diseases. J Mammary Gland Biol Neoplasia 2005; 10:325.

[12] Hughes LE, Mansel RE, Webster DJ. Aberrations of normal development and involution (ANDI): a new perspective on pathogenesis and nomenclature of benign breast disorders. Lancet 1987; 2:1316.

[13] Gadd MA, Souba WW: Evaluation and treatment of benign breast disorders, in Bland KI, Copeland EM III (eds): *The Breast: Comprehensive Management of Benign and Malignant Diseases.* Philadelphia: WB Saunders, 1998, p 233.

[14] Marchant DJ: Benign breast disease. *Obstet Gynecol Clin North Am* 29:1, 2002. [PubMed: 11892859]

[15] Agoff SN, Lawton TJ. Papillary lesions of the breast with and without atypical hyperplasia. Can we accurately precict benign from core needle biopsy? Am J clin pathol 2004;122:440-443

[16] Gill H.K, Loffe OB, Berg WA. Whin is a diagnosis of sclerosing adenosis acceptable at core biopsy? Radiol 2003;228:50-57

[17] Ellis IO. Intraductal proliferative lesions of the breast: morphology, associated risk and motecular biology. Modern pathology 2010;23:s1-s7.
[18] Schnitt SJ. Benign breast disease and breast cancer risk: potential role for antiestrogens. Cancer Res 2001;7:44195-44225
[19] Siegel R, Ward E, Brawley O, Jemal A. Cancer statistics, 2011: The impact of eliminating socioeconomic and racial disparities on premature cancer deaths. CA Cancer J Clin 2011; 61:212
[20] American cancer society. Breast cancer. Statistics. http://www.cancer.org/Cancer/BreastCancer/DetailedGuide/breast-cancer-key-statistics
[21] Leonard GD, Swais SM. Ductal carcinoma in situ, complexities and challenges. J natl cancer inst 2004;96:906-20
[22] Pinder SE. Ductal carcinoma in situ (DCIS) : Pathological features, differential diagnosis, prognostic factors and specimen evaluation. Mod pathol 2010;23:58-13
[23] Ueng SH, Mezzetti T, Tavassoli FA. Papillary neoplasms of the breast. A review. Arch pathol lab med 2009;133:893-907
[24] Collins LC, Schnitt SJ. Papillary lesions of the breast: Selected diagnostic and management issues. Histophathol 2008;52:20-29
[25] Gastellano I, Marchio C, Tomatis M, Porti A, Gasella D , Bianchi S, et al. Micropapillary ductal carcinoma in situ of the breast: An inter-institutional study. Mod pathol 2010;23:260-269
[26] Sullivan ME, Khan SA, Sullu Y, Schiller C, Sunik B. Lobular carcinoma in situ variants in breast cores. Arch pathol lab med 2010;134:1024-1028
[27] Sneige N, Wang J, Baker BA, Krishnamurthy S, Middleton LP. Clinical, histopathologic, and biologic features of pleomorphic lobular (ductal-lobular) carcinoma in situ of the breast: A report of 24 cases. Mod phathol 2002;15:1044-1050
[28] Hanby AM, Hughes TA. In situ and invasive lobular neoplasia of the breast. Histopathol 2008;52:58-66
[29] Mitrick JS, Gianutsas R, Pollack AH, Susman M, Baskin BL, KO WD, press man PI, Feiner HD, Roses DF. Tunular carcinoma of the breast: sensitivity of diagnostic techniques and correlation with histopathology, AM J roentgenol 1999; 172:319-23
[30] Winchester DJ, Sahin AA, Tucker SL, Singletary SE. Tubular carcinoma of the breast. Predicting axillary nodal metastases and recurrence. Ann Surg 1996;342-47
[31] Fein Messer M, Sulkes A, Mergenstern S, Sulkes J, Stern S, Okon E. HLA-DR and B2 microglobulin expression in medullary and atypical medullary carcinoma of the breast: Histopathologically similar but biologically distinct entities. J clin pathol 2000;53:286-291
[32] Rapin V, Contesso G, Mouriesse H, Bertin F, Lacombe MJ, Piekarski JD, Travagli JP, Gadenne C, Friedman S. Medullary breast carcinoma. A reevaluation of 95 cases of breast cancer with inflammatory stroma. Cancer 1988;61:2503-2510

[33] Gunhan-Bilgen I, Memis A, Ustun EE, Zekioglu O, Ozdemir N. Metaplastic carcinoma of the breast: Clinical, mammographic and sonographic findings with histopathologic correlation. Am J roentgenol 2002;178:1421-5

[34] Wargotz ES, Norris HJ. Metaplastic carcinoma of the breast cancer 1989;64:1490-1499

[35] Wargotz ES, Norris HJ. Metaplastic carcinoma of the breast. IV. Squamous cell carcinoma of ductal origin. Cancer 19901;65:272-276

[36] Adsay NV, Merati K, Nassar H, Shia J, Sarker F, Pierson C, Cheng J, Vischer D, Hruban R, Klimstral D. Pathogenesis of colloid (pure mucinous) carcinoma of exocrine organs: coupling of gel-forming mucin (muc2) production with altered cell polarity and abnormal cell-stroma interaction may be the key factor in the morphogenesis and indolent behavior of colloid carcinoma in the breast and pancreas. Am J Surg Pathol 2003;27:571-578

[37] Fentimas IS, Millis RR, Smith P, Ellul JPM, Lanpejo O. Mucoid breast carcinomas: Histology and prognosis. Br J Cancer 1997;75:1061-1065

[38] Tavassoli FA, Norris HJ. Secretory carcinoma of the breast. Cancer 1980;45:2402-2413

[39] Kavalakat AJ, Corilakam RK, Culas TB. Secretory carcinoma of breast in a 17-years old male. World J Sugr Oncol 2004;2:17

[40] Arce C, cortes-padilla D, Hunstman DG, Miller MA, Duennas – Gonzalez A, Alvardo A, Perez V, Gallardo-rincon D, Lara-Mediaa F. Secretory carcinoma of the breast containing the ETV6-NTRK3 fusion gene in a male: Case report and review of the literature. World J Surg Oncol 2005;3:35

[41] Kothari AS, Beechey-Newman N, Hamed H, Fentiman IS, D'Arrigo C, Hanby AM, Ryder K, Paget disease of the nipple. A multi focal manifestation of higher-risk disease. Cancer 2002;95:1-7

[42] Burke ET, braeuning MP, Mclelland R, Pisano ED, Cooper LL. Paget disease of the breast. A pictorial assay. Radiographics 1998;18:1459-640

[43] Arpino G, Barsou VJ, Clark GM, Elledge RM. Infiltrating lobular carcinoma of the breast. Tumor characteristics and clinical outcome. Breast Cancer Bes 2004;6:R149-R156

[44] Esposito NN, Moham D, Brufsky A, Lin Y, Kapali M, Dabbas DJ. Phyllodes tumor. A clinicopathologic and immunohistochemical study of 30 cases. Arch Pathol Lab Med 2006;130:1516-1521

[45] Lae M, Vincent-salmon A, Sarignoni A, Huon I, Freneaux P, Sigal – Zafrani B, Aurias A, Sastre-Garau X, Couturier J. Phyllodes tumors of the breast segregate in two groups according to genetic criteria. Mod Pathol 2007;20:435-444

[46] Tan PH, Jayabaskar T, Chuah KL, Lee HY, Tan Y, Hilmy M, Hung H, Selvarajan S, Bay BH. Phyllodes tumors of the breast. The role of pathologic parameters. Am J Clin Pathol 2005;123:529-540

[47] Taira N, Takabatake D, Aoji K, Ohsumi Sh, Takashima Sh, Nishimura R, Teramoto N. Phyllodes tumor of the breast: Stromal overgrowth and histological classification are useful prognosis predictive factors for local recurrence in patients with a positive surgical margin. Jpn J Clin Oncol 2007;37:730-736

Chapter 4

On the Bone Tumours: Overview, Classification, Incidence, Histopathological Issues, Behavior and Review Using Literature Data

Alina Maria Sisu, Loredana Gabriela Stana, Codruta Ileana Petrescu, Romulus Fabian Tatu, Roxana Folescu and Andrei Motoc

Additional information is available at the end of the chapter

http://dx.doi.org/10.5772/52969

1. Introduction

1.1. Classification of bone tumours

According to World Health Organization, bone tumours can be divided into primary and secondary, [7]. Primitive bony tumours are classified using histo-genetic criteria and malignancy anatomic-clinical criteria.

1.1.1. Tumours that form bones

Benign: osteoma, osteoid osteoma, benign osteoblastoma;

Malignant: osteosarcoma (osteogenic sarcoma) with subtypes: conventional, chondroblastic, fibroblastic, osteoblastic, telangiectatic, small cell, low-grade central, secondary, parosteal, periosteal, high-grade surface,[8].

1.1.2. Tumours that form cartilage

Benign: chondroma, osteochondroma, chondroblastoma, chondromixoid fibroma;

Malignant: chondrosarcoma with subtypes: central, primary and secondary, peripheral, dedifferentiated, mesenchymal, clear cell;

a. **Medullar tumours:** Ewing sarcoma/ primitive neuroectodermal tumour;
   It is the third most common bone cancer. Most Ewing tumors start in bones, but they can start in other tissues and organs. This cancer is most common in children and teenagers. It is rare in adults over age 30.

b. **Giant cell tumours,** malignant giant cell tumours, osteoclastoma;
c. **Fibrogenic tumours:** fibrosarcoma;
d. **Fibrohistiocystic tumours:** malignant fibrous histiocytoma;
e. **Haematopoietic tumours**: plasma cell myeloma, malignant lymphoma;
f. **Notochordal tumours**: chordoma;
g. **Vascular tumours**: angiosarcoma;
h. **Smooth muscle tumours**: leiomyosarcoma;
i. **Lipogenic tumours**: liposarcoma;
j. **Miscellaneous tumours**: adamantinoma;

Tumour type	Age	Location	Histologic aspect
Osteoma	41-50	Skull bones	Matured lamellar bone
Osteoid osteoma	11-20	Short and long bones diaphysis	Osteiod outlined by osteoblasts, incorporated in a fibrous stroma
Osteosarcoma	10-25	Long bones metaphysis	Osteoid and bone formed of malignant osteoblasts and fibroblasts.
Chondroma	11-40	Feet, hands	Maturated hyaline cartilage (enchondroma/ecchondroma), preserving lobulation
Chondrosarcoma	30-60	Long bones metaphysic, axial skeleton	Immature cartilage, no preserving lobulation, cells arranged in groups of two or four, with atypia and mitosis
Ewing sarcoma	5-25	Long bones diaphysis	Small, round, undifferentiated cells, no stroma, a lot of capillary arrangement.
Giant cells tumour	20-40	Knee	Multinucleated giant cells, fusiform cells, mononuclear cells.
Metastases	50-90	Anywhere	Frequently adenocarcinomas

Table 1. Overview on tumours

Our study revealed 198 cases of benign tumours , with a male/female ratio=1.2/1, with an average age of 41 years, ages between 15-78. The most afected were 21-30 and 51-60 age groups. A male predominance in males in 21-30 group was revealed. In 11-40 age group were highlighted 69 out of 108 cases (63.88%). In 51-60 age group was a female predominance, 27 cases. The most frequent osseous benign tumour in our study was osseous cyst followed by giant cell tumour(Table 1).

In 2009-2011 in our clinic we treated 87 tumour osseous cases. Out of these, 19 were treated using surgical biopsy and 68 were entirely excised. Sites, morphological types of the bone tumours stated during the histopathological examination and their frequency are shown in Tables 2, 3.

Anatomical site	Number of cases
Hip bone	6
Proximal extremity of femur	8
Distal extremity of femur	13
Fibula	3
Proximal extremity of tibia	8
Middle 1/3 of tibia	7
Distal 1/3 of tibia	3
Synovial cyst of the leg (synovialoma)	9
Superior surface of the foot	4
Radiocarpal cyst	18
Humerus	5
Proximal 1/3 ulna	3

Table 2. Anatomical sites of the bone tumours

Tumour	Number of cases
Epidermal cyst	4
Synovialoma	9
Osteochondroma	49
Osteoclastoma	7
Osteosarcoma	7
Lipomiosarcoma	1
Giant cell tumour	8
Solitary osseous mieloma	2

Table 3. Histopathological examination

1.2. Benign tumours

1.2.1. Solitary osseous cyst

From microscopically point of view, is a dense osseous tissue which outlines a well -blood supplied connective tissue, sometimes macrophages filled with hemosiderin and colesterol.

1.2.2. Giant cell tumour or mieloplaxe tumour or osteoclastoma

Is composed of mononucleated stroma, with fusiform cells, well- blood supplied, and of giant multinucleated cells, resembling osteoclasts. Microscopically cells are multinucleated, giant, having a mesenchymal origin, with dimensions 10-50 microns, with 20-30 nuclei central situated, in a basophile cytoplasm and a fibrous stroma.

1.2.3. Osteoid osteoma

Is a solitary benign tumour which produces dense osseous tissue with a particular entity, nidus. Microscopically, the central zone contains osteoid tissue with osteoblasts, osteoclasts and fibroblasts, in a network of well -blood supplied osteoid travee. These are anastomosed each other and have a progressive calcification, making a final image of osteosclerosis.

1.2.4. Osteoma

Is a unique or multiple benign tumour, formed by bones osteoforming proliferation with membranous origin. Microscopically is slighty different from adult osseous tissue. It has irregular osseous travee, located around the haversian spaces.

On 198 cases of benign tumours discovered and treated in Romania, we had the following distribution: solitary osseous cyst 66 cases, giant cell tumour 63 cases, osteoid osteoma 36 cases, osteoma 33 cases.

1.3. Malignant tumours

1.3.1. Osseous metastases incidence

In Sweden, in 10 years from a group of 832 cases of malignant primary bone tumours 242 were osteogenic sarcoma (28.8%), 193 chondrosarcoma (22.9%) and 74 cases Ewing's sarcoma (8.8%). All three tumours showed a predilection for males,[9].

In Ethiopia in 2003-2008 were treated 216 bone tumour patients with a male/female ratio=1. Of these, 36% (74/205) were malignant. The commonest was osteosarcoma, 52/182, 28.5%, [10].

According to Marugame et al,[11], the distribution of histological type for primary bone cancer in Japanese populationfor 1993–2001 was: osteosarcoma, the most frequenthistological type, accounting for approximately 40%. Chondrosarcoma was the second-most frequent, accounting for approximately 25%. Ewing sarcoma was the third-most frequent, accounting for approximately 10%. Malignant fibrous histocytoma and giant cell tumor accounted for approximately 6and 2%, respectively.

In North America and Europe, the incidence rate for bone sarcomas in males is approximately 0.8 new cases/100,000 populations. Higher incidence rates have been observed on males in Argentina and Brazil (1.5-2/1=M/F) and Israel (1.4/1=M/F). From histological point of view osteosarcoma is the most common primary malignant tumour of bone, accounting for approximately 35%, chondrosarcoma (25%), Ewing sarcoma (16%) ,[12].

The most frequent cancers that give osseous metastases are: breast carcinoma, small cell pulmonary carcinoma, renal carcinoma, thyroid carcinoma, prostate carcinoma.

Once the tumour metastases in the bone it becomes incurable. 20% of patients suffering from breast cancer live 5 years after discovering a bony metastasis. Breast and prostate cancers spread especially in bones.

Osteosarcoma is the most frequent malignant primary bone tumour, with a higher incidence in 15-20 year old group. Male/female ratio is 1.4-1.5-1. Ewing sarcoma is the second most common primary malignant bone cancer, seen most frequently on children and adolescents.

Chondrosarcoma occurs mostly in adulthood, with a male/female ratio=1. Our data showed an increased percentage in males in Romania, but a 3/1 female/male ratio in Timisoara,[13].

1.3.2. Osteosarcoma

Site and incidence

Osteosarcoma is the most common primary malignant tumour of bone, more common in males. The incidence is 3/1,000,000 population. It accounts for <1% of all malignant neoplasm. The most frequent site is the distal femur, followed by the proximal tibia and the proximal humerus.

In Romania field 2005-2010 were treated 468 cases of osteosarcomas with a male/female ratio=1.3/1, with some variability in clinics (in our clinic 7 out of 18 cases were osteosarcomas. Ratio F/M=3/1.) Out of these 468, 198 were benign (42.30%) and 189 malignant (40.38%). Out of these malignant, with a male/female ratio =1.2/1, 168 were malignant (88.88%). As benign tumours on the first place was osseous cyst and secondary the giant cell tumour. As age groups, 21-30 and 51-60 years were equal, 45 case each, with a significant difference: in the first group 27 cases were females and in the last one 27 cases were males.

From primary malignant tumours point of view a ratio male/female=1.33/1. Most of these tumours after the histopathological examination were osteosarcomas.

From secondary malignant tumours point of view a ratio male/female=1/1. 51 were carcinomas, 42 malignant fibrous histiocytomas, and 27 fibrosarcomas.

Locations of osteosarcomas are: osseous, central, surface, gnathic, multifocal, soft tissue, intramuscular.

The most frequent location was femur (50%), followed by tibia 19.6%, humerus 15.2% and distal fibula 2.2%.

Accidentally, osteosarcomas could be found in hyoid bone or nasal septum.

Histology - Microscopically types

- Central: high-grade, conventional, telangiectatic, small cell, epitheloid, osteoblastoma-like, chondroblastoma-like, fibrohistiocystic, giant cell;
- Low-grade: low-grade central, fibrous dysplasia-like, desmoplastic fibroma-like;
  Surface: low-grade, parosteal, intermediate-grade, periosteal, high-grade, dedifferentiated parosteal, high-grade surface;
- Intracortical;
- Gnathic;
- Extraskeletal: high-grade, low-grade;

Diferent types

- **Conventional Osteosarcoma** is also divided into osteoblastic, chondroblastic and fibroblastic subtypes according to histological feature, even from treatment and response point of view there is no difference between them. Grading the osteosarcoma is important from oncologic point of view, because based on this could be found the best treatment, especially the type of surgery.

Using Broders schema, the grade of tumour is numbered from 1 to 4, depending on the percentage of anaplasia, the cytologic atypia of the cells being the most important factor in grading tumours (Figure 1).

- **Telangiectatic Osteosarcoma** is an osteosarcoma in which take place local destructions with replacement of anatomic spaces. New formed aneurismal bone cyst and production of osteoid bone can establish diagnosis.
- **Giant cell-richosteosarcomas** contain osteoclast-like giant cells.
- **Small cell osteosarcoma** represents a rare histological combination of osteosarcoma and Ewing sarcoma, until 2% of osteosarcomas.
- **Epithelioid osteosarcoma** has the cell tumour poorly differentiated, for this reason being difficult to distinguish if is a sarcoma or a carcinoma.
- **Osteoblastoma-like and chondroblastoma-like osteosarcoma** resembles osteoblastoma with atypical osteoblasts and having different histological feature. These tumours are extremely rare, but are important to be established a precise diagnosis; these could metastasize (Figure 2).
- **Giant cell-rich osteosarcoma** contains benign multinucleated giant cells, but sometimes could contain lot of benign giant cells that cover the real malignant elements (Figure 3).
- **Gnathic osteosarcomas** appear in maxilla and mandible bone. They are chondroblastic, osteoblastic, fibroblastic, small cell type concerning the matrix production.
- **Low-grade central osteosarcomas** have been reported as very rarely, resembling the low-grade parosteal sarcoma, fibrous dysplasia and other benign lesions **(**Figure 4).
- **Surface osteosarcomas** consist of osteosarcoma whose epicentres are out of the cortex of the bone outlines. According to some criteria (anatomic location, predominant pattern of matrix, histological grade) there are several types of surface osteosarcomas: parosteal osteosarcoma, periosteal osteosarcoma, dedifferentiated parosteal osteosarcoma, high-grade surface osteosarcoma.

i. **Parostealosteosarcoma** is the most common form of surface osteosarcomas, frequently been confused with osteochondroma and osteoma. Is credited with < 0.5% of osteosarcomas, 70-83% out of them are located on distal posterior femur.

ii. **Periosteal osteosarcoma** is rarely than parosteal osteosarcoma and has a cartilaginous matrix component. As histological grade is between I grade parosteal osteosarcoma and III/IV grade osteosarcoma.

iii. **Dedifferentiated parosteal osteosarcoma** is composed of low-grade parosteal osteosarcoma and high-grade conventional parosteal osteosarcoma. According to Rizzoli Institute, dedifferentiation occurs in 25% of low-grade parosteal osteosarcomas.

iv. **High-grade surface osteosarcoma** is microscopically high-grade. It could be possible to have a high-grade surface osteosarcoma that is a dedifferentiated parosteal osteosarcoma in which the high-grade component has replaced the low-grade component.

- **Intracortical osteosarcoma** is very rare high-grade osteosarcoma that from histological point of view is osteoid or maybe bone formation. It is treated like conventional osteosarcoma (Figures 5,6).

- **Multifocal osteosarcoma** is unusual, affect children, young adults. It is a high-grade sarcoma, very aggressive, without escape in terms of surviving.
- **Extraskeletal osteosarcoma** is credited with <2.2% of all soft tissue sarcomas. From histological point of view it resembles all types of osteosarcoma, even it has grown as soft tissue in low-grade central osteosarcoma. ¾ of patients are dying in the first 5 years of diagnosis.

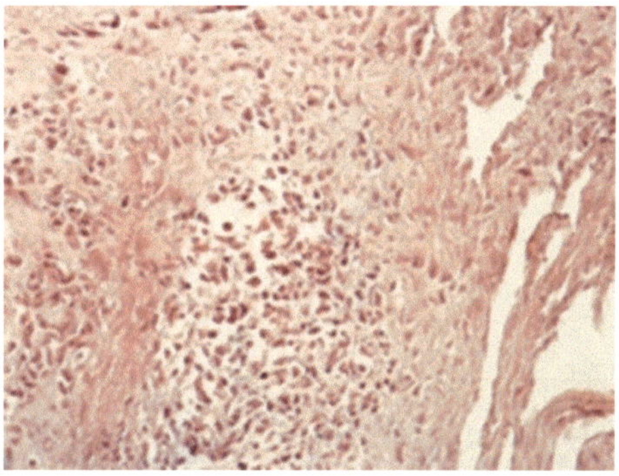

Figure 1. Conventional osteosarcoma with abundance of hyper chromatic nuclei, polyhedral tumour cells, sarcomatous vessels; HE staining X 100 (microscopic aspect)

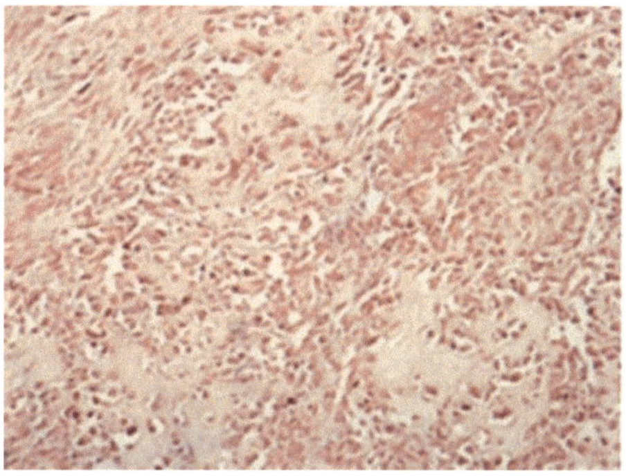

Figure 2. Chondroblastic osteosarcoma - compact groups of malignant tumour cells, areas with cellular hyaline cartilage and osteiod formation; HE staining X 100 (microscopic aspect)

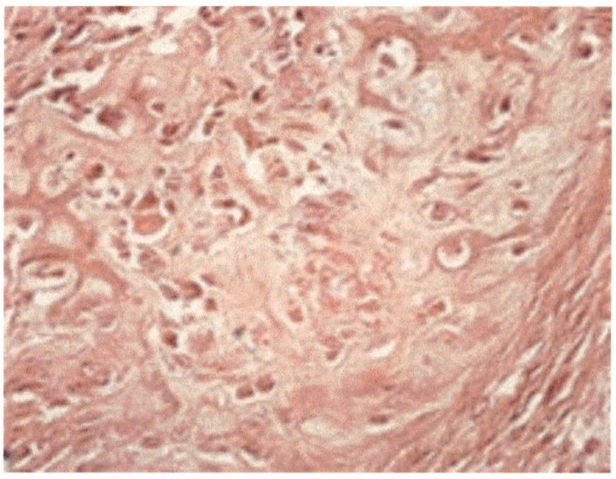

Figure 3. Classic osteosarcoma with an abundant production of tumour osteoid areas and bone matrix, enclosing giant malignant tumour cells; HE staining X400 (microscopic aspect)

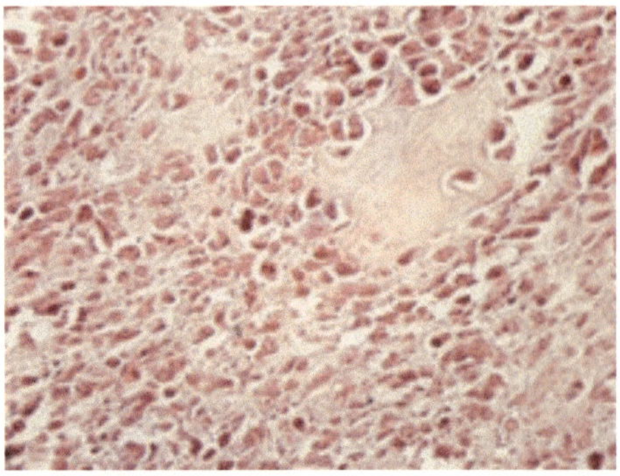

Figure 4. Osteoid osteosarcoma- polyhedral tumour cells, with atypical mitosis, little bone and osteoid matrix; HE staining X 200 (microscopic aspect)

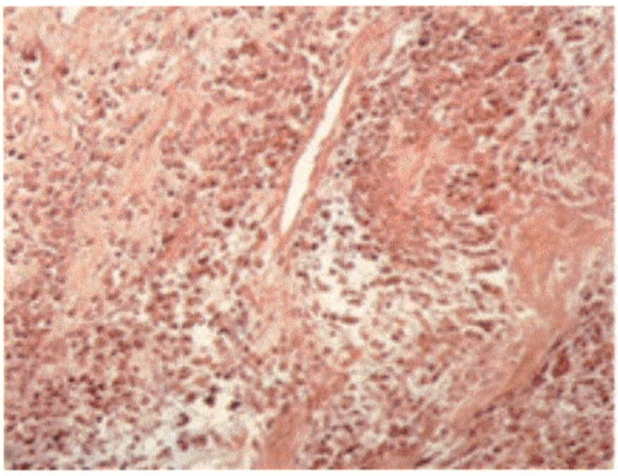

Figure 5. Osteosarcoma-tumour cells having sizes and shapes variable with hyper chromatic nuclei and mitosis areas; HE staining X 100 (microscopic aspect)

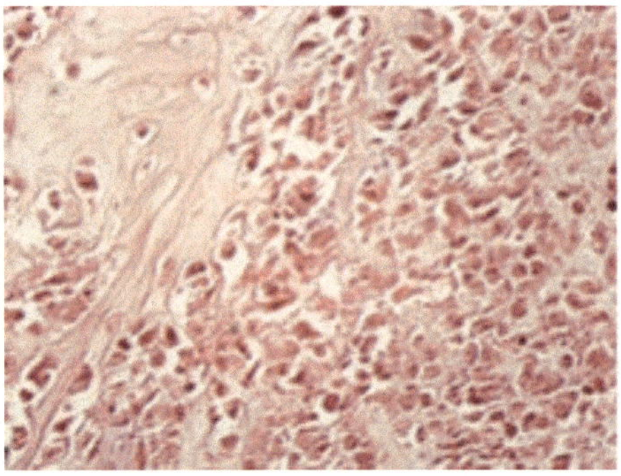

Figure 6. Osteosarcoma- polymorph tumour cells having a big size nucleus, prominent nucleolus and osseous matrix; HE staining X 200 (microscopic aspect)

1.3.3. Staging bone tumours

As Enneking et al have stated,[14], there is a system for staging bone sarcomas, according to correlation of the tumour location and metastases presence(Table 4);T1 - the tumour is intra compartmental; T2 - the tumour is extra compartmental; M0 - no regional or distant metastasis; M1 - regional or distant metastasis; G1 - low grade; G2 - high grade.

Stage	Tumour	Metastases	Grade
I A	T1	M0	G1
I B	T2	M0	G1
II A	T1	M0	G2
II B	T2	M0	G2
III	T1 or T2	M1	G1 or G2

Table 4. Enneking staging system for primary malignant tumours of bone

According to American Joint Committee on Cancer Staging System [15,16] it has been used a new, more complex classification of the primary malignant osseous tumours, where also is taken into consideration the lymphatic nodes existence (Table 5), a criterion which states the following:Tx - primary tumour cannot be assessed; T0 - no evidence of primary tumour; T1 - tumour 8 cm or less in greatest dimension; T2 - tumour more than 8 cm in greatest dimension; T3 - discontinuous tumours in the primary bone; Nx - regional lymph nodes not assessed; N0 - no regional lymph node metastases; N1 - regional lymph node metastases; Mx - distant metastasis cannot be assessed; M0 - no distant metastasis; M1 - distant metastasis; M1a - lung; M1b - other distant site; Gx - grade cannot be assessed; G1 - well differentiated (low grade); G2 - moderately differentiated (low grade); G3 - poorly differentiated (high grade); G4 - undifferentiated (high grade).

Stage	Tumour	Lymph Node	Metastases	Grade
IA	T1	N0	M0	G1 OR G2
IB	T2	N0	M0	G1 OR G2
IIA	T1	N0	M0	G3 OR G4
IIB	T2	N0	M0	G3 OR G4
III	T3	N0	M0	ANY G
IVA	ANY T	N0	M1a	ANY G
IVB	ANY T	N1	ANY M	ANY G
IVB	ANY T	ANY N	M1b	ANY G

Table 5. Staging of the primary malignant osseous tumours

1.3.4. Chondrosarcoma

Site and incidence

In 1994-2007 were assessed 62 cases of chondrosarcomas in Romania, with a slightly decreasing for the next two years.

Out of these 62 patients 46 were males (74.2%) and 16 females (25.8%). Male/female ratio=2.88/1. On age groups distribution was the following: average age of all patients was 48.8 years, 16-81. On gender groups' distribution was the following: average age in females was 59.10, 16-78; average age in males was 45.26, 16-71. On gender and age groups the highest frequency is on 45-56 years in males, almost 20%. 66-75 group age in females, 9.8%.

As example, in 2001-2007, in Russian Federation were examined 77 patients with chondrosarcoma . The dedifferentiated form of the tumor was confirmed in 10 (13%) cases.

The most common place is femur, 41.9%, followed by tibia, 16.1% and humerus 9.7%. Less frequent chondrosarcoma is highlighted in hip bone, 16.2%, phalanges 6.5%, and 3.1% in calcaneus, scapula and vertebrae. From 41.9% chondrosarcomas located on the femur 53.8% has a distal location. On tibia and humerus the location of a chondrosarcoma is 100% proximal.

Histology

From histological feature point of view, chondrosarcomas are divided in following groups:

- **Well differentiated chondrosarcoma** (differential diagnosis with rich-cell chondroma);
- **Clear cell chondrosarcoma** (with a "broken glass" cytoplasm);
- **Myxoid chondrosarcoma** – II grade (differential diagnosis with chondromyxoid fibroma);
- **Dediferentiated chondrosarcoma** (has a different sarcomatous area);
- **Mesenchymal chondrosarcoma.**

In order to have a precise diagnosis are followed some criteria: cellular density, cellular atypia, mitosis, according to these being described the grade of malignancy. Radiologic imaging is the first that could put a screening diagnostic, followed by MRI and RMN.

Magnetic Resonance Imaging (MRI) can be helpful in differentiating between benign and malignant lesions in several ways. Greater than 90% medullar involvement can be suggestive of chondrosarcoma, while the absence of 90% medullar involvement of non-contiguous areas of cartilage within the bone can suggest the presence of an enchondroma.

In addition, the timing and progression of gadolinium contrast enhancement patterns may help direct a clinician toward or away from a diagnosis of malignancy. Many surgeons consider MRI critical for surgical planning because it can illustrate the tumour extension involved in bone and soft tissues [17,18].

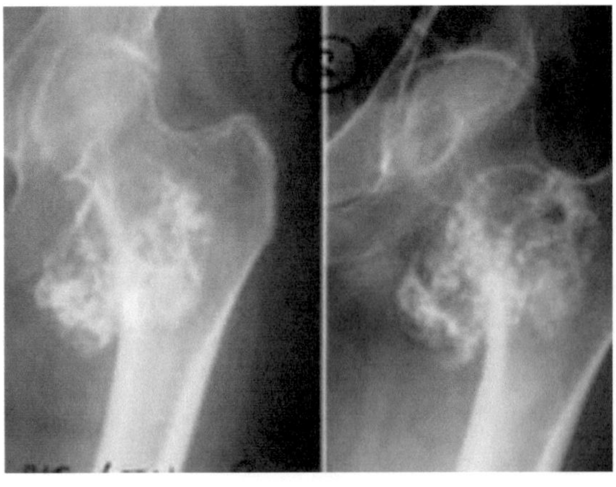

Figure 7. Large hip joint tumour on the inferior surface of the lesser trochanter of the femur (radiologic images)

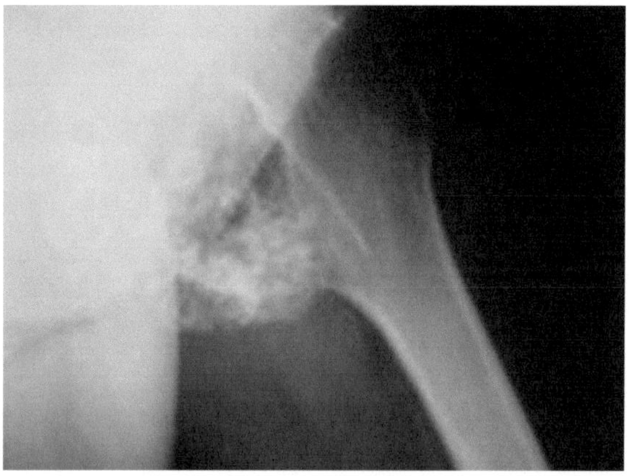

Figure 8. X- ray: Hip joint tumour, with clear, obvious, inhomogeneous outline

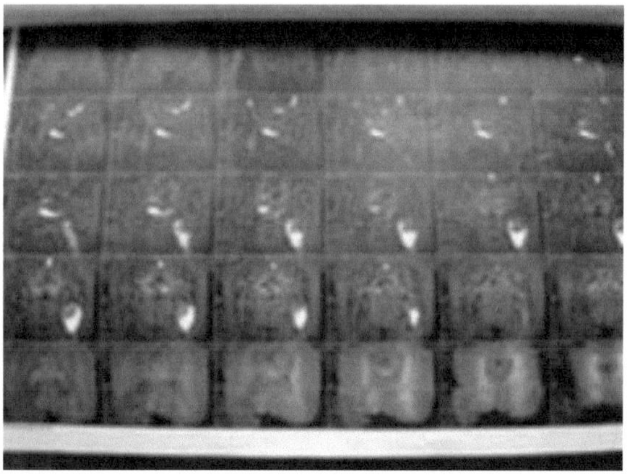

Figure 9. MRI sagittal section: shows an important tumour, 80/50/60 mm with a lot of liquid

On macroscopic examination, chondrosarcoma is seen like a grayish-white, lobulated mass. It has focal calcification and muriform aspect (Figure 10). The bigger one (2/1, 5 cm) is decalcified.

Histological, the tumour is stained HE. Could be found tumour fragments with lobulated pattern composed of cartilage matrix which supports many chondroplasts congested with focal loss of arranging symmetrical character and containing not a strong polymorphism (Figures 11, 12, 13, 14).

It was associated blades oblong of bone compact tissue. These were deformed and fragmented by the invasion of tumour tissue. Histological aspects are in favour for well-differentiated chondrosarcoma, [19-21].

1.4. Survival rate

Based on the literature data for 1995-2001, the overall 5-year relative bone cancer survival rate was calculated 69.4%. By rase and gender groups it was: 67.5% for Caucasian men;

72.1% for Caucasian women; 70% for Afro-American men; 68.4% for Afro-American women.

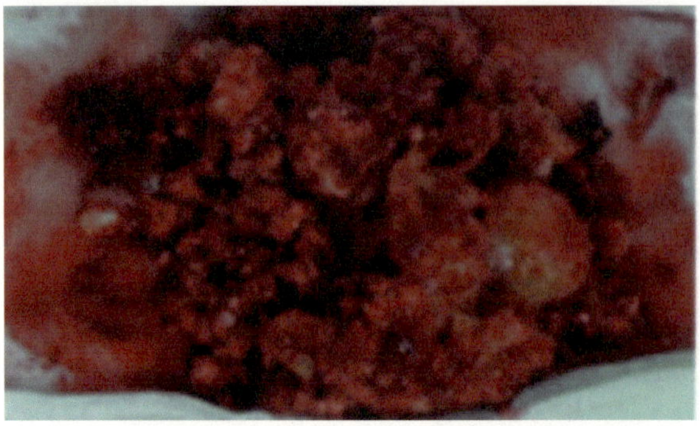

Figure 10. Macroscopic aspect; exophytic sarcoma, with calcified areas and haemorrhage

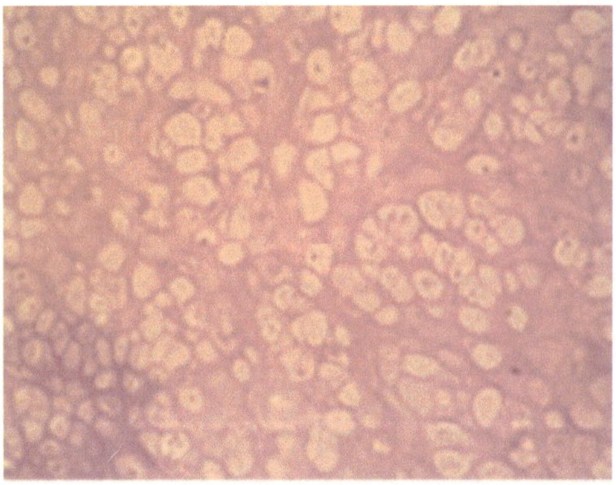

Figure 11. Well-differentiated chondrosarcoma consisting of pale hyaline matrix; HE staining X 40 (microscopic aspect)

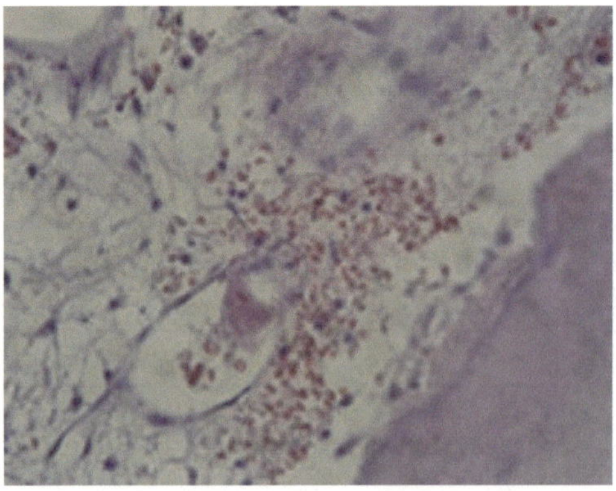

Figure 12. Malignant chondrocytes, large, atypical, with large nuclei; HE staining X 40(microscopic aspect)

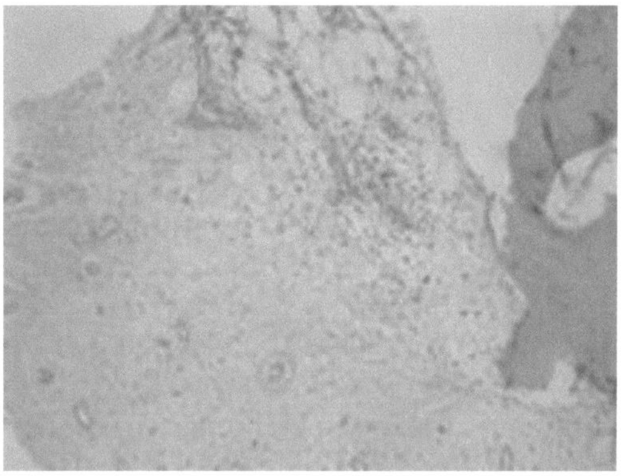

Figure 13. Well-differentiated chondrosarcoma consisting of nodules hyaline matrix; lymphoplasmocytes infiltrate; HE staining x 10 (microscopic aspect)

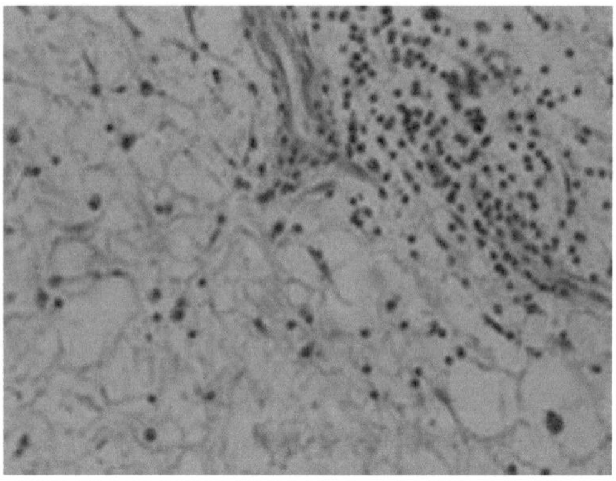

Figure 14. Well-differentiated chondrosarcoma consisting of nodules hyaline matrix; lymphoplasmocytes infiltrate; HE staining X 40 (microscopic aspect)

1.5. Bone cancer statistics on stages

This is very important for the prognosis.

- 41% of bone cancer cases are diagnosed while the cancer is still confined to the primary site, so it is a localized stage.
- 36% of bone cancers are diagnosed after the cancer has spread to regional lymph nodes or directly beyond the primary site.
- 15% of bone cancer cases are diagnosed after the cancer has already metastasizes, so it is a distant stage.
- 8% of bone cancer cases had staging unknown.
- In literature cases the corresponding 5-year relative bone cancer survival rates were:
- 84.5% for localized stage; 69.4% for regional stage; 30.6% for distant stage; 62.2% for unknown stage.

2. Conclusions

The most important thing in dealing with a bone tumour is a correct and full diagnosis. This include: clinical staging, a right excision, with 5 cm limits around tumour, a very precise histopathological examination and, not for the last, a post surgery treatment (radiotherapy, hormonal therapy, immunotherapy, chemotherapy). All these have in common an increase of 5-year survival rate.

Taking into account that malignant primary bone tumours are few, the secondary ones, meaning the metastases, are the dangerous. So, besides the treating of the metastases, is also essential to treat, and sometimes to find, the primary tumour. It is very true that the secondary tumour is discovered when the primary is in an advanced stage and the rate survival decreases very much.

Metastases behaviour is different from the primary tumour behaviour. Histopathological feature is different on breast tumours successive metastases, suggesting molecular changes depending on the tissue where the tumour is growing. Tumour cells preserve the initial pattern of the origin tissue, but the malignant phenotype is modified, depending on the metastazing area,[22].

Conventional radiography is very useful for diagnostic information. Magnetic resonance imaging (MRI) is recommended over computed tomography (CT) scanning for delineation of tumour extent before surgery.

Nuclear imaging is limited in providing diagnosis for bony lesions. Angiography is useful when a compression on the vessels is suspected. Of course, is also important the location of the tumour on the bone.

Histopathological examination of the biopsy sample provides with certainty the type of the tumour, but in some cases the tumour feature so resembles to others that is very difficult, even for an old specialist, to put without any doubt, a correct diagnosis.

A longer survival of cancer patients leads to a higher risk of population to develop bone metastases and pathological fractures. For this reason, reconstructive procedure requires a guarantee longer term, in order to avoid mechanical problems during the life of the patient,[23]. The follow-up of the patients is multidisciplinary, including oncology, orthopaedics, radiology, geriatrics, endocrinology, intensive care, physiokinetotherapy.

Author details

Alina Maria Sisu, Loredana Gabriela Stana, Codruta Ileana Petrescu,
Roxana Folescu and Andrei Motoc
Department I Anatomy and Embryology, Faculty of Medicine, "Victor Babes"University of Medicine and Pharmacy Timisoara, Romania

Romulus Fabian Tatu
Department of Orthopaedics, Traumatology, Urology and Imagistics, Faculty of Medicine, "Victor Babes"University of Medicine and Pharmacy Timisoara, Romania

3. References

[1] Von Schulthess Ch, Zollikofer L. In G.K. von Schulthess Ch.L. Zollikofer, editor, Musculoskeletal Diseases Springer Milan Berlin Heidelberg, New York; 2005.

[2] Coleman RE, Rubens RD. The Clinical Course of Bone Metastases from Breast Cancer. Breast Journal Cancer 1987; 55:61-66.

[3] Anderson BO, Shyyan R, Eniu A et al. Breast Cancer in Limited-Resource Countries: An Overview of the Breast Health Global Initiative 2005 Guidelines. Breast Journal 2006; 12 S3-15.

[4] Mundy GR. Metastasis to Bone: Causes, Consequences and Therapeutic Opportunities. National Review Cancer 2002; 48(2):584-593.

[5] Cancer Stats: Worldwide Cancer London: Cancer Research UK; 2005.

[6] Cancer Stat Fact Sheets. Cancer of the Breast. Bethesda: National Cancer Institute 2005.

[7] World Health Organization. Fact Sheet No. 297 In Cancer WHO, Geneva; 2006.

[8] World Health Organization: WHOSIS (WHO Stastistical Information System) 2006: A Guide to Statistical Information at WHO- World Health Statistics 2006; http://www.who.int/whosis/en/ (accessed November, 10, 2011).

[9] Larsson SE, Lorentzon R. The Geographic Variation of the Incidence of Malignant Primary Bone Tumors in Sweden. Journal of Bone and Joint Surgery 1974; 56-A, 592-600.

[10] Negash BE, Admasie D, Wamisho WE, Tinsay MW. Bone Tumors at Addis Ababa University, Ethiopia: Agreement Between Radiological and Histopathological Diagnoses, A -5-year Analysis at Black-Lion Teaching Hospital. International Journal of Medicine and Medical Science 2009; 1(4),119-125.

[11] MarugameT, Katanoda K, Matsuda T, Hirabayashi Y, Kamo K, Ajiki W and Sobue T. The Japan Cancer Surveillance Research Group, The Japan Cancer Surveillance Report: Incidence of Childhood, Bone, Penis and Testis Cancers. Japanese Journal of Clinical Oncology 2007;37(4)319–323.

[12] American Cancer Society: Information and Resources for Cancer 2000-2008.

[13] Poenaru DV, Raica M, Ouassim D. In Metastazele osoase, Editura Mirton; 2009.

[14] Enneking WF, Spanier SS, Goodman MA. A System for the Surgical Staging of Musculoskeletal Sarcoma. Clinical Orthopaedics 1980; 153:106–120.

[15] American Joint Committee on Cancer Bone. In: Fleming ID, Cooper JS, HensonDE, et al. AJCC Cancer Staging. 1997:143–147.

[16] American Joint Committee on Cancer Bone. In: GreeneFL, Page DL, Fleming ID, et al. AJCCCancer Staging Manual New York Springer- Verlag; 2002.

[17] Sandberg AA, Bridge JA. Updates on the Cytogenetics and Molecular Genetics of Bone Soft Tissue Tumors: Chondrosarcoma and Other Cartilaginous Neoplasms. Cancer Genetics Cytogenetics2003; 143:1–31.

[18] Wehrli BM, Huang W, de Cromrugghe B, Ayala AG, Czerniak B. Sox 9, A Master Regulator of Chondrogenesis, Distinguishes Mesenchymal Chondrosarcoma From Other Small Blue Round Cell Tumors. Human Pathology2003; 34:263–269.

[19] Mitchel A, Ruda NJR, Fenton PV. Juxtacortical Dedifferentiated Chondrosarcoma from a Primary Periosteal Chondrosarcoma. Modern Pathology1996; 9:279–283.

[20] Rosenberg AE, Neilsen GP, Keel SB., Renard LG, Fitzek MM, Munzenrider JE, et al. Chondrosarcoma of the Base of the Skull: A Clinicopathologic Study of 200 Cases with Emphasis on Its Distinction from Chordoma. American Journal of Surgical Pathology1999; 23:1370–1378.

[21] Kalil RK, Inwards CY, Unni K, Bertoni F, Bacchini P, Wenger DE, et al. Dedifferentiated Clear Cell Chondrosarcoma. American Journal of Surgical Pathology 2000; 24:1079–1086.

[22] Peh WCG, Muttarak M. Bone Metastases. Retrieved July 27, 2005; http://emedicine.com/radio/topic88.htm (accessed December, 11, 2011).

[23] Greenberg HS, Deck MD, Vikram B, et al. Metastasis to the Base of the Skull; Clinical Finding in 43 Patients. Neurology 1981; 31:530-537.

Chapter 5

Nocardiosis: Clinical and Pathological Aspects

Sharmila P. Patil, Nitin J. Nadkarni and Nidhi R. Sharma

Additional information is available at the end of the chapter

http://dx.doi.org/10.5772/52376

1. Introduction

1.1. Taxonomy and history

Nocardiosis is an opportunistic, localized or disseminated granulomatous infection caused by an aerobic actinomycete most commonly found in soil, decomposing vegetation, and other organic matter, as well as in fresh and salt water [1]. Infection most commonly occurs through the respiratory tract. Manifestations of disease range from cutaneous infection caused by traumatic inoculation of the organism in a normal host to severe hematogenous spread to pulmonary or central nervous system (CNS) disease in an immunocompromised host [2].

Taxonomy of nocardia has undergone many revisions. Aerobic actinomycetes are bacteria belonging to the order Actinomycetales, *Nocardia* is a genus in the family Nocardiaceae. As Nocardiaceae branch into filaments they were misclassified as fungi. Like members of the genus *Mycobacterium*, the nocardiae contain tuberculostearic acids, but in contrast to mycobacteria, they also possess short-chain (40 to 60 carbon) mycolic acids and usually exhibit characteristic branching on Gram staining [3,4,5,6]. More than 50 species have been identified by phenotypic and molecular methods. Originally referred to as *Nocardia asteroides* was later found to be a group of bacteria named *N asteroides* complex which was responsible for most of the human infections[1]. On the basis of drug susceptibility patterns *N asteroides* complex was later separated into different species: *Nocardia abscessus, Nocardia brevicatena-paucivorans* complex, *Nocardia nova* complex, *Nocardia transvalensis* complex, *Nocardia farcinica* and Nocardia *asteroids*[7]. *Nocardia cyriacigeorgica* was recently differentiated from *N asteroids* [8].

Some species are more prevalent in geographical locations with a specific climate. *Nocardia brasiliensis,* usually associated with cutaneous infection and mycetoma, is more commonly isolated in areas with tropical or subtropical climates and is often encountered in the southwestern or southeastern United States [9,10]. Saubolle and Sussland recently reported that nocardial infections in the United States seem to be more prevalent in the arid, warm climates of the southwest [11].

The taxonomic history of the genus *Nocardia* is fraught with confusion and controversy. The organism initially placed in the genus *Nocardia* was isolated by veterinarian Edmond Nocard in 1888 from a case of bovine[12]. One year later, Trevisan characterized the organism and named it *Nocardia farcinica.* Taxonomic studies by Gordon and Mihm in 1962 found no phenotypic differences between Nocardia strain and strains of isolates known as "*N. asteroides*"[13,14]. Because of the uncertain taxonomic status of the *N. farcinica* type strain and because *N. asteroides* had become the most common designation of isolates of this genus, the name *N. asteroides* was chosen to replace *N. farcinica* as the type species of the genus *Nocardia.*

Nocardia exhibits varying degrees of acid-fastness, depending on the mycolic acid composition in the cell wall and type of stain used [3]. The modified Kinyoun acid-fast stain uses 1% sulfuric acid as a decolorizer (instead of the more potent hydrochloric acid used in the decoloration step in the Ziehl- Neelsen staining procedure), which enhances the ability of *Nocardia* to retain the colored fuchsin[15]. Unlike mycobacteria, *Nocardia* has a "beaded" acid-fast appearance on microscopy. *Nocardia* can resemble *Actinomyces* species on Gram stain; however, *Actinomyces* species are not acid-fast and grow under anaerobic conditions[1].

2. Epidemiology

It has a universal distribution, affecting people mainly between 20-50 years of age [16]. Males are more affected than females. Pathogenic species of *Nocardia* can be found in house dust, beach sand, garden soil, and swimming pools [15]. Despite the occurrence of nocardiosis in many animals (e.g. cats, dogs, guinea pigs, and cattle), there is no evidence of respiratory spread from infected animals to humans[17]. There is also no evidence of person-to-person transmission. Patients with depressed cell-mediated immunity especially are at high risk for infection, including those with lymphoma, other malignancies, human immunodeficiency virus infection and solid-organ or hematopoietic stem cell transplant and those receiving long-term treatment with steroids or other immunosuppressive medications like azathioprine and cyclosporine[18,19]. Among stem cell transplant patients, nocardiosis can develop at varying time periods, which range from 2 to 3 months to 1 to 2 years after transplant. Among solid organ transplant recipients, *Nocardia* infection has a frequency of 0.6% to 3% and has been well described in kidney, heart, and liver recipients[20,21]. A case control study of 5126 solid organ transplant recipients, *Nocardia* infection was found highest among lung transplant recipients, followed by recipients of heart, small bowel, kidney, and liver transplants[22,23,24]. Risk factors in these patients include the early rejection of grafts and intensive immunoupuppressive therapy. Use of azathioprine and prednisone or high-dose prednisone alone may pose a greater risk of development of nocardiosis than combination therapy with cyclosporine and prednisone together[25,26].

With the comparatively recent advent of HIV infection, the incidence of nocardiosis has comparatively risen. It affects mainly rural more than the urban population and occurs in patients with CD4 T cell count less than 100 cells/µl. Such patients are more likely to develop pulmonary and extra pulmonary disease [2]. Host resistance to nocardiosis depends on the number and phagocytic/lytic capability of the polymorphonuclear cells and the status of the cell mediated immunity. The last of this fails in AIDS patients and predisposes to severe forms of nocardiosis. However, low frequency of this complication in patients with advanced HIV can be attributed to sulphonamide therapy and the leading role of neutrophils in immune response to nocardia[2]. Intravenous drug abusers can be predisposed to cutaneous nocardiosis since direct inoculation through injections sites can occur, leading to abscesses[2]. Surgical wound infections due to N. farcinica has been described[27].

3. Microbiology

The genus *Nocardia are branched* gram-positive (Figure 1), variably acid-fast, strictly aerobic bacteria, as they age, they fragment into rod-shaped or coccoid elements[15]. Nocardiosis bacteria induces abscess and granulomatous response in the skin. In hematoxilin & Eosin staining of nocardiosis shows abscess (collection of neutrophils) and granules (grains) (Figure 2). Grains are closely aggregated with a peripheral radial deposition of intensely eosinophilic material – a Hoeppli – Splendore (HS) reaction (Figure 3a and 3b). H&E stains demonstrate the bacilli poorly. They are 1 micrometer diameter , gram positive, Grocott silver positive, usually positive with Zeihl Neelson stain, this differentiate nocadiosis from actinomyces and related bacilli. The Grocott silver method is the most sensitive screening stain for nocardiosis.

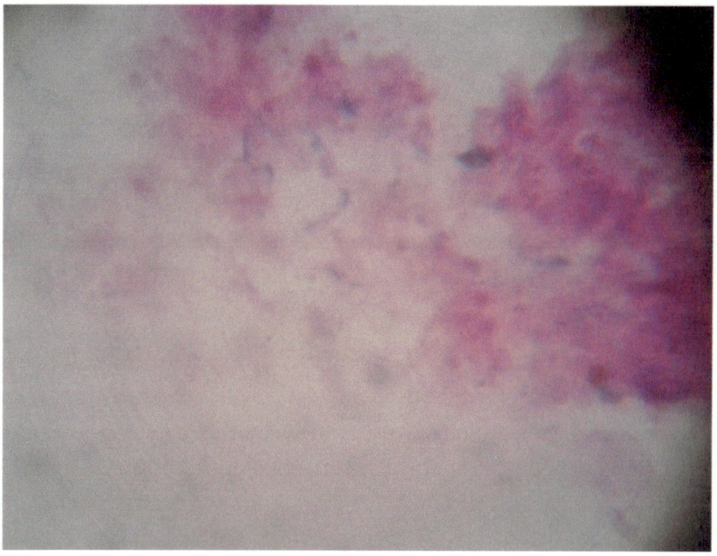

Figure 1. Gram positive filamentous bacteria showing branching, consistent with N.braziliense

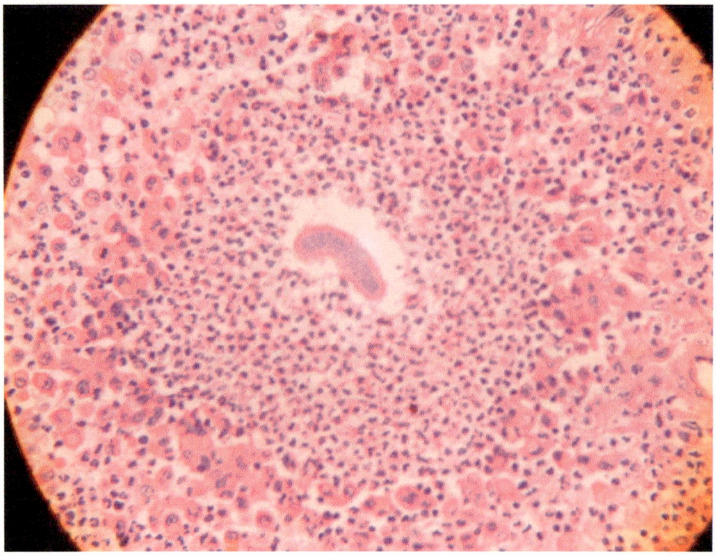

Figure 2. Histopathology of nocardiosis showing grains with neutrophils around it

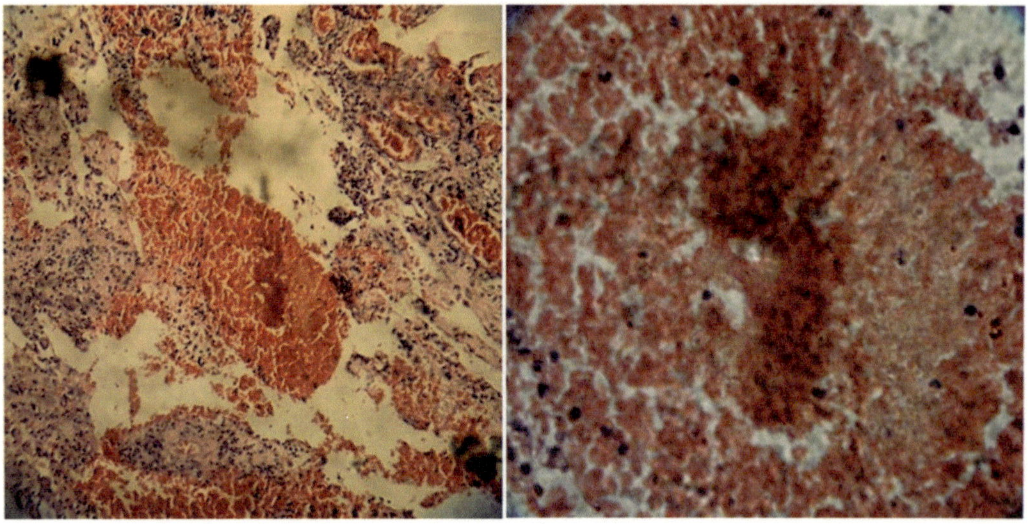

Figure 3. a. Histopathology of nocardiosis with inflammatory cells around it (10x)
b. 40x magnification showing irregularly staining granular structure surrounded by RBCs and necrotic tissue with few neutrophils disease

On blood agar, filamentous colonies have a chalky white or cotton-ball appearance. Unlike *Actinomadura,* and *Streptomyces* species the catalase-positive nocardiae grows in a nutrient broth. They grow readily over most of the simple media e.g. Sabouraud's glucose agar, blood agar, brain-heart infusion agar, and Lowenstein-Jensen agar[15]. More vigorous growth is achieved by adding 10% carbon dioxide. On agar, colonies are usually rough with velvety surface because of the aerial hyphae (Figure 4). Most of the primary isolates are white or light orange and have a characteristic moldy or earthy odour. Optimum temperature for growth is 37⁰C but growth is slow and pure colonies are visible only after 48-72 hours of incubation. Before discarding, the culture should be observed for 2 weeks[28].

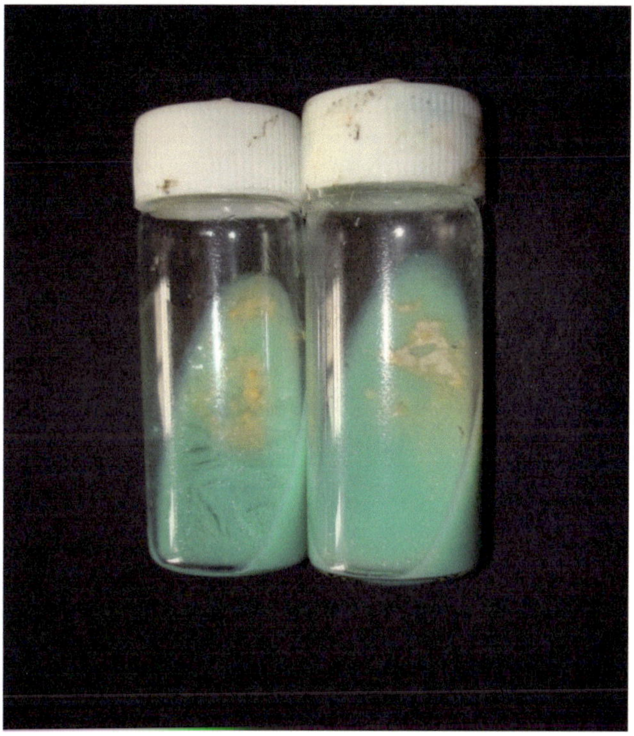

Figure 4. Powdery yellow colonies of N.braziliences on LJ medium

Microscopic examination of gram-stained clinical specimens are thin, delicate, weakly to strongly gram-positive, irregularly stained or beaded branching filaments. A modified Ziehl-Neelsen stain, which decolorizes with 1% sulphuric acid instead of acid alcohol is the best technique for demonstrating nocardia[17]. There are multiple species, existing mainly in the soil, but human disease is mostly caused by Nocardia asteroides (so called because of star shaped colonies it produces in cultures). *Nocardia* are not visualized on hematoxylin and eosin stain of tissue or periodic acid-Schiff (PAS) stain for fungi. Methenamine silver preparations may reveal the organism in some instances. Routine blood cultures are not usually positive, but nocardia can be isolated from blood if biphasic blood culture systems are inoculated and incubated aerobically for up to 30 days[15,17]. Blood specimens are processed by centrifugation. Exudate, joint, CSF specimen and homogenized tissue specimens should be inoculated directly into media such as thioglycollate broth, trypticase soy broth or chopped-meat glucose broth. Serological methods including hemagglutination, precipitin, and complement-fixing antibody testing have a limited value because of a high degree of shared antigens and serological cross-reactivity among the heterogeneous pathogenic *Nocardia* species and other actinomycetes, especially *Rhodococcus, Streptomyces,* and *Corynebacterium* species [29].

Other Biochemical and molecular methods: DNA probing, PCR, PCR-RFLP. PCR analysis of 16S rDNA is a useful tool to identify the species of nocardia. The application of this method has enabled the identification of nocardia in pathological specimens. It usually takes about 2 weeks for microbiological isolation and antibiotic susceptibility tests in cases of nocardiosis, but real-time PCR analysis of 16S rDNA can be completed in a few hours. This is relatively rapid, because amplification is carried out in capillary glass tubes, which are used only in the lightcycler instrument.

In RFLP analysis, the DNA sample is broken into pieces (digested) by restriction enzymes and the resulting *restriction fragments* are separated according to their lengths by gel electrophoresis. RFLP methodologies are a means for the rapid and accurate identification of clinical isolates of *Nocardia* species and far surpass the conventional biochemical methods in their discriminatory capabilities.

4. Pathogenesis

After entry of the organism response begins in the reticuloendothelial system with early mobilization of neutrophils, thus limiting the spread of infection [30]. Later cell mediated immunity comes into a role and is triggered by activated macrophages, T cell population which causes direct lymphocyte-mediated toxicity to the organism. The interactions of phagocytic cells with nocardia depends on the virulence of the strain and with the growth phase of the nocardial cells. Virulent nocardia is attributed to complex cell wall glycolipids which inhibits phagosome - lysosome fusion and decreases lysosomal enzyme activity in macrophages, neutralizes phagosomal acidification, and even resists the oxidative killing mechanisms of phagocytes. In chronic granulomatous disease, neutrophils and macrophages fail to generate a burst of oxidative metabolism during phagocytosis, thus impairing the intracellular killing of catalase- positive bacteria such as *Nocardia* species [30]. The host must ultimately mount a lymphocyte response and subsequently release antibody and/or lymphocyte signals enabling the phagocytic cells to kill *N asteroides*. Immune T cells effectively clear *Nocardia* species organisms from the lung and prevent extrapulmonary dissemination. Neutrophils predominate in the early lesions of nocardiosis, and infection progresses unless antimicrobial agents are given or CMI takes over.

5. Clinical features

5.1. Lung

Pulmonary nocardiosis is the most common clinical presentation of infection because inhalation is the primary route of bacterial exposure[17]. Occasionally the gastrointestinal tract is penetrated, especially the appendix[31]. Rarely, pulmonary infection follows a dental or periodontal infection due to ingestion of contaminated food or raw vegetable material. Infection occurs in persons of all ages, even neonates. Men are affected three times as commonly as women [17]. Patients on immunosuppressive drugs, chronic granulomatous disease [32,33,34], chronic alcoholism, diabetes mellitus, and human immunodeficiency virus infection are also more susceptible to pulmonary infections with *Nocardia*. The onset of symptoms may be acute, subacute or chronic and untreated pulmonary nocardiosis can have several features similar to tuberculosis, including fever, weight loss, nonproductive cough, anorexia, night sweats, dyspnea, hemoptysis. Acute forms are particularly seen in the compromised host.

Patients can exhibit pneumonia, abscess formation, bronchopneumonia, total consolidation (lobar or even multilobar), pleural involvement or even empyema which has been seen in up to 25% of cases.

Pleural thickening or effusion can be seen radiologically. Pleural effusions can develop in up to one-third of patients. It can be very difficult clinically and radiographically to differentiate *Nocardia* from filamentous fungi (eg, aspergillosis, mucormycosis) or mycobacterial disease [17]. Chronic long standing lung lesions can lead to sinus formation. Chest X ray can also show cavitation, consolidation, abscess formation or even miliary lesions. Rarely, *Nocardia* species organisms invade preexisting lung cavities, producing a "fungus ball" appearance.

Tissues usually exhibit a mixed cellular response with polymorphonuclear leukocytes, macrophages, and lymphocytes. However, on occasion, tissue sections reveal a granulomatous reaction with central necrosis.

Other uncommon features include tracheitis, bronchitis, pleuropulmonary fistula, mediastinitis with superior vena cava syndrome and sinusitis.

6. Cutaneous involvement

Primary cutaneous and soft tissue nocardiosis can result from traumatic injury to the skin that involves contamination with soil[35]. It can be clinically evident or self limiting. Many cases go underdiagnosed as gram stains and culture are not routinely done for most superficial skin infections. After skin inoculation, a superficial abscess, localized cellulitis,pustules, pyoderma, ulcerations or paronychia can develop healing with variable scarring (Figure 5a and 5b).

Cutaneous nocardiosis can resemble indolent soft tissue infections as caused by *Staphylococcus aureus* or streptococci. The infection can spread to the regional lymph nodes and produce a single or linear chain of nodular lesions resembling sporotrichosis. This lymphocutaneous nocardiosis is often called *sporotrichoid nocardiosis*. In more advanced cases, a mycetoma with a sinus tract development can occur. Mycetoma is a chronic, granulomatous, subcutaneous tissue infection caused by both bacteria (actinomycetoma) and fungi (eumycetoma). This chronic infection was termed Madura foot and eventually mycetoma, owing to its etiology. The hallmark triad of the disease includes tumefaction, fistulization of the abscess and extrusion of colored grains. The color of these extruded grains in the active phase of the disease offers a clue to diagnosis. The "dot-in-circle" sign has recently been proposed as a highly specific magnetic resonance imaging (MRI) and ultrasonography (USG) sign of mycetoma, which may allow a noninvasive as well as early diagnosis. At least half of the mycetomas are caused by aerobic actinomycetes, mostly *Nocardia* species, whereas members of the genus *Actinomadura* are frequently recorded only in certain geographic locations [15]. *N brasiliensis* is the most frequently recognized cause *Nocardia* induced mycetomas, but *N asteroides, N otitidiscaviarum,* and *N transvalensis* can also be etiologic organisms.

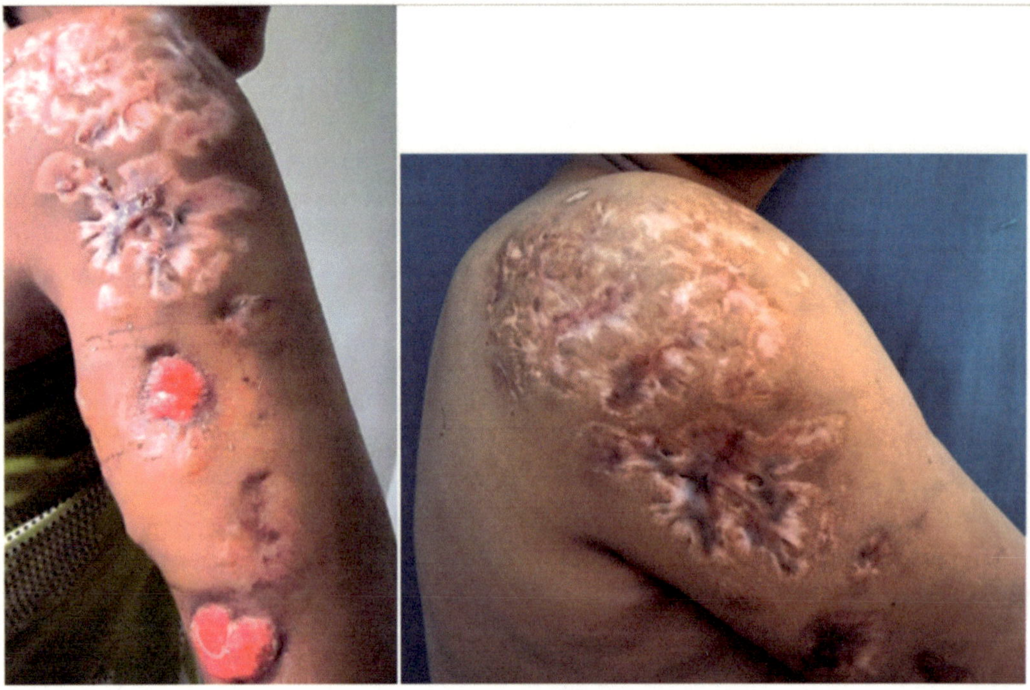

Figure 5. a. Primary cutaneous nocardiosis with ulcerated lesions and scarring
b. Photograph of the same patient with all lesions healing with scarring

Cutaneous nocardiosis is characterized by one of two manifestations: primary cutaneous infection or disseminated infection with skin involvement. The two forms have different microbiological, clinical and prognostic features which is illustrated in table number 1[36].

Nocardia bacteremia is not occasionally present but if occurs it can lead to infection in the eyes (keratitis), heart valves, liver, spleen, adrenal glands, thyroid gland, and other organ tissues. In a review of *Nocardia* bacteremia done in USA, 64% patients had concurrent pulmonary nocardiosis, 28% had concurrent cutaneous disease, and 19% had concurrent CNS disease and poor outcomes are correlated with acute onset of nocardiosis (duration less than 1 month), late identification of nocardia, involvement of more than 2 sites and lack of proper treatment.

Post traumatic keratitis and endophthalmitis with compound-fracture infection or poststemotomy mediastinitis and postoperative nosocomial *N farcinica* wound infections following cardiac, blood vessel, or transplantation surgery have recently been described.

Rarely, *Nocardia* species organisms can be inoculated directly into the bloodstream during iv drug abuse or accidentally into a vein, producing local septic thrombophlebitis.

7. Systemic involvement

The most common sites for dissemination include the CNS (brain), skin and subcutaneous tissues, eyes (especially the retina), kidneys, joints, bones, and the heart. Unlike the primary pulmonary infection, lesions of disseminated or systemic nocardiosis progress unless treated. Self - limited or subclinical disease is not recognized frequently, although some CNS infections may evolve slowly over a period of many months or even years.

CNS – Central nervous system involvement is a well-described complication of nocardial infection[36]. Most reviews of this problem have focused on nocardial brain abscess, whose typical clinical presentation is an intracranial space-occupying lesion. Recently, *Nocardia* has been cited as a cause of persistent neutrophilic pleocytosis resembling other subacute or chronic forms of meningitis in its clinical presentation and CSF findings. In a typical case of pyogenic brain abscess, headache is clearly the most common presenting compliant. The nature of the headache is characterized by dull aching that is poorly localized. Depression, schizophrenia, dyslexia and amnesia have also been recorded [37].

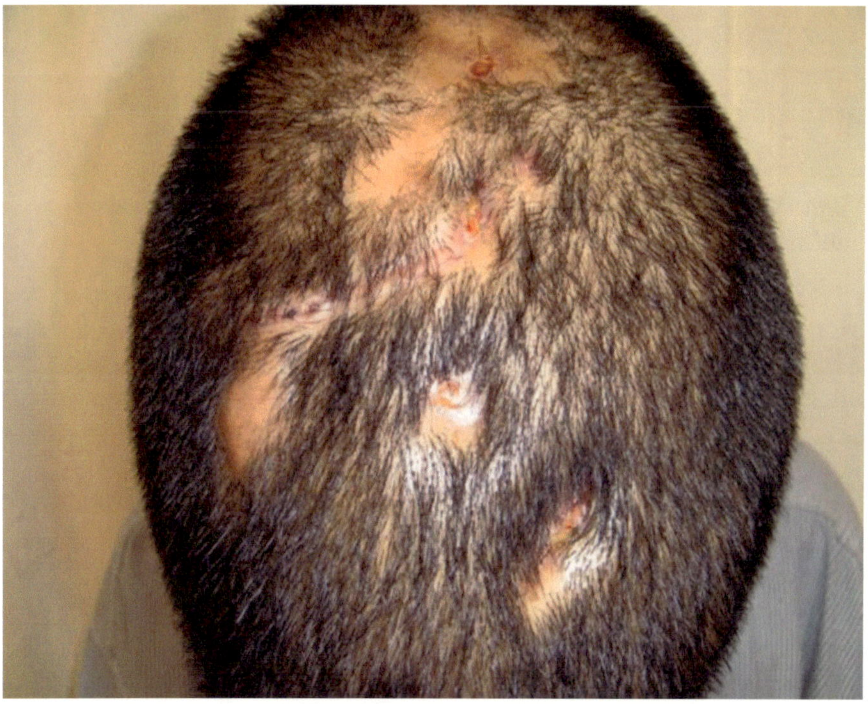

Figure 6. Primary cutaneous nocardiosis with cranial and cerebral extension

The most common source of microbial infection remains direct or indirect cranial infection (Figure 6) arising from the paranasal otogenic brain sinuses, middle ear, and teeth. Seeding of the brain presumably occurs via transit of infecting bacteria through the valveless organ transplant. Although dental and sinus infections remain an important source of brain abscess. The typical presentation was subacute to chronic meningitis characterized by fever, stiff neck, and headache. CSF studies revealed neutrophilic pleocytosis, hypoglycorrhachia, and elevated protein level. CT and MRI scanning can help in diagnosis and management of brain abscess. CT scan with intravenous contrast of the brain with abscess will demonstrate ring-enhancing lesion. Needle aspiration or biopsy of a cerebral mass is not confirmatory for the diagnosis.

Cerebral nocardiosis commonly accompanies pulmonary disease, but isolated CNS disease may occur. In immunocompetent patients, cerebral nocardiosis is less common and may resemble a brain tumor or vascular infarct [38,39]. Central nervous system imaging should be considered for patients with any adverse neurologic symptoms, severe pulmonary nocardiosis, or significant immunosuppression.

Other systemic involvement includes peritonitis, epididymo-orchitis, iliopsoas, ischiorectal and perirectal abscess, hematogenous endophthalmitis and retinitis, pericarditis, endocarditis, aortitis, septic arthritis and bursitis, peritonitis in chronic peritoneal dialysis, osteomyelitis, and a disseminated miliary picture with diffuse organ abscesses.

Eye involvement like retinal infection or endophthalmitis, keratoconjunctivitis can occur.

8. Nocardiosis and HIV

Systemic *Nocardia* infections occur more frequently in immunocompromised patients. *Nocardia* species is recognized as an opportunistic pathogen for patients with impaired host defense mechanisms.

Lymphoreticular malignancies, organ transplantation, corticosteroid or other immunosuppressive therapy, and underlying pulmonary disease are important predisposing factors [40,41,42]. Uttamchandani et al. found a strong association of *Nocardia* infection with injection drug use [43]. Nocardiosis occurred among patients with advanced HIV disease. The clinical features of nocardiosis in these HIV-infected patients were similar to those described in other immunocompromised patients. The duration of illness was typically chronic, and the signs and symptoms reflected the sites involved. The lung was the most commonly affected site. The chest radiographic features were variable and not specific for nocardiosis. The diagnosis of nocardiosis is often delayed because none of the clinical, laboratory or radiographic features are pathognomonic. The diagnosis therefore relies on the isolation of *Nocardia* species, which can be difficult, particularly when the specimens are contaminated with other microorganisms. Nocardiosis caused or contributed to the death of two thirds of the patients. The high fatality rate could be attributed to three factors: dissemination of the infection due to delayed institution of therapy, relapse of nocardiosis due to discontinuation of treatment, and severe immune dysfunction of the host.

9. Treatment

Sulfonamides, including sulfadiazine and sulfisoxazole, have been the antimicrobials of choice to treat nocardiosis for the past 50 years despite bacteriostatic activity [44]. Sulfadiazine can induce oliguria, azotemia, and crystalluria in patients who fail to maintain a high fluid intake. This complication can be prevented by alkalinizing the urine with oral sodium bicarbonate. Sulfisoxazole is equally effective and much less likely to cause oliguria.

Trimethoprim-sulfamethoxazole (TMP-SMZ) is now most frequently used to treat this infection. Divided doses of 5 to 10 mg/kg per day of the trimethoprim component or 25 to 50 mg/kg per day of sulfamethoxazole are recommended to produce sulfonamide serum concentrations between 100 and 150 g/mL. Adverse reactions to high-dose TMP-SMX therapy are frequent and include myelosuppression, hepatoxicity, and renal insufficiency. Trimethoprim-sulfamethoxazole is active against most *Nocardia* species; however, *N otitidiscaviarum* is commonly resistant to TMP-SMX [43]. 90%-95% of pleuropulmonary infections respond favourably. However, in patients with disseminated disease, especially of the CNS, and/or patients with depressed CMI, certain factors may complicate the picture. Most important is the frequent occurrence of side effects in HIV-infected persons or organ transplant recipients: 44%-80% experience fever, skin rash, and/or neutropenia. HIV-infected patients require long-term maintenance suppressive therapy and are particularly intolerant of the TMP-SMZ combination, manifesting severe hypersensitivity reactions, hepatotoxicity, and/or prolonged myelosuppression. In organ transplantation patients treated with the anti rejection medication cyclosporine, TMP-SMZ may cause reversible cyclosporine-induced nephrotoxicity. Daily TMP-SMX prophylaxis most reliably prevents nocardiosis compared to intermittent therapy with oral TMP-SMX (2 double-strength tablets twice weekly or 1 single strength tablet 3 times weekly) [45]. Non immunosuppressed patients with pulmonary or systemic nocardiosis (excluding CNS involvement) should be treated for a minimum of 6-12 months and hose with CNS infection should be treated for 12 months. In one study of the efficacy of TMP-SMZ, relapse occurred rarely when patients received therapy for > 3 months [46]. Parenteral therapy need not be continued beyond a period of 3-6 weeks, as determined by response in individual patients.

Alternatives to sulfonamides include amikacin, imipenem, meropenem, ceftriaxone, cefotaxime, minocycline, moxifloxacin, levofloxacin, linezolid, tigecycline, and amoxicillin - clavulanic acid [47,48].

Linezolid is an oxazolidinone that has activity against most gram-positive bacteria, including in vitro activity against all *Nocardia* species and strains [49,50]. Linezolid binds to a site on the bacterial 23S rRNA of the 50S subunit and prevents the formation of a functional 70S-initiation complex, which is an essential component of the bacterial translation process. Dose is 600 mg orally or iv twice daily. CNS nocardiosis is associated with significant morbidity and mortality. A number of recent reports have highlighted the excellent penetration of the CSF by linezolid after intravenous administration of the drug every 12 h.

Tigecycline, a glycylcycline, appears to be active in vitro against most *Nocardia* species. Of the fluoroquinolones, moxifloxacin is fairly active in vitro against *asteroides* complex.

Combination therapy with imipenem and cefotaxime, amikacin and TMP-SMX, imipenem and TMP-SMX, amikacin and cefotaxime, or amikacin and imipenem may provide enhanced activity. Alternative oral drug therapy for nocardial infections theoretically might include dapsone because its mechanism of action (folate antagonism) is identical to that of the sulphonamides.

Surgical intervention can be advised for the drainage or excision of abscesses or an empyema.

	Primary Cutaneous	Disseminated with skin Involvement
Species	N. brasiliensis	N. asteroids
Risk Factors	Local trauma related to plants And soil	Immunosuppression
Primay site	Skin	Lung
Skin manifestations	Acute: Lymphocutanoeus Superficial skin infections Chronic : Mycetoma	Pustules Nodules Abscesses
Diagnosis	Direct Smear: Gram and acid fast stainin. Culture: Standard or Special media. Biochemical and molecular methods: DNA probing, PCR, PCR-RFLP, Gene sequencing, ribotyping	
Treatment	TMP-SMX; alternatives are amikacin, minocycline, imipenem, 3rd generation cephalosporins, linezolid	
Duration of treatment	Lymphocutaneous/ superficial: 2-4 months Mycetoma: 12 months	No CNS involvement or immunio- Suppression: 6-12 months CNS involvement or immunoi- Suppression: 12 months
Prognosis	Good but can recur	Poor, mortality rate 44-85%

Table 1. PCR: polymerase chain reaction. RFLP- fragment length polymorphism, TMP-SMZX trimethoprim- sulphomethoxazole

10. Conclusion

The spectrum of subcutaneous and deep mycoses is a very wide one. Of these, nocardiosis is becoming increasingly important especially in the era of HIV infections. Nocardiosis can present in diverse clinical manifestations, including cutaneous nodules, ulcerations, subcutaneous abscesses, pyoderma like lesions, lymphangitis (sporotrichoid pattern), mycetoma like lesions. Moreover, the systemic spectrum of nocardiosis is also wide, including, pulmonary, central nervous system, eye, bone, and solid organs. Hence, unless a high index of suspicion is kept, nocardiosis can be either underdiagnosed or misdiagnosed. The usual diagnostic methods are histopathology and culture, though the gold standard remains PCR. Clinico pathological correlation is important for diagnosis. The treatment of nocardiosis essentially involves long term administration of chemotherapeutic agents like sulphonamides, cotrimoxazole, linezolid and amikacin. Early initiation of chemotherapy can avoid surgical excision which may be required in late or complicated cases.

Author details

Sharmila P. Patil, Nitin J. Nadkarni and Nidhi R. Sharma
Dr. D.Y.Patil Medical College, Nerul, Navi Mumbai, Maharashtra, India

Acknowledgement

Acknowledgement to Dr. Vishalakshi Vishwanath, Head of department, Rajiv Gandhi Medical College and Hospital, Thane, Mumbai for histopathology photographs of Nocardiosis no. 6a and 6b.

11. References

[1] Wilson JW .Nocardiosis: Updates and Clinical Overview. Mayo Clin Proc. 2012;87:403-407.
[2] Corti ME, Fiotti, MFV. Nocardiosis: A review. Int J Infect Dis 2003;7: 243-250 .
[3] Brown-Elliott BA et al. Clinical and Laboratory Features of the Nocardia spp. Based on Current Molecular Taxonomy. Clin Microbiol Rev. 2006;19: 259–282 .
[4] Goodfellow, M., and T. Pirouz.. Numerical classification of sporoactinomycetes containing meso-diaminopimelic acid in the cell wall. J. Gen. Microbiol.1982; 128:503-507 .
[5] Mordarska, H., M. Mordarski, and M. Goodfellow. Chemotaxonomic characters and classification of some nocardioform bacteria. J. Gen. Microbiol.1972; 71:77-86.
[6] Pijper, A., and B. D. Pullinger. South African nocardioses. J. Trop. Med. Hyg. 1972; 30:153-156.
[7] Wallace RJ Jr, Steele LC, Sumter G, Smith JM. Antimicrobial susceptibility patterns of Nocardia asteroides. Antimicrob Agents Chemother. 1988;32:1776-1779.
[8] Schlaberg R, Huard RC, Della-Latta P. Nocardia cyriacigeorgica, an emerging pathogen in the United States. J Clin Microbiol. 2008;46:265-273.
[9] Fergie, J. E., and K. Purcell. Nocardiosis in south Texas children. Pediatr. Infect. Dis. J. 2001; 20:711-714

[10] Wallace RJ, Jr., Brown BA, Blacklock Z, Ulrich R, Jost K et al . New Nocardia taxon among isolates of Nocardia brasiliensis associated with invasive disease. J. Clin. Microbiol.1995; 33:1528-1533
[11] Saubolle MA, and Sussland D. Nocardiosis: review of clinical and laboratory experience. J. Clin. Microbiol.2003;41:4497-4501.
[12] Nocard E. Note sur la maladie des boeufs de la Gouadeloupe connue sous le nom de farcin. Ann. Inst. Pasteur 1888; 2:293-302.
[13] Gordon, R. E., and J. M. Mihm. A comparative study of some strains received as nocardiae. J. Bacteriol. 1957; 73:15-27.
[14] Gordon, R. E., and J. M. Mihm. The type species of the genus Nocardia. J. Gen. Microbiol. 1962;27:1-10.
[15] McNeil MM, Brown JM. The medically important aerobic actinomycetes: epidemiology and microbiology. Clin Microbiol Rev. 1994;7:357-417.
[16] Reed RC. Nocardiosis and actinomycosis. Medicine 2005;33: 114-115
[17] Lerner PI. Nocardia species, in Manedll GL, Douglas RG Jr., Bennett GE, editors: Principles and practice of infectious diseases, New York, 1985, John Wiley & Sons, Inc. pp 1423-1427
[18] Young LS, Rubin RH. Mycobacterial and nocardial diseases in the compromised host. In: Rubin RH, Young LS, eds. A Clinical Approach to Infection in the Compromised Host. 4th ed. New York, NY: Kluwer Academic; 2002:257-261.
[19] Long PF. A retrospective study of Nocardia infections associated with the acquired immune deficiency syndrome (AIDS). Infection. 1994;22:362-364
[20] Choucino C, Goodman SA, Greer JP, Stein RS, Wolff SN, Dummer JS. Nocardial infections in bone marrow transplant recipients. Clin Infect Dis. 1996;23:1012-1019.
[21] Van Burik JA, Hackman RC, Nadeem SQ, et al. Nocardiosis after bone marrow transplantation: a retrospective study. Clin Infect Dis. 1997;24:1154-1160.
[22] Forbes GM, Harvey FA, Philpott-Howard JN, et al. Nocardiosis in liver transplantation: variation in presentation, diagnosis and therapy. J Infect. 1990;20:11-19.
[23] Wilson JP, Turner HR, Kirchner KA, Chapman SW. Nocardial infections in renal transplant recipients. Medicine (Baltimore). 1989;68:38-57.
[24] Peleg AY, Husain S, Qureshi ZA, et al. Risk factors, clinical characteristics, and outcome of Nocardia infection in organ transplant recipients: a matched case-control study. Clin Infect Dis. 2007;44:1307-1314.
[25] Arduino RC, Johnson PC, Miranda AG. Nocardiosis in renal transplant recipients undergoing immunosuppression with cyclosporine. Clin Infect Dis. 1993;16:505-512.
[26] Roberts SA, Franklin JC, Mijch A, Spelman D. Nocardia infection in heart-lung transplant recipients at Alfred Hospital, Melbourne, Australia, 1989-1998. Clin Infect Dis. 2000;31:968-972.
[27] Blumel J. Blumel E, Yasin AF, Schmidt-Rotte H, Sehaal KP. Typing of Nocardia farcinica by pulse filed gel electrophoresisa and randomly amplified polymorphic DNA PCR. J Clin Microbiol 1998; 36: 118-122
[28] Curry WA. Human nocardiosis.A clinical review with selected case reports. Arch Intern Med 1980; 140: 818-826

[29] Beaman BL, Boiron P, Beaman L, Brownell GH, Schaal K, Gombert ME. Nocardia and nocardiosis. J Med Vet Mycoll992; 30(suppl1):317-31.

[30] Beaman BL, Beaman L. Nocardia species: host-parasite relationships. Clin Microbiol Rev 1994;7:213-64.

[31] Lerner PI. Nocardiosis. State-of-the-art clinical article. Clin Infect Dis .1996; 22:891-903

[32] Chapman, S. W., and J. P. Wilson. 1990. Nocardiosis in transplant recipients. Semin. Respir. Infect. 5:74-79.

[33] Jonsson, S., R. J. Wallace, Jr., S. I. Hull, and D. M. Musher. 1986. Recurrent Nocardia pneumonia in an adult with chronic granulomatous disease. Am. Rev. Respir. Dis. 133:932-934.

[34] Lopes, J. O., S. H. Alves, J. P. Benevenga, A. Salla, and I. Tatsch. 1993. Nocardia asteroides peritonitis during continuous ambulatory peritoneal dialysis. Rev. Inst. Med. Trop. Sao Paulo 35:377-379.

[35] Patil SP, Gautam MM, Sodha AA, Khan KJ. Primary cutaneous nocardiosis with craniocerebral extension: A case report Dermatol Online J. 2009; 15:8

[36] Dodiuk-Gad R, Cohen E, Ziv M, Goldstein LH, et al. Cutaneous nocardiosis: report of two cases and review of literature. Int J. Dermatol 2010; 49: 1380-1385

[37] Beaman BL, Beaman L, Kjelstrom JA, Ogata SA. Bacteria and neurodegeneration In: Calne D, ed. Neurodegenerative diseases. Orlando, Florida: WB Saunders, 1994:319-38.

[38] Borm W, Gleixner M. Nocardia brain abscess misinterpreted as cerebral infarction. J Clin Neurosci. 2003;10:130-132.

[39] Menku A, Kurtsoy A, Tucer B, Yildiz O, Akdemir H. Nocardia brain abscess mimicking brain tumour in immunocompetent patients: report of two cases and review of the literature. Acta Neurochir (Wien). 2004;146:411-414

[40] Murray JF. Finegold SM. Froman S. Will DW. The changing spectrum of nocardiosis: a review and presentation of nine cases. Am Rev Respir Dis 1961;83:315-30.

[41] Frazier AR. Rosenow EC III. Roberts GD. Nocardiosis: a review of 25 cases occurring during 24 months. Mayo Clin Proc 1975;50:657-63.

[42] Ambriosioni J, Lew D, Garbino J. Nocardiosis: Updated Clinical Review and Experience at a Tertiary Center. Infection 2010; 38: 89-97

[43] Uttamchandani RB, Daikos GL, Reyes RR, Fischl MA et al. Nocardiosis in 30 patients with advanced human immunodeficiency virus infection: clinical features and outcome. Clin Infect Dis. 1994 Mar;18:348-53.

[44] McNeil MM, Brown JM, Hutwagner LC, Schiff TA. Evaluation of therapy for Nocardia asteroides complex infecton: CDN/NCID report. Infect Dis Clin Pract. 1995;4:287-292

[45] Peterson PK, Ferguson R, Fryd DS, Balfour HH Jr, Rynasiewic J, Simmons RL. Infectious diseases in hospitalized renal transplant recipients: a prospective study of a complex and evolving problem. Medicine (Baltimore). 1982;61:360-372.

[46] Wallace RJ Jr, Septimus EJ, Williams TW Jr, et al. Use of trimethoprimsulfamethoxazole for treatment of infections due to Nocardia. Rev Infect Dis 1982;4:315-25.

[47] Garlando F, Bodmer T, Lee C, Zimmerli W, Pirovino M. Successful treatment of disseminated nocardiosis complicated by cerebral abscess with ceftriaxone and amikacin: case report. Clin Infect Dis 1992; 15: 1039–40.

[48] Yew WW, Wong PC, Kwan SY, Chan CY, Li MS. Two cases of Nocardia asteroides sternotomy infection treated with ofloxacin and a review of other active antimicrobial agents. J Infect 1991; 23:297–302
[49] Diekema DJ, Jones RN. Oxazolidinone antibiotics. Lancet 2001; 358: 1975–82.
[50] Moylett EH, Pacheco SE, Brown-Elliott BA, et al. Clinical experience with linezolid for the treatment of Nocardia infection.Clin Infect Dis. 2003;36:313-318.

Chapter 6

Cytopathology of Canine Mammary Gland Affections

Shivani Sangha and Amarjit Singh

Additional information is available at the end of the chapter

http://dx.doi.org/10.5772/52437

1. Introduction

Mammary gland of dogs is the most common site for development of various neoplastic and non-neoplastic affections like tumors, mastitis, steatitis, galactostasis, galactorrhea, agalactia etc. It has been postulated that inflammatory and non proliferative breast diseases do not increase risk of cancer [1]. However, proliferative breast diseases with or without atypia confers mild and moderate risk respectively, whereas carcinoma in situ is associated with substantial risk of life if left untreated [2].The carcinomas often have a poor prognosis due to high rate of local recurrence as well as metastasis, necessitating surgery in some cases adjuvant to chemotherapy [3].The canine mammary tumor (CMT) account for between 25 to 50 percent of all the tumors occurring in the canines [4-6] and are only second to skin tumors [7]. Considering the rate of occurrence of mammary tumors among various species, breast cancer is most frequent in women (32%), the highly occurring neoplasia (52%) in bitches and ranks third most common neoplasia (17%) in queens after lymphohaemopoietic and skin tumors [8-10]. Keeping in view, the high rate of occurrence, rapid onset of growth, and poor survival statistics of the patients, a quick and early diagnosis of mammary tumor is required.

Today, the worldwide tendency is to look for quick and inexpensive method of tumor diagnosis as the routinely used histological method requires invasive sampling and long hours for processing of the tissue samples. Such a quick, inexpensive, less painful and easily repeatable technique is cytology. It refers to microscopic evaluation of cells which have either naturally exfoliated or has been artificially removed from the body or tissue mass. The technique was first used in the United States by Guthrie in 1921 [11]. The technique requires minimal of sophisticated instruments and is relatively non-invasive technique that obviates the need of open biopsy. Furthermore, implantation of cancer cells after this technique is very rare [12]. Diagnostic cytology has recently been employed for diagnosis of some of the tumors in the veterinary medicine [13-15]. When applied to mammary gland tumors, the method showed low sensitivity and specificity [13, 16, 17].The reasons have been assumed to be heterogeneous composition of mammary tumors [18, 19]. More recently, valuable additional information with improved diagnostic accuracy has been provided by cytological features of fine needle aspirates or from imprints of tissue sections [20, 21]. Both palpable (solid or cystic) or non palpable benign or malignant mammary gland lesions can be diagnosed through this technique. In some studies, combination of cytology, radiology and clinical assessments has resulted in accurate diagnosis in 99%of cases [22]. Thus, this chapter focus on application of various techniques in evaluating cytological samples from affected mammary gland of canine and feasibility of cytology in differentiating benign and malignant neoplastic lesions.

2. Techniques of sample collection for cytology of mammary gland

2.1. Solid tissue cytology

2.1.1. Fine needle Cytology

Fine needle aspirates are obtained with 10-20 ml disposable syringe bearing 21-25 gauge needle. The softer the tissue, the smaller the needle and syringe used whereas firm tissues like fibroadenomas require larger syringe to maintain adequate pressure [23]. Generally, a 10 ml syringe yield adequate cytological sample from mammary gland of dogs. The mass is located clinically and stabilized in position. The skin over the puncture site is cleaned with alcohol or spirit and the samples are collected using aspiration or non-aspiration procedure.

Aspiration procedure

After cleaning the mass with some antiseptic solution, the needle with syringe attached is introduced into the centre of mass. Strong negative pressure is applied by withdrawing the plunger to about 3/4th of the volume of syringe. The needle is moved through the mass three or four times in different directions. Still with the needle in the mass, suction is slowly released. The needle is then removed from the mass and the syringe from the needle. The syringe is then filled with little air and then reconnected to the needle. Finally, the contents of the needle are blown on to one or more clean dry slides, which are rapidly air dried.

Non-aspiration procedure (Capillary technique/ Stab technique)

This technique is similar to the standard fine needle aspiration technique, except no negative pressure is applied during collection. Here the plunger of syringe is filled with air before the collection attempt so as to allow rapid expulsion contents onto a glass slide.

Caution: Usually in both the cases, the aspirate may not be visible in the syringe. However, when the air pressure is applied to syringe for expulsion of contents on the slide, the needle will contain sufficient tissue for cytological smear preparation.

2.1.2. *Tissue imprints or Impression smears*

Tissue imprints can be obtained by pressing the glass slide over the lesion from live animal or from the surface of the tissue excised during surgery. Do this several times, to have multiple impressions over one slide. Samples collected through touch impression contain tissue cells, superficial inflammatory cells and greater microbial contamination as compared to aspirates or swabs.

To minimize microbial or cellular contamination, clean the area of the lesion with cotton swab moistened with saline solution. Do not use water to prevent osmosis induced cell rupture. In case, imprints are to be obtained from the tissue excised during surgery, the surface of excised tissue is cut to get a fresh surface for impression smear. Next, the excess blood and tissue fluid is swabbed/ dabbed from the area to be imprinted by blotting paper, and the surface of lesion is pressed hard against the clean glass slide. No further smearing of the material is done to avoid cellular distortion and the slides are simply air dried.

2.2. Fluid Cytology

In case if fluid is filled in the syringe during fine needle aspiration, collect it in a sterile tube. Quickly, make few smears from the fluid. To avoid coagulation, keep a portion of specimen in some anticoagulant (preferably EDTA) containing vial and other portion of sample in sterile capped test tube (for the purpose of microbial culture, if required, as anticoagulant prevents microbial growth).

2.2.1. *Tissue imprints or Touch Impression smears*

Teat of affected mammary gland occasionally shows fluid on squeezing. For making touch impressions, teat orifice is cleaned with spirit swab and then pressed hard against the clean dry glass slide to get the touch impression. If fluid is found enough, a smear can also be drawn.

2.2.2. *Swabs*

These are collected in case of purulent lesions or fistulous tracts. Before collection of sample, the lesion should be cleaned with moist and sterile cotton. The swab is directly introduced into the lesion and then gently rolled on the glass slide to make the smear. Dry the smears in air. Do not rub the swab over the slide as it will result in distortion of cell size and shape thus leading to misdiagnosis.

3. Choice of technique for sample collection

Choice of technique for collection of cytological sample depends on nature of lesion as mention below:

Solid lesions: Fine needle aspirates are preferred for obtaining samples from solid lesions. Aspiration procedure is commonly used, however, Non-aspiration procedure is recommended for highly vascular lesions. Touch impressions can also be made in addition to aspirates.

Ulcerative superficial lesions: Impression smears should be made both before and after cleaning the ulcerated surface.

Teat fluids and secretions: Touch impressions or swabs are useful.

4. Preparation of Slides

A minimum of four to six slides from multiple sites within the lesion are made using following techniques

4.1. Slide-over-slide smears (Squash Preps)

The technique is useful in case aspirated material is thick. The material collected from the fine needle cytology procedure is expelled near one end (0.5 inch) of a clean glass slide ("sample" slide). A second glass slide ("spreader" slide) is placed on top of and perpendicular to the slide containing the sample. The spreader slide is then lightly drawn out across the length of bottom slide, spreading the sample. No downward pressure is applied to the spreader slide while making the smear as this usually result in rupturing of cells. Squash preps result on fine spreading of the cells and yield better cytological diagnosis in case of samples containing flecks of particulate matter.

4.2. Blood smear technique

To prepare the smear by blood smear technique, a small drop of sample is placed on the glass slide approximately 0.5 inch from the end. Another slide is moved over it at an angle of 30°-40° until it contacted the drop. When the sample fluid fills the crease between the slides, gently slide the second slide forward until the sample fluid drains away from the second slide. This results in a cytological smear with feathered edge.

4.3. Starfish preparation

Here the aspirate is dragged peripherally in several directions with the point of a syringe needle, producing a starfish shape. This technique tends not to damage fragile cells but allows a thick layer of tissue fluid to remain around the cells.

4.4. Sediment smear

For making sediment smear, centrifugation of the fluid is done for 5 minute at 165-360 G to concentrate the cells. A drop from this cellular concentrate is taken to make the smear just like blood smear. Further analysis of cellular concentrate for the physical (specific gravity) and chemical properties (total protein, calcium etc) can be helpful to determine the pathogenesis of the disease.

4.5. Combination technique

Here, one drop of the aspirate is taken on the slide (specimen slide). A spreader slide is kept on the one third of the aspirate and squash prep is made. Next, a slide tilted at angle of 30 degree is placed on the end opposite to squash prep portion. As this slide comes in to contact with one third of the aspirate, the slide is moved forward and slid like making a blood smear. Now, the smear is having one third area spreaded like blood smear, middle one concentrated and untouched and the other one-third area spreaded by squash prep method.

4.6. Line smear concentration technique

When the aspirated fluid contains few cells which do not sediment upon centrifugation, line smear technique is useful. Here, a drop of fluid is taken at one end of the clean slide. A spreader slide is used to spread the drop on previous slide in a manner similar to blood smear technique except that the spreader slide is raised directly upwards after covering three fourth of the smear. This results in a smear with line containing higher concentration of cells than the rest of slide.

5. Precautions while slide preparation for cytology

One should proceed to prepare the slide for cytological examination as soon as possible after collection of the specimen. This will prevent the sample from clotting or drying out on the slide before preparation of the smear. Another caution to be kept in mind is always use tip of the needle to spread the sample to avoid distortion in cellular shape. Also, avoid making too thick smears so that blood or other exfoliated cells do not dominate the main cell type by controlling the amount of sample being expelled from the syringe. While making squash smears, gently pull the two slides apart as too much pressure will cause cellular disruption. Always prepare at least four to five smears from one specimen in order to increase diagnostic sensitivity and specificity. Frosted or colored edged slides are preferred for cytological studies as labeling of these slides help in permanent marking and easy identification of upward side of slide containing usually colorless sample and hence prevents wipe off sample in error during staining procedure. During cytological examination of fluids, always make few smears immediately after collection of fluids as quality of cells from sample kept in EDTA containing vials is not as good as fresh sample.

6. Staining of Cytologic Smears

Cytologic smears can be stained with Papanicolaou stains and it's derivatives like Sano's trichome or Romanowsky type stains like Wright stain, Leishman stain, Diff- quick, Dipstat etc.

6.1. Papanicolaou stains

These stains use wet smears (i.e. the smear needs to be fixed before staining) and provide excellent nuclear and cell structural details but do not stain the cytoplasm and many organisms well. The staining with these stains involves multiple steps and thus requires considerable time also. These factors restrict the use of papanicolaou stains in the veterinary cytology.

6.2. Romanowsky type stains

Romanowsky type stains are the preferred stains for the cytological studies in veterinary practice. These are permanent stains and use air dried smears. Different stains like Wright stain, Leishman stain, Giemsa stain etc. come under this category and staining is done as per their standard protocols. Wright-Leishman combination can also be used which is made by mixing 3 parts of Wright stain with 1 part of Leishman stain [24]. Slides are stained in similar manner as for the standard Wright's technique except that the staining time is extended to 6-8 minutes. When there is a confusion to decide exact time limit between time range given for staining, keep in mind that thicker the smear or more the protein content in the aspirate, more is the time required for the stain [23]. So, select for higher value from the time range in case of thicker aspirates.

Romanowsky stains excellently stain the cytoplasm and the other micro-organisms present in the smear but due to smudging effect of these stains on the nucleus, nuclear and nucleolar details are not much appreciable. However, the detail is sufficient enough for differentiating neoplastic lesions from inflammatory lesions. These stains dissolve cellular lipids leaving vacuolated areas in the smear after staining. To overcome this problem, new methylene blue (NMB) stain can be used in combination to Romanowsky stains which outlines the lipid droplets and the fungi. Also, staining with New methylene blue stain is useful in diagnosis of blood contaminated samples as NMB do not stain RBC hemoglobin. As this stain is wet mount, non-permanent stain, the smears can be counter stained with Wright or Giemsa stain to get permanently stained smears.

To conclude, being quick, inexpensive, easily available and readily staining the cytoplasm and most of the organisms in the cytological smears, Romanowsky stains remain first choice of the cytologists on veterinary side. These stains help to screen inflammatory lesions from non-inflammatory mammary gland lesions, to diagnose causative agent in case of inflammatory lesions like streptococcal mastitis or tuberculosis and further assessing the malignancy potential of the mammary tumors. In particular cases, if further nuclear detailing is required, papanicolaou stains can be used.

7. Microscopic examination of slides

7.1. Cell count

The issue of specimen adequacy in breast FNAs remains controversial and has been addressed by several authors. It is advocated that a minimum number of epithelial cells be required for diagnosis and the samples containing fewer than the specified minimum be reported as non-diagnostic. Interpretations based on inadequately cellular specimen may not contain a representative sample of the lesion, giving a false impression of normalcy, or, even worse, may result in a false impression of a neoplasia that is not really present [23]. The published recommendation for the minimum number of cells in the cytological smear is of at least six clusters of cells with a minimum of 5-10 cells per group [25, 26].

7.2. Type of cells

After getting an idea for sufficient number of well stained cells in the cytologic smear from mammary gland aspirate, observe for the cell type to judge whether the lesion is inflammatory or neoplastic in nature.

7.2.1. Inflammatory cells

Neutrophils, macrophages, lymphocytes, eosinophils and epitheliod cells are commonly encountered inflammatory cells from the aspirates of mammary lesions. Neutrophils are multinucleated and are usually characterized by mild nuclear alterations like nuclear swelling, chromatin hyalinization, foamy cytoplasm etc. to severe degenerative changes like karyorrhexis and karyolysis. Eosinophils dominate during allergic response to some foreign body. The cells like monocytes/macrophages, lymphocytes and epitheloid cells dominate during chronic inflammatory lesions like granulamatous mastitis.

7.2.2. Non-Inflammatory cells

Epithelial cells

These cells are variable in size from small (basal cells) to large with particular feature of cell to cell adhesion. This adhesion causes cells to be present in form of sheets or clumps. Epithelial cells generally contain round to oval nuclei with clear cytoplasmic boundaries.

Mesenchymal cells

These are usually elongated cells with round to rod shaped nuclei and the cytoplasm tapering in one or more directions. Characteristically, mesenchymal cells have indistinct cytoplasmic boundaries that blend with the background. Due to cohesive nature of connective tissue from which the mesenchymal cells originate, cellular smears are sparsely populated.

Note: Mixture of inflammatory and non-inflammatory cells suggest neoplastic lesion with secondary inflammation.

7.3. On the basis of observing the cell type, the mammary gland lesions can be broadly classified as

7.3.1. Inflammatory lesions

Inflammatory breast aspirate shows low cellularity with epithelial cells arranged in clusters and small groups with the presence of myo-epithelial cells. Cytological atypia and nuclear changes are minimal [27, 28].The Inflammatory lesions can be cytologically classified as:

Acute Inflammatory lesions

Mainly neutrophils dominate the smear (>90%) and usually show degenerative changes like nuclear swelling, foamy cytoplasm etc. Extracellular, eosinophilic material is usually present in considerable amount. For example: Purulent mastitis, udder abscess etc.

Mixed (Chronic-Active) Inflammatory lesions

It is an intermediate stage with cellular smears showing mixture of neutrophils (50-70%) and mononuclear cells like monocytes and lymphocytes. Macrophages and epitheloid cells can also be observed. The cellular smears taken from the animals suffering from affections like fat necrosis, organized hematoma, steatis etc. also exhibit mixed inflammatory lesions.

Chronic Inflammatory lesions

This category of lesions present cellular smears dominated by mononuclear inflammatory cells like lymphocytes, macrophages, multinucleated giant cells and or numerous epithelial macrophages. For example: Granulamatous mastitis, tuberculous mastitis.

7.3.2. Non-Inflammatory lesions

7.3.2.1. Hyperplastic / Dysplastic lesions

Hyperplasia and dysplasia are the proliferative lesions that make normal tissue resembles neoplastic cells. Like aspirates from neoplastic lesions, aspirates from epithelial or mesenchymal hyperplastic lesions do not present good nuclear criteria of malignancy like variable nuclear to cytoplasmic ratio, macronucleoli and abnormal chromatin patterns. Rather, the hyperplastic cells present a constant nuclear to cytoplasmic ratio as they are proliferating under controlled mechanism. Dysplastic and hyperplastic lesions include lobular hyperplasia, adenosis etc.

Note: A mixture of inflammatory and tissue cells suggest neoplasia with secondary inflammation or inflammation with secondary tissue cell dysplasia.

7.3.2.2 Neoplastic lesions

The type (benign or malignant), grade and tissue of origin of various neoplastic lesions of mammary gland can be diagnosed from cytological smear by studying the nuclear and cytoplasmic details and chromatin patterns as described in section 7.4.

7.4. Cytological and nuclear criteria of malignancy: Mammary gland tumors

On basis of nuclear and cytoplasmic details, cellular smears of mammary gland tumors can be classified in the following manner:

a. On the basis of behavior of tumor as benign or malignant [29].
b. On the basis of tissue of origin as epithelial, mesenchymal or mixed type [30].
c. On the basis of severity of tumor as grade I, II or III [31].

7.4.1. On the basis of behavior of tumor: Benign or malignant

Tumors can be classified as benign or malignant according to following criteria [29]:

General criteria	
1. Anisocytosis	Variations in the cells sizes
2. Pleomorphism	Variations in the shapes of cells of the same type
3. Hypercellularity	Increase in the number of exfoliated cells
Nuclear criteria	
1. Macrokaryosis	Increase in size of nuclei
2. Anisokaryosis	Variations in size of nuclei
3. Multinucleation	Increase in the number of nuclei
4. Nuclear / Cytoplasm ratio	Increased
5. Nuclear molding	Deformation of the nuclei
6. Mitotic figures	Increased and abnormal
7. Chromatin pattern	Coarse pattern
8.Macronucleoli	Increase in the size of the nucleoli.
9. Angular nucleoli	Presence of angular nucleoli
10. Anisonucleosis	Variation in size of nucleoli

Table 1. Classification of mammary tumors according to behavior of tumor (Benign or Malignant)

If three or more of the below mentioned tumor criteria are present, tumor is of malignant type otherwise benign type.

Various terms are used to assess abnormal chromatin pattern in the nucleus like strippled, reticular or lacy, coarse, clumped or smudged chromatin. The fine smooth chromatin shows uniform pattern of thin chromatin strands with fine borders. Strippled pattern refers to smooth pattern of chromatin with small aggregates of chromatin dispersed in whole of the nucleus. When the chromatin strands appear thicker than normal, the term reticular or lacy chromatin is used. When the chromatin strands become very thick, giving ropy or chord-like appearance, coarse chromatin pattern is indicated. When large aggregates of reticular or coarse chromatin are dispersed throughout the nucleus, the clumped chromatin pattern is visible. Further, if the boundaries of chromatin strands or clusters are not very discrete and become vague, it leads to smudged pattern of the chromatin.

7.4.2. *On the basis of tissue of origin (Histogenic classification)*

According to type of tissue from which tumor originated, the tumors can be classified as epithelial, mesenchymal or mixed type of tumor [30].

7.4.2.1. *Epithelial tumors*

These are epithelial in origin and often exfoliate in clumps or sheets. Cytologically, the smears contain clusters, clumps or sheets of cells with round to oval nuclei and clear cytoplasmic boundaries (Fig.1). Adenomas, adenocarcinomas and mixed mammary adenocarcinoma are grouped as epithelial tumors. In case of adenoma or adenocarcinoma the cells may get arranged in acinar or ductular pattern with central lumen. In case of papillary or cystic adenomas, cytoplasm may appear distended by secretory product.

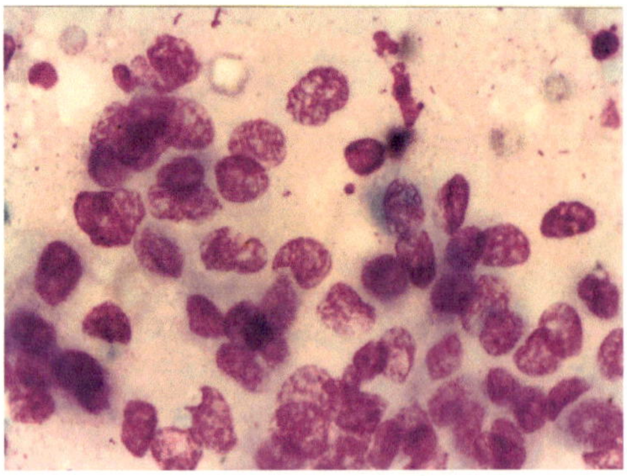

Figure 1. Epithelial tumor: Fine needle aspirate smear consist of cells situated in separate groups with round to oval nuclei and lined by clear cytoplasmic boundaries, Wright-Leihman x 750.

7.4.2.2. *Mesenchymal Tumors*

These originate from connective tissue. In contrast to epithelial tumors, mesenchymal tumors do not exfoliate regularly and are found as individually settled polygonal/elliptical/stellate or spindle shaped cells with poorly defined cell membrane (Fig.2). Lipoma and liposarcoma are classified under this category.

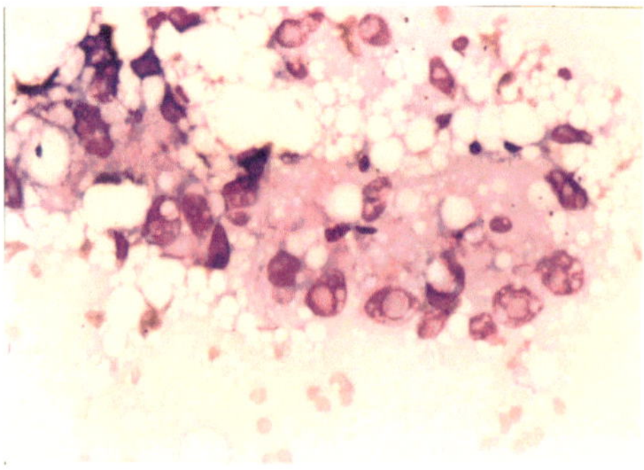

Figure 2. Mesenchymal tumor: Consist of individually settled pleomorphic cells with scarce cytoplasm and poorly defined cell membrane, Wright- Leishman x 150.

7.4.2.3. *Mixed type of Tumors*

Mixed type of tumors reveal cellular elements of both epithelial and mesenchymal type (Fig.3). Thus, clusters of cells with round to oval nuclei and clear cytoplasmic boundaries as well as individually settled polygonal/elliptical/stellate or spindle shaped cells with poorly defined cell membrane are found in the cellular smear. Mixed mammary adenoma and mixed mammary adenocarcinoma are included in this group.

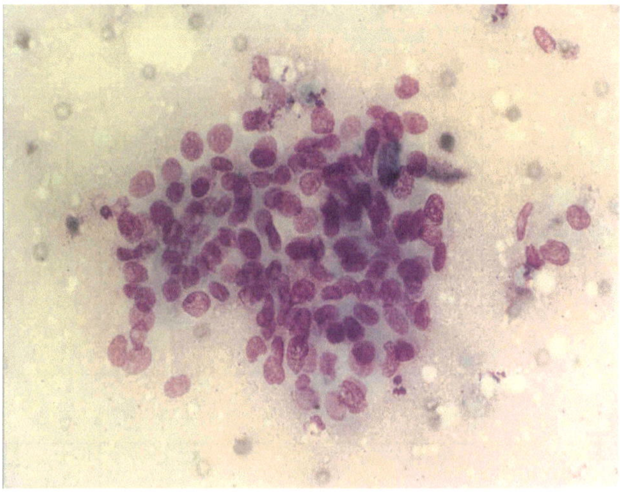

Figure 3. Mixed tumor: Touch impression composed of oval stellate cells located in clusters as well as individually settled in the smear. Cells are hyperchromatic, contain intracytoplasmic vacuoles and have increased nuclear to cytoplasmic ratio, Wright-Leishman x 300.

Types of tumor	Characteristics
1. Epithelial	Cells in separate groups or together with clear cytoplasmic boundaries and round/oval nuclei.
2. Mesenchymal	Individually settled cells mixed with extra cellular matrix, poorly defined cell membrane scarce cytoplasm, oval/ elliptical nuclei, polygonal, fusiform/ stellate or elliptical cells.
3. Mixed	Both epithelial and mesenchymal cellular elements in variable number.

Table 2. Classification of mammary tumors according to tissue of origin (Histogenic classification)

7.4.3. *On the basis of severity of tumor (Cytoprognostic Classification)*

The smears can be graded into three types in order of increasing severity. A simple numerical system is applied to both topographic and cytology criteria as shown in the table below [31].

	Morphology	Score
Cells	Isolated	3
	In clusters	0
	Large size	3
Nuclei	Anisokaryosis	2
	Naked	3
	Budding	2
	Hypochromasia	3
	Hyperchromasia	2
Enlarged Nucleoli	Red	3
	Blue	2
Mitosis	>3/slide	1
	>6/slide	3

Table 3. Cytoprognostic classification of mammary gland tumors

Grade is obtained by adding the different scores obtained

Grade I: Score <5
Grade II: Score 5-9
Grade III: Score >10

When a double malignant cell population is found in same tumor, the most anaplastic cells are taken in to account for scoring purpose.

8. Diagnostic interpretation of fine needle aspirates (FNAs)

Fine needle aspirates from the neoplastic lesions often present smears with variety of confusing cell population and it is very difficult to give concise and clear interpretation. Following the Guidelines of the Papanicolaou Society of Cytopathology for Fine-Needle Aspiration Procedure and Reporting, the smears can be interpreted in a very clear and concise manner tabulated below [32].

Interpretation	Characteristics of cellular smear
1. Inadequate / Unsatisfactory	Acellularity / hypocellularity, poor fixation, poor staining, poor preparation (crush artifact), excessive blood, necrosis or debris.
2. Benign a). Aspirates in which diagnosis can be given	Benign cells with characteristic cytological features.
b). Aspirates in which only a negative narrative diagnosis is possible	No malignant cell population is seen in given specimen but clinician is advised to correlate the lesion with clinical findings or to do re-sampling from multiple sites of the lesion.
3. Malignant	Smears contain cells diagnostic of malignancy.
4. Suspicious for malignancy	a). Sample contain few poorly preserved malignant cells or obscured by blood or inflammatory. b). Only some features of malignancy are present but clinical history show indication for malignancy. c). Cytological criteria of malignancy overlap with benign lesions.
5. Atypical cells present	Adequate sample containing mostly benign cells but few atypical cells which are unlikely to be malignant.

Table 4. Diagnostic Categories of Fine Needle Aspirates

9. Common misleading artifacts and contaminants in cytological smears

Stain precipitates, glove powder, keratin bars, talc crystals, air drying artifact, lubricant jelly artifact and formalin fume artifacts usually lead to misinterpretation of cytological slides. Cytology slides should not be even kept near formalin jars as the formalin fumes partially fix the cells of air dried smears and interfere with the staining of slides.

10. Clinico-cytological observations of mammary gland affections

10.1. Mastitis

In bitches affected with acute mastitis (Fig. 4), cytologic examination of secretions from inflamed mammary glands reveals bacteria and numerous degenerative neutrophils (Fig.5). Samples of milk taken from affected mammary gland of bitches show gel formation during sodium lauryl sulphate reagent test (Fig. 6) and color change of milk sample from yellow to green occur on addition of bromothymol blue reagent to it. Both these tests confirm the presence of high degree of mastitis in affected animals diagnosed cytologically.

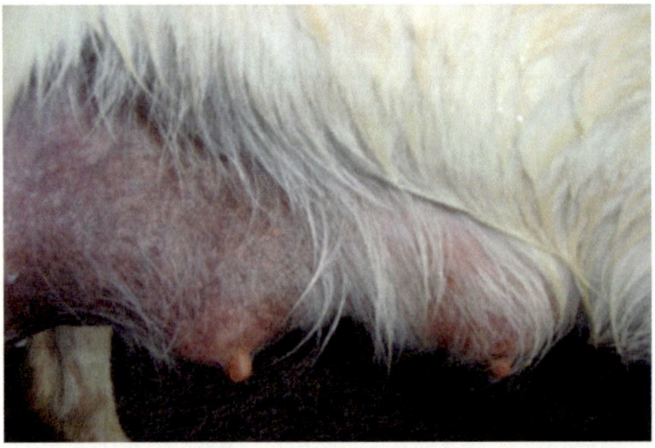

Figure 4. Mastitis: Red, hot, inflamed mammary gland of 4 year old Labrador Retriever bitch.

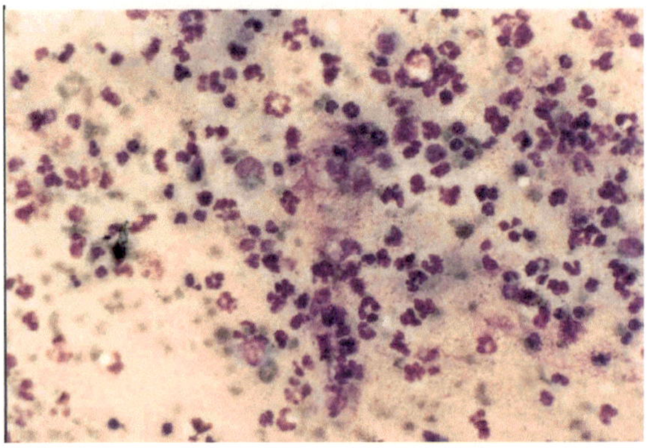

Figure 5. Mastitis: Fine needle aspirate showing numerous degenerative neutrophils and bacteria, Wright-Leishman X 300.

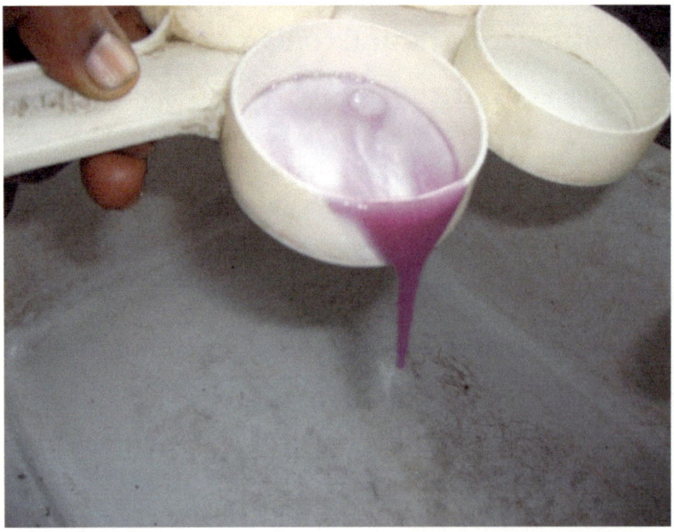

Figure 6. Milk sample from inflamed mammary gland undergoes dense gel formation on addition of sodium lauryl sulphate reagent which confirms mastitis.

10.2. Steatitis

Steatitis is inflammation of subcutaneous adipose tissue. Cytologically, the aspirate reveals inflammatory cells (neutrophils, monocytes) infiltrating the adipose tissue (Fig. 7).

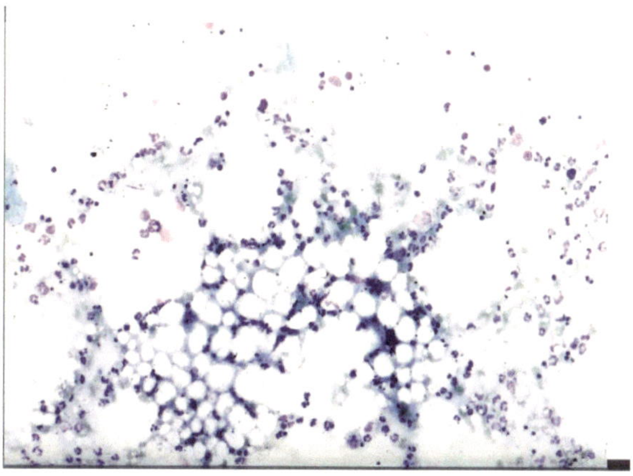

Figure 7. Steatitis: Fine needle aspirate consisting of inflammatory cells infilterating the adipocytes, Wright- Leishman x 150.

10.3. Lipoma

Mature lipocytes containing abundant fat usually rupture during aspiration of lipomas and yield oily smears containing free fat with few lipocytes. These smears do not dry in air and the fat get washed off on staining with alcohol based stains leaving behind few lipocytes with clear empty areas. Cytologically, smears reveal single or group of large fat cells containing large volume of pale cytoplasm and outlined by a single thin membrane. The nucleus is small, dense and pushed to periphery of cell (Fig. 8). Stains like Sudan IV, Oil Red O, New Methylene blue may be used to visualize fat cells directly on fresh smears before alcohol fixation.

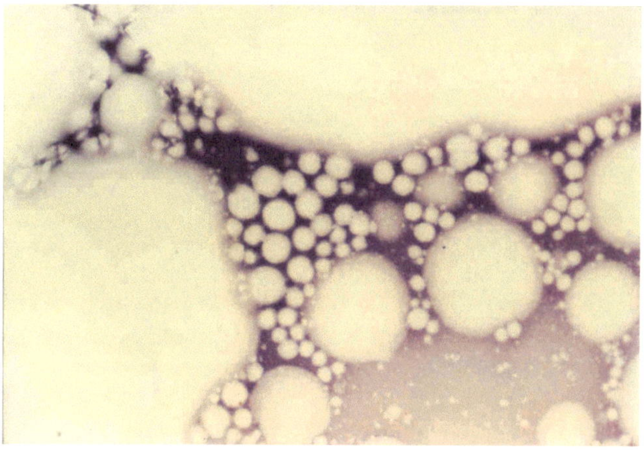

Figure 8. Lipoma: Poorly cellular fine needle aspirate smear with abundant free lipid residue from disrupted adipocytes, Wright x 150.

10.4. Liposarcoma

In comparison to lipomas, fine needle aspirates of liposarcoma are characterized by abundant lipocytes or lipoblasts, free fat and thus appear greasy. Sometime the smears contain abundant lipoblasts and lipocytes but very little free fat may not give oily appearance. Cytologically, the aspirates are characterized by hypercellularity, pleomorphism, anisokaryosis, cells with vacuolated cytoplasm and nuclei displaced to periphery of cells (Fig.2).Small to large fat vacuoles may be observed in background of smear. In general, the more immature and anaplastic cells have fewer and smaller fat globules. Typically, the lipoblast nucleus is round and variation in nuclear size and multinucleation is seen.

10.5. Adenocarcinoma

Adenocarcinomas appear as hard, solitary well encapsulated, round or discoid growths which measure up to 10 cm in diameter (Fig.9). Cytologically fine needle aspirates are characterized by anisocytosis, macrocytosis, hypercellularity, multinucleation, increased nuclear to cytoplasmic ratio and prominent nucleoli (Fig.10).

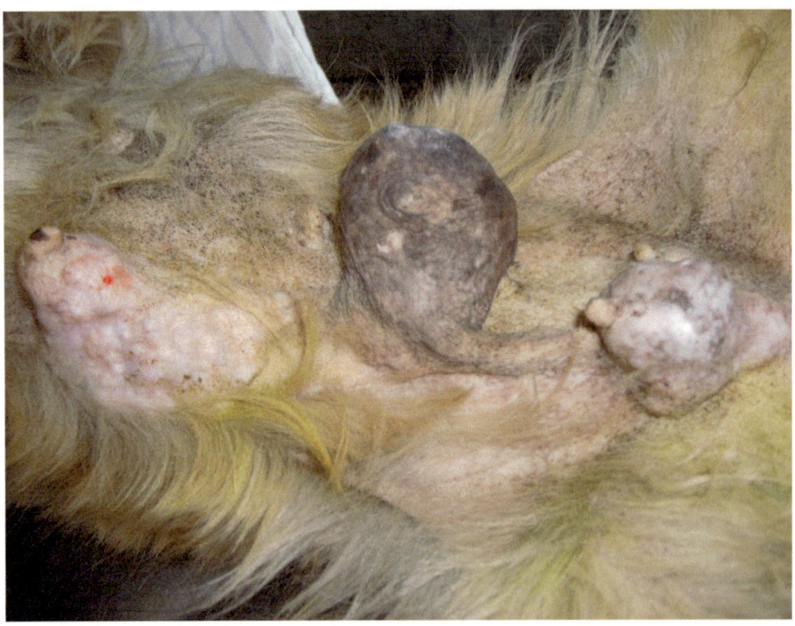

Figure 9. Adenocarcinoma: Three year old Golden Retriever with hard pendulous globate masses involving multiple pair of mammary glands.

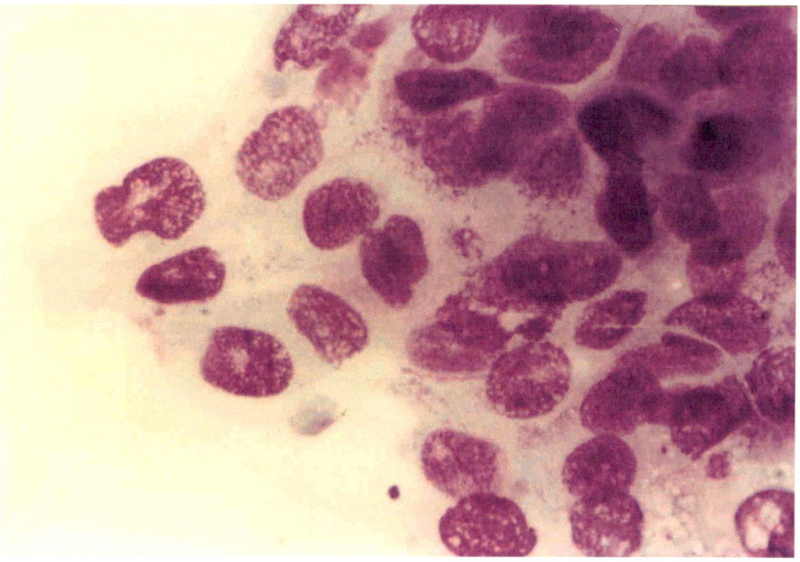

Figure 10. Adenocarcinoma: Fine needle aspirate with hypercellular pleomorphic, large hyperchromatic naked cells with coarse chromatin and prominent nucleoli, Wright x 750.

10.6. Inflammatory adenocarcinoma

Fine needle aspirates of inflammatory adenocarcinoma reveal isolated or clusters of hyperchromatic epithelial cells with enlarged nuclei, prominent nucleoli and coarse chromatin. Inflammatory cells like neutrophils and lymphocytes infiltrate the surrounding tissue (Fig.11). Grossly, the growths are about 2 to 10 cm in diameter, fixed to body wall and vary from soft to hard in consistency.

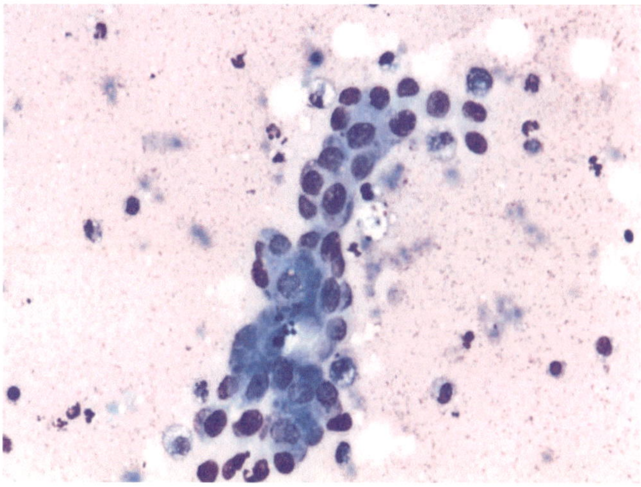

Figure 11. Inflammatory adenocarcinoma: Touch impression consisting of hyperchromatic cells with enlarged nuclei having prominent nucleoli, more basophilic cytoplasm and intracytoplasmic vacuoles. Inflammatory cells infilterate the surrounding area, Wright-Leishman x 150.

10.7. Mixed mammary adenoma/adenocarcinoma

The mixed tumors are usually multiple, occasionally solitary. They appear as small circumscribed nodules of about 2 cm in diameter and as pendulous, globate masses up to 10 cm in diameter. Grossly the affected areas are well encapsulated, hard, fibrous, and cartilaginous and may show glistening white lobules of fibrous tissue with multiple cysts filled with straw colored fluid and irregular areas of glandular tissue. In some cases, gritty sound can be observed on excision of the affected tissue. Cytologically, the aspirates contain both epithelial and stromal elements. The smears are hypercellular containing hyperchromatic spindle shaped connective tissue cells (Fig.12) and clusters of epithelial cells as described in adenocarcinomas.

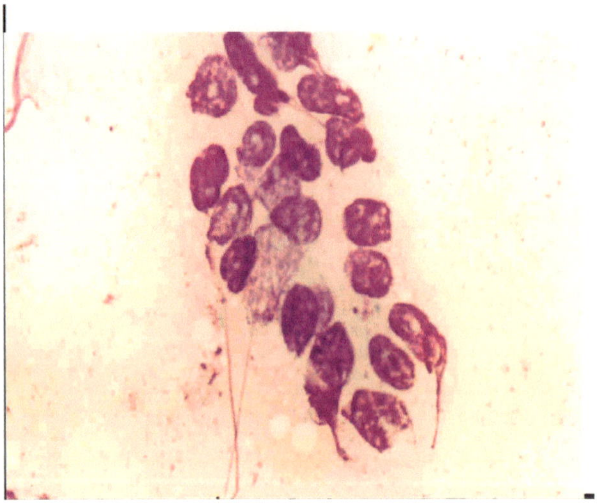

Figure 12. Mixed mammary tumor: Fine need aspirate containing oval to spindle shaped pleomorphic cells, Wright-Leishman x 750.

10.8. Squamous cell carcinoma

These are epithelial tumors characterized by variation in cell shape from round to polygonal to tadpole to linear to rectangular. There are large cells with abundant cytoplasm that have retained large functional non-pyknotic nucleus and coarse to marginated chromatin. The nuclei may be encircled by vacuoles or vacuoles may be scattered throughout the cell [23]. Neutrophils are commonly seen in the smear as the carcinoma lesions are usually ulcerated and infected.

10.9. Adenoma

Grossly, the growths are hard to soft in consistency varying from 2 to 10 cm in diameter (Fig. 13). In contrast to adenocarcinomas, fine needle aspirates of adenomas yield clusters of morphologically uniform population of well differentiated cells with little or no pleomorphism (Fig.14).

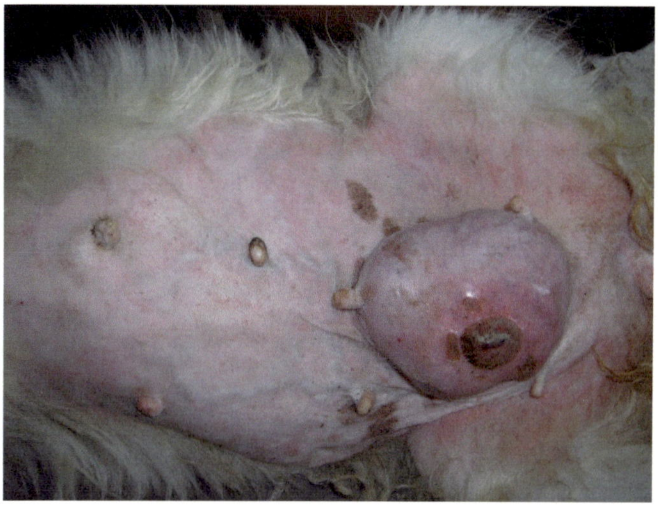

Figure 13. Adenoma: Localized small nodular growth on right inguinal mammary gland of a nine year old female Pomerian dog.

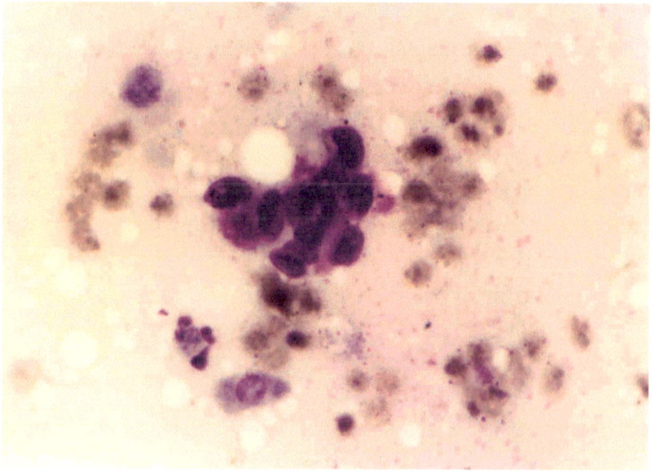

Figure 14. Adenoma: Fine needle aspirate composed of clusters of clusters of cells with highly basophilic cytoplasm, variable shaped nuclei and increased nuclear to cytoplasmic ratio, Wright-Leishman x 300.

10.10. Fibroadenoma

Fibroadenomas are benign skin lesions and are usually found solitary on the body. Cytologically, the smears are hypercellular with sheets of epithelial cells mixed with fusiform to stellate shaped pleomorphic myoepithelial cells. The nuclear to cytoplasmic ratio is increased, nuclear chromatin is fine to lacy and the cells have tail of cytoplasm that appear to trail away from the nucleus in one or two directions. The added presence of large number of bipolar/naked nuclei in the background of the smear is the reliable cytological feature in favor of fibroadenoma [33].

10.11. Papillomas

These are benign epithelial growths varying from cauliflower like to papillary projections with thin stalks. Aspiration yields uniform, large, polygonal cells with round to ovoid nuclei having low nuclear to cytoplasmic ratio. The abundant cytoplasm is lightly basophilic and foamy to eosinophilic and granular. Neutrophils may be prominent [23].

10.12. Fat necrosis/ organized hematoma

Aspirates of fat necrosis/organized hematoma show inflammatory cells, hemosidrin laden macrophages, multinucleated cells with or without cholesterol crystals and a necrotic background [34]. Fat necrosis can also occur in combination with cancer. However, the fat necrosis will resolve with time, so a series of aspirates taken at monthly intervals can help in ruling out neoplasia.

11. Conclusions

11.1. Best sample collection technique

Among different cell retrieval techniques, tissue imprints or impression smear technique is found to be best followed by fine needle biopsy and teat discharge smears. The reason could be the fact that while making impression, the wider area of affected tissue came in contact with slide and thus enhanced obtaining of cellular material. Moreover the specimen can be easily collected from exact site of affected tissue (visible grossly) many a times without any difficulty like sudden movement of animal or bending of needle in hard tissue etc. However, obtaining of cellular material by means of fine needle aspiration combined with simultaneous preparation of tissue imprints is recommended.

11.2. Limitations of cytology

Inspite of expanding true positive cases of cytological testing, the diagnostic value of this method has many limitations. One of the major imperfections is "geographic miss" i.e. puncturing the lesion from inappropriate site and thus leading to misdiagnosis, so multiple aspirates by adequately trained hands are needed from multiple site of lesion in order to improve diagnostic value. Certain disadvantages of fine needle aspiration biopsy technique like sampling of low amount of tumor mass or inadequate tissue can be minimized by preparation of multiple aspirates from various areas of the lesion and the sampling should be performed from the peripheral areas instead of the center of the mass in which fluid and necrotic debris accumulate especially in big tumor formations [35]. Baker and lumsden 2000 [36] also encouraged preparation of more aspirates in order to increase the number of representative cells as cell types and tumor morphology differ beneath lesions.

The entry of blood in syringe while taking aspirate or entry of tissue fluid on pressing slide hard over the excised tissue while making touch impression contribute to contamination of smear and thus diminished diagnostic accuracy of cytology. In order to increase the precision of the cytological results, the application of "triple test" is recommended i.e., the combination of physical examination, imaging findings and the cytologic examination.

Cytological interpretation is most successful in slide preparations with one cell layer thickness and not broken. However, in such slides one can go to edge of smear for thin layer of cells. Artifacts like stain precipitates are commonly observed during smear examination as purple dots and mistaken for bacteria. To minimize the problem, stains should be changed weekly as many of the wright-giemsa stains favor fungal and bacterial growth also. Also, the precipitates are less observed in "dip" type stains like diff-quick stain.

Further, in cytologic preparations of hyperplasia and adenoma, differential diagnosis is very difficult and histological examination is required in consensus for accurate characterization and establishing medical prognosis or treatment.

However, as already shown by other studies in veterinary medicine, fine needle aspiration cytology had an edge over histopathological examination in terms of providing immediate diagnosis and thus timely determination of plan of action [37].

11.3. Diagnostic value of cytology in mammary gland affections

To conclude, cytology is most useful in diagnosis of neoplastic lesions followed by hyperplastic or inflammatory lesions. Even in cases in which diagnosis is not definitive, the fine needle aspiration features may guide the clinical and surgical management [38].

In case of inflammatory breast lesions, FNAC combined with microbiological studies can be helpful in identifying the causative agents and thus directs towards quick appropriate therapy. The presence of negative culture does not exclude infection; however, positive culture can direct therapy [28, 39]. In tune to this, workers like Das et al [39] and Nemenqani and Yaqoob [34] propagated fine needle aspiration technique to be useful in diagnosis of inflammatory breast lesions and their classification into acute mastitis/breast abscess, tuberculous mastitis, chronic non-specific mastitis and miscellaneous conditions.

Being non expensive and requiring minimal use of sophisticated instruments, we advocate the fine needle aspiration technique to be first hand choice for diagnosis in areas with economic constraints. Furthermore, the cytologic diagnosis is significantly associated with post operative patient outcome in univariate survival analysis [40].

Thus, the cytological interpretation is quiet helpful in rapid screening of the mammary gland affections, establishing diagnosis, identifying the pathogenesis, prognosis and directs towards what type of treatment should be opted in case of mammary gland affections.

Author details

Shivani Sangha*

Incharge, Civil Veterinary Hospital Dakoha, Gurdaspur, Punjab, India

* Corresponding Author

Amarjit Singh
Animal Disease Research Centre,
Guru Angad Dev Veterinary and Animal Sciences University, Ludhiana, Punjab, India

Acknowledgement

Authors are thankful to editor of Brazilian Jjournal of Veterinary Pathology for allowing to publish some of the pictures and data already published in the Brazilian Journal of Veterinary Pathology, 2011, 4 (1): 13-22, in the research paper entitled "Sensitivity and specificity of cytological techniques for the diagnosis of neoplastic and non neoplastic lesions of canine mammary gland".

12. References

[1] Shrestha A, Chalise S, Karki S, Shakya G. Fine needle aspiration cytology in a palpable breast lesion. Journal of Pathology of Nepal 2011; 1:131-135.
[2] Fausto KA. Robbins and Cortan Pathological basis of disease. Robbins, Cortan. (ed). 7th edition, Elsevier. Philadelphia; 2004. p1121-1130.
[3] Karayannopoulou M, Kaldrymidou E, Constantinidis TC. Adjuvant post-operative chemotherapy in bitches with mammary cancer. Journal of Veterinary Medical Association Physiology Pathology Clinical Medicine 2001; 48:85-96.
[4] Anderson AC. Parameters of mammary gland tumors in ageing beagles. Journal of American Veterinary Medical Association 1965; 147:1653-1654.
[5] Fidler IJ, Abt DA, Brodey RS. The biological behavior of canine mammary neoplasia. Journal of American Veterinary Medical Association 1967; 151:1311-1318.
[6] Schneider R, Dorn CR, Taylor Don. Factors influencing canine mammary cancer development and post surgical survival. Journal of National Cancer Institute 1969; 43:1249-1261.
[7] Moulton JE. Tumors of mammary gland. In: Moulton JE. (ed.) Tumors in domestic animals. 3rd edition. University of California press, Berkley and Los Angeles; 1990. p518-552.
[8] Hayes HMJR, Milne KL, Mandell CP. Epidemiological features of feline mammary carcinoma. Veterinary Record 1981; 108(22):476-479.
[9] Hayes AA, Mooney S. Feline mammary tumors. Journal of Veterinary Clinics of North America Small Animal Practice 1985; 15(3):513-520.
[10] Macewen EG. Spontaneous tumors in dogs and cats: Models for the study of cancer biology and treatment. Cancer Metastasis Review 1990; 9(2):125-136.
[11] Guthrie CJ. Gland puncture as a diagnostic measure. Bull Johns Hopkins Hospital 1921; 32:264-269.
[12] Engzell J, Jackobosan PA, Sigurson A, Zajicek J. Aspiration biopsy of metastatic carcinoma in lymph nodes of neck. Acta Otolaryngyol (Stockholm) 1971; 72:138-147.

[13] Stockhaus C, Schoon HA, Grevel V, Oechtering G, Teske E. The diagnostic value of cytology in the diagnosis of soft tissue sarcoma in the dog and cat. Tieraztl prax 2003; 31:148-153.
[14] Stockhaus C, Teske E. Clinical experiences with cytology in the dog. Schweiz Arch Tierheilkd 2001; 143:233-240.
[15] Reinhardt S, Stockhaus C, Teske E, Rudolph R, Brunnberg L. Assessment of cytological crieteria for diagnosing osteosarcoma in dogs. Journal of Small Animal Practices 2005; 46:65-70.
[16] Hellmen E, Lindgren A. The accuracy of cytology in diagnosis and DNA analysis of canine mammary tumors. Journal of Comparative Pathology 1989; 101:443-450.
[17] Allen SW, Prasse KW, Mahaffey EA. Cytologic differentiation of benign from malignant canine mammary tumors. Veterinary Pathology 1986; 23:649-655.
[18] Misdrop W, Hart AA. Canine mammary cancer. I. Prognosis. Journal of Small Animal Practices 1979; 20:385-394.
[19] Rutterman GR. Mammary tumors in the dog. In: Kessler M (ed.) Small Animal Oncology. Berlin, Germany:Parey; 2000. p261-272
[20] Roglic M, Mouriquand J. Classification cytopronostique des tumeurs du sein. *Senalogia* 1980; 5:151-154.
[21] Wallgren A, Zajicek J. The prognostic value of the aspiration biopsy in mammary carcinoma. Acta Cytology 1976; 20:479-485.
[22] Verhaeghe M, Cornillot M, Herbeau J, Wintz A, Verhaeghe G. Le triplet diagnostic radioclinique dans les tumeurs due sein. A propos de 2460 cas. Memoire Academie Chirugi 1969; 95:48-61.
[23] Meinkoth JII, Cowell RL. Sample collection and preparation in cytology: Increasing diagnostic yield. Journal of Veterinary clinics small animal practice 2002; 32:1187-1207.
[24] Coles EH. Veterinary Clinical Pathology. 4th edition. W.B. Saunders Company, Philadelphia, London; 1986.
[25] Abendroth CS, Wang HH, Ducatman BS. Comparative features of carcinoma in situ and atypical ductal hyperplasia of the breast on fine needle aspiration biopsy specimens. American Journal of Clinical Pathology 1991; 96:654-659.
[26] Sneige N, Staerkel GA, Caraway NP. A plea for uniform terminology and reporting of breast fine needle aspirates. The MD Anderson Cancer Center Proposal. Acta cytology 1994; 38:971-972.
[27] Masood S. Inflammatory breast lesions in Cytopathology of the breast. In: ASCP Theory and Practice of Cytopathology 5th edition. USA ASCP Press Chicago; 1996. p51-76.
[28] Demay RM. Diseases and condition of the breast In: The Art and Science of Cytopathology: Aspiration Cytology. USA ASCP Press Chicago; 1996. p856-859.
[29] Tyler R, Cowell R, Tyler D, Baldwin C, Morton R. Introduction In: Cowell R, Tyler D, Meinkoth J, Mosby. (ed.) Diagnostic Cytology and Haematology of the Dog and Cat; 1999. p1-19.
[30] Alleman A, Bain P. Diagnosing neoplasia: The cytologic criteria for malignancy. Veterinary Medicine 2000; 3:204-222.

[31] Mouriquand J, Fior MG, Villemain D, Bouchet Y, Sage JC, Mermet MA, Bolla M. Value of cytoprognostic classification in breast carcinomas. Journal of Clinical Pathology 1986; 39(5):489-496.

[32] Guidelines of the Papanicolaou Society of Cytopathology for Fine-Needle Aspiration Procedure and Reporting. Diagnostic Cytopathology 1997; 17(4):239-247.

[33] Mendoza P, Lacambra M, Tan PH, Tse GM. Fine needle aspiration cytology of the breast: The Non-malignant catagories. Journal of Pathology Research International 2011, Article ID 547580, p1-8.

[34] Dalal Nemenquani, Nausheen Yaqoob. Fine needle aspiration cytology of inflammatory breast lesions. Journal of Pakistan Medical Association 2009; 59(3):167-169.

[35] Henson K.L. Reproductive system. In: Raskin R, Meyer D.J (eds): Atlas of canine and feline cytology, W.B Saunders company, Philadelphia, 2001;277-289.

[36] Baker R, Lumsden JH. The mammary gland. In: Baker R, Lumsden JH (ed.) Color Atlas of Cytology of the Dog and Cat, Mosby, St Louis; 2000. p253-262.

[37] Larkin HA. Veterinary cytology fine needle aspiration masses or swellings on animals. Veterinary Journal 1994; 47:65-73.

[38] Haziroglu R, Yard B, Aslan S, Yildrim MZ, Yumusak N, Beceriklisoy H, Agaoglu R, Kucukaslan I. Cytological evaluation of canine mammary tumors with fine needle aspiration biopsy technique, Revue Medical Veterinary 2010; 161(5):212-218.

[39] Das DK, Sodhani P, Kashyap V, Parkash S, Pant JN, Bhatnagar P. Inflammatory lesions of the breast: Diagnosis by fine needle aspiration cytopathology 1992; 3:281-289.

[40] Simon D, Schoenrock D, Baumgartner W, Notle I, Barron R, Mischker. Cytological examination of fine needle aspirates from mammary gland tumors in dog: Diagnostic accuracy with comparison to histopathology and association with post operative outcome. Journal of Veterinary Clinical Pathology 2009; 38(4):521-528.

Ossifying Fibromas of the Craniofacial Skeleton

Bruno Carvalho, Manuel Pontes,
Helena Garcia, Paulo Linhares and Rui Vaz

Additional information is available at the end of the chapter

http://dx.doi.org/10.5772/51030

1. Introduction

Ossifying fibromas (OF) of the craniofacial skeleton, as described in WHO classification of odontogenic tumors (2005)(Barnes L 2005), are benign fibro-osseous neoplasms characterized by the replacement of normal bone by a fibrous cellular stroma containing foci of mineralized bone trabeculae and cementum-like material that vary in amount and appearance.(Brannon and Fowler 2001; El-Mofty 2002; Cruz, Alencar et al. 2008) The accurate nature and classification of OF has undergone considerable debate among pathologists, resulting in a confusing evolution of competing nomenclatures.(Brannon and Fowler 2001; Sarode, Sarode et al. 2011) Contemporary reviews have classified benign fibro-osseous lesions of the craniofacial complex into neoplasms, developmental dysplastic lesions and inflammatory/reactive processes. [Table 1](Eversole, Su et al. 2008) In this reviews, subtypes vary with regard to behavior and propensity for recurrence after surgical excision. The definitive diagnosis can rarely be rendered on the basis of histopathological features alone and is usually dependent upon assessment of microscopic, clinical and imaging features together. This review will discuss the clinical, microscopic, radiological and therapeutic aspects of ossifying fibromas in this localization.

2. Definition and histological subtypes

Neoplasms with a fibro-osseous histology are represented by the ossifying fibroma group of lesions. These are neoplasms in the true sense, exhibiting progressive proliferative capabilities with boney expansion and, importantly, well defined margins radiologically. According to their pattern of mineralization, four overlapping clinicopathological entities have been historically identified: juvenile psammomatous ossifying fibroma (JPOF), juvenile trabecular ossifying fibroma (JTOF), gigantiform cementoma (GC) and cemento-ossifying fibroma (COF) not otherwise specified (NOS), implying that the clinicopathologic features do not conform to the other types of ossifying fibromas. GC may show an autosomal dominant genetic or "familial" underpinning. Most ossifying fibromas are single focal lesions; however gigantiform cementoma is typically multifocal and may occur in all four jaw quadrants in a single patient. There are also reports of lesion multiplicity in the other forms of ossifying fibroma yet such occurrences are quite rare. Notwithstanding these entities, it must be emphasized the contrast of OF with the much more common fibrous dysplasia (FD), a developmental hamartomatous fibro-osseous lesion, from which the differential is difficult based solely on clinical or radiographic criteria (Brannon and Fowler 2001; El-Mofty 2002; Noudel, Chauvet et al. 2009).

I. Bone dysplasias
- **a. Fibrous dysplasia**
  - **i. Monostotic**
  - **ii. Polyostotic**
  - **iii. Polyostotic with endocrinopathy (McCune-Albright)**
  - **iv Osteofibrous dysplasia[a]**
- **b. Osteitis deformans**
- **c. Pagetoid heritable bone dysplasias of childhood**
- **d. Segmental odontomaxillary dysplasia**

II. Cemento-osseous dysplasias
- **a. Focal cemento-osseous dysplasia**
- **b. Florid cemento-osseous dysplasia**

III. Inflammatory/reactive processes
- **a. Focal sclerosing osteomyelitis**
- **b. Diffuse sclerosing osteomyelitis**
- **c. Proliferative periostitis**

IV. Metabolic Disease: hyperparathyroidism

V. Neoplastic lesions (Ossifying fibromas)
- **a. Ossifying fibroma NOS**
- **b. Hyperparathyroidism jaw lesion syndrome**
- **c. Juvenile ossifying fibroma**
  - **i. Trabecular type**
  - **ii. Psammomatoid type**
- **d. Gigantiform cementomas**

[a]Osteofibrous dysplasia is found in the fibula and tibia only

Table 1. Classification of fibro-benign lesions of the cranio-facial complex

3. Epidemiology

According to WHO classification (2005) OF most commonly occurs in the 2nd to 4th decades and shows a predilection for females. The mean age of the histological subtypes varies. In patients with JPOF it is about 20 years compared to 35 years in cases of conventional ossifying fibroma. JTOF has a still lower mean age range (8.5-12 years).

4. Clinical and imagiological features

The commonest fibrous-osseous lesions of the orbit and sinonasal tract are OF and FD. The diagnosis between these two entities may be challenging, because they share similar features. There are four main clinical subtypes of FD: monostotic (affects one bone, and accounts for 85% cases of FD), polyostotic (affects multiple bones), McCune–Albright syndrome in which multiple disseminated lesions of bone are accompanied by skin hyperpigmentation and endocrine disturbances; and osteofibrous dysplasia (Brannon and Fowler 2001; Smith, Newman et al. 2009).

The juvenile variants of ossifying fibromas share many similarities, but they have been distinguished on the basis of their histopathological features, site, and age of recurrence (Shields, Peyster et al. 1985; Noudel, Chauvet et al. 2009; Smith, Newman et al. 2009). Their location is also different: JPOF arises mainly around paranasal sinuses and orbits, whereas JTOF usually affects the maxilla. The last entity, COF, is an odontogenic neoplasm arising from the periodontal ligament and affects the tooth-bearing areas of the jaws, mandible, and the maxilla; the cementicles are the characteristic feature instead of the bone elements. JTOF also known as trabecular desmo-osteoblastoma affects mainly the jaws of children and adolescents. Only 20% of the patients are over 15 years of age. In a review of a number of case series the mean age range was found to be 8.5–12 years (Slootweg and Muller 1990; Slootweg, Panders et al. 1994; El-Mofty 2002). Origin in extragnathic locations is extremely rare. Clinically, it is often characterized by a progressive and sometimes rapid expansion of the affected area; pain is a rare symptom. Cystic degeneration and aneurysmal bone cyst formation has been reported in a few cases. Radiographically, JTOF is an expansive lesion and may be fairly well demarcated, with cortical thinning and perforation. Depending on the amount of calcified tissue produced, the lesion will show varying degrees of radiolucency or radiodensity. Ground-glass as well as a multilocular honeycomb appearance has been described.

Differing from JTOF, JPOF is a lesion that affects predominantly the extragnathic craniofacial bones, particularly centered on the periorbital, frontal, and ethmoid bones (El-Mofty 2002). First described by Gogl in 1949 and Margo in 1985, JPOF seems to stand out as a separate clinicopathologic entity different from the gnathic cemento-ossifying fibroma.(Gogl 1949; Margo, Ragsdale et al. 1985) Patients are young, although the average age of incidence has varied in different studies from 16 to 33 years with an age range of 3 months to 72 years (in general a few years older than those with JTOF). The greatest majority of the reported cases of JPOF originated in the paranasal sinuses, particularly frontal and ethmoid. About 10% have been reported in the calvarium. Around 7% may occur in the mandible. Orbital extension of sinonasal tumors may result in proptosis, and visual complaints including blindness, nasal obstruction, ptosis, papilledema, and disturbances in ocular mobility. Radiographic examination of JPOF shows a round, well-defined, sometimes corticated osteolytic lesion with a cystic appearance. Sclerotic changes are evident in the lesion which may show a ground-glass appearance (Su, Weathers et al. 1997). The lesions appear less dense than normal bone. **Figure 1** and **figure 2** show an example of a JPOF invading the left periorbit and ethmoid sinus.

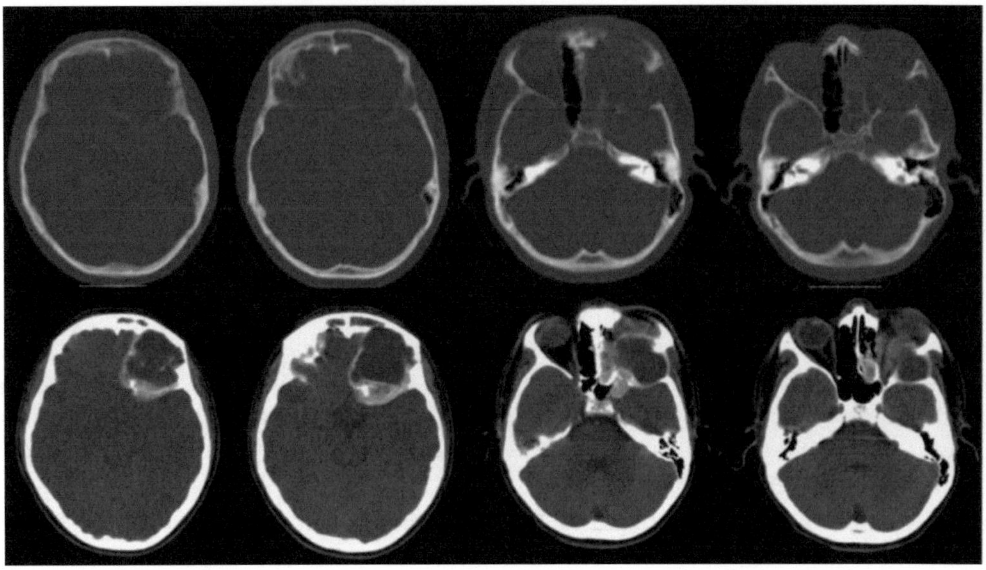

Figure 1. Axial CT scan showing a fibrous-osseous lesion (JPOF) of the left orbit and ethmoid sinus.

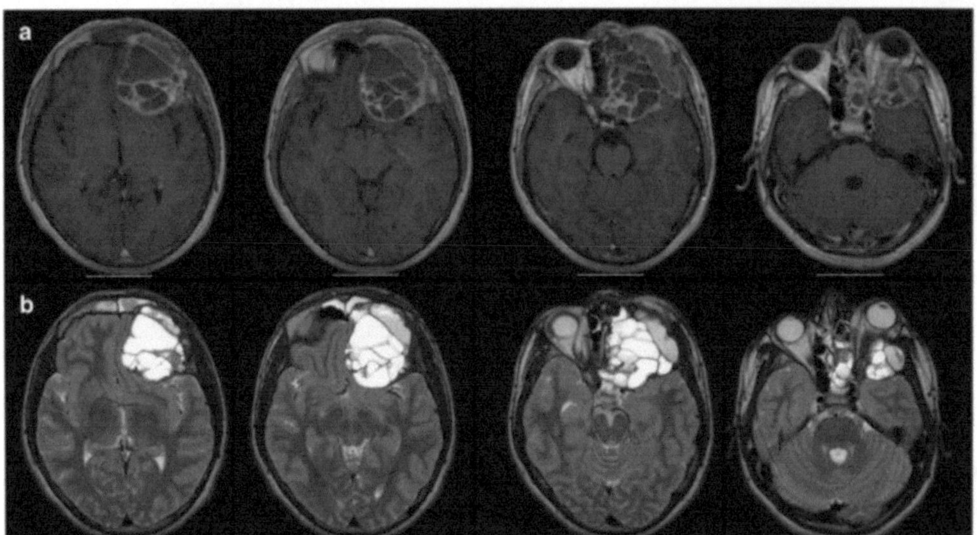

Figure 2. Gadolinium-enhanced axial T1-weighted (a) and T2-weighted (b) magnetic resonance imaging (MRI) showing an expansive cystic lesion (JPOF) invading the left periorbit and ethmoid sinus.

Gigantiform cementoma is an extremely rare form of ossifying fibroma, usually multifocal with tumors that are often massive. Lesions arise during childhood and progressively expand to cause facial deformity during early adult years (Young, Markowitz et al. 1989; Rossbach, Letson et al. 2005).

Table 2 summarizes some of the clinical, radiographic and microscopic characteristics of these entities.

Disease	Clinical features	Radiologic findings	Histopathology
Fibrous dysplasia	Expansion of bone Unilateral, painless Alk phosphatase Mono/Polyostotic	Diffuse radiolucent/ ground glass	Trabecular "Chinese/Hebrew"
Ossifying fibroma Not otherwise specified	Expansile, painless Rarely multifocal Jaws	Circumscribed lucent or target lesion Root divergence	Trabecular Cementifying
Ossifying fibroma Trabecular variant	Expansile, painles Root divergence Aggressive	Circumscribed lucent Floccular opacities	Trabecular Giant cell foci Fibroplasia
Ossifying fibroma Psammomatoid	Expansile Facial bone Aggressive	Circumscribed Dense floccular opacities	Psammoma
Gigantiform cementoma	Massive, expansile Multiquadrant Often familial	Well delineated lucent with floccular opacities	Trabecular Cementifying

Table 2. Clinical, radiographic and microscopic parameters that distinguish among Ossifying Fibromas and Fibrous Dysplasia.

5. Etiopathogeny

The etiology of OF is unknown but odontogenic, developmental and traumatic origins have been suggested, (Caylakli, Buyuklu et al. 2004; Noudel, Chauvet et al. 2009; Mohsenifar, Nouhi et al. 2011) and thought to be of periodontal ligament origin because of their capacity to produce cementum and osteoid material (Slootweg and Muller 1990).

It has been hypothesized that JPOF originates from overproduction of the myxofibrous cellular stroma normally involved in the growth of the septa in the paranasal sinuses as they enlarge and pneumatize. These stromal cells secrete hyaline material that ossifies and connective tissue mucin that initiates the cystic areas (Sarode, Sarode et al. 2011).

6. Macroscopical and microscopical analysis

6.1. Ossifying fibromas

Ossifying fibroma NOS shows three histologic patterns or a mixture of these patterns:

(1) Ossifying form: common, similar to fibrous dysplasia, shows a pattern with small irregular osteoid trabeculae that are typically rimmed by osteoblasts (**figure 3a**). The stromal element is

hypercellular and the fibroblastic cells are devoid of atypical cytologic features. Early formative tumors show woven bone patterns when assessed under polarized light, and in mature lesions osteoblastic rimming is minimal and the irregular trabeculae are often lamellar.

(2) Cementifying form: is similar to the psammomatoid variant. Most also contain more typical osseous trabeculae in addition to the cemental structures which are ovoid or droplet in shape. These ovoid calcifications resemble normal cementicles that are present in the periodontal ligament. In previous publications the ovoid lesions have been referred to as cementifying fibromas while those with both osseous and cementoid calcifications are labeled as cemento-ossifying fibromas.

(3) Storiform form: typified by streaming of the fibroblastic stromal elements in a pinwheel configuration similar to benign fibrous histiocytoma (**figure 4**). Dispersed throughout are wispy calcifications that appear like dystrophic bone and many also show an ovoid configuration (Eversole, Su et al. 2008).

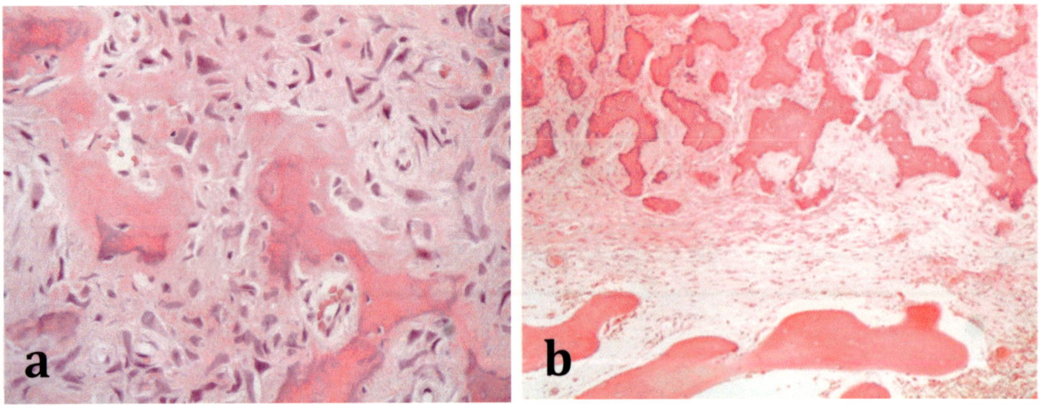

Figure 3. Ossifying fibroma NOS (**a**) irregular osteoid rimmed by osteoblasts and a fibrous stroma; (**b**) interface between an ossifying fibroma (up) and normal bone (down).

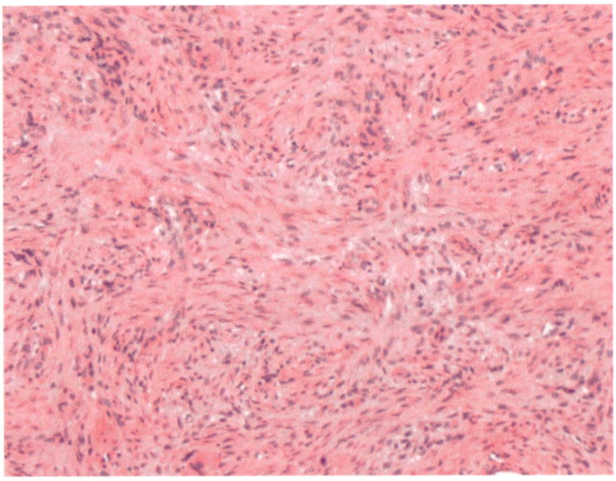

Figure 4. Ossifying fibroma NOS showing areas of fibrous stroma with a storiform pattern. Courtesy of Manuel Jácome, MD, Department of Pathology of IPOFG-Porto.

6.2. Juvenile ossifying fibromas

Two distinct clinicopathologic entities are known:

(1) Trabecular juvenile ossifying fibroma (JTOF): well-defined but unencapsulated lesion that infiltrates surrounding bone, composed of a cell-rich fibrous stroma containing bundles of cellular osteoid and bone trabeculae without osteoblastic rimming, and aggregates of giant cells (**figure 5**). Stromal cells are spindle or polyhedral and produce little collagen and the fibrillary osteoid matrix gives the tumor a characteristic loose structure. Cellular, immature osteoid, with plump eosinophilic osteoblastic cells, forms strands that may be long and slender or plump ("paint brush strokes"). The immature cellular osteoid is not always easily distinguished from the cellular stroma. Irregular mineralization takes place at the center of the osteoid strands, and progressive calcification results in anastomosing trabeculae of immature woven bone. Maturation to lamellar bone is not observed. Local aggregates of multinucleated giant cells are commonly seen in the stroma. Mitotic activity of the stromal cells may be present but is never numerous. Cystic degeneration and aneurysmal bone cystformation has been reported in a few cases.

Collagen is usually not observed, yet older lesions may show some collagenisation (Eversole, Leider et al. 1985; El-Mofty 2002; Eversole, Su et al. 2008).

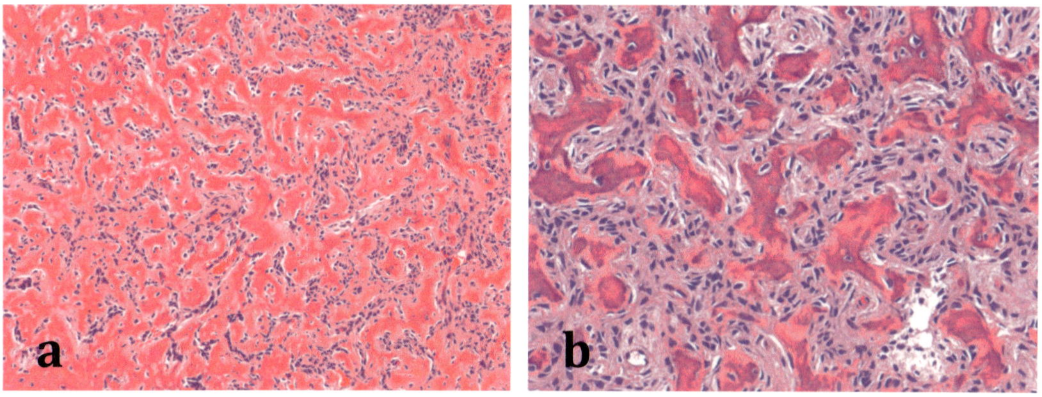

Figure 5. Juvenile trabecular ossifying fibroma (**a**) trabecular strands of immature osteoid; (**b**) immature osteoid with irregular mineralization and cellular stroma. Courtesy of Manuel Jácome, MD, Department of Pathology of IPOFG-Porto.

(2) Psammomatoid juvenile ossifying fibroma (JPOF)

On gross examination, the tumor is described as firm to hard in consistency and tan-white, grayish-white or grayish-brown in color and well demarcated from the surrounding bone, though not encapsulated. On sectioning, the cut surface is typically a tan-white, rubbery, homogeneous mass with a firm-to-gritty consistency and also displays large cystic areas (Sarode, Sarode et al. 2011).

On light microscopic examination, the tumor has multiple small acellular calcified structures, round and uniform and with concentric lamellar calcification, called ossicles/psammomatoid bodies; they are homogenously distributed in a relatively cellular stroma that may have whorled appearance, composed of uniform, stellate, and spindle shaped cells. In some cases the stroma is myxoid and may undergo cystic change with edema, hemorrage and clusters of multinucleated giant cells, where one can also find acellular mineralized deposits with bizarre shape (Noudel, Chauvet et al. 2009; Linhares, Pires et al. 2011; Sarode, Sarode et al. 2011). Occasionally, shrunken cells become embedded in the calcified matrix of the ossicles. The psammomatoid bodies are basophilic and bear superficial resemblance to dental cementum, but may have an osteoid rim. Mitotic activity is extremely rare in the stromal cells. At the periphery of the lesion, the ossicles may be very closely packed with little intervening stroma, or coalesce and form irregular thin bony trabeculae that may become thicker, with numerous reversal lines. A shell of normal bone is usually present and may show osteoclastic resorption endosteally associated with osteoblastic activity on the periosteal surface. Cystic degeneration and aneurismal bone cyst formation is commonly reported (El-Mofty 2002; Eversole, Su et al. 2008; Linhares, Pires et al. 2011).

6.3. Gigantiform cementoma

This entity is often multifocal, with expansile masses of the maxilla and/or mandible; microscopic examination displays a benign hypercelular stroma with monomorfic appearing fibroblasts showing no mitosis, mature collagen fibers and scattered ovoid, often laminated, psammomatoid calcifications with variable size, many of them very large (Young, Markowitz et al. 1989; Abdelsayed, Eversole et al. 2001).

7. Differential diagnosis

Ossifying fibroma (OF) is often confused with focal cementoosseous dysplasia (FCOD). Importantly, the later is an endosseous nonneoplastic process that occurs around the roots of mandibular teeth and fails to expand bone. Alternatively, OF is a potentially aggressive lesion that causes cortical expansion and often causes divergence of contiguous teeth. Both lesions may show similar histological features with trabecular bone and cementifying areas. Older lesions of FCOD may show dense corticated bone islands, a finding that is not present in OF.

While fibrous dysplasia (FD) and OF may share microscopic features, the clinicoradiologic differences are now widely accepted (Linhares, Pires et al. 2011).

In contrast to FD, JPOF shows osteoclasts and osteoblasts typically lining the trabeculae, which are composed of entrapped lamellar bone. The entities can be distinguished from one another on the basis of molecular detection of activating missense mutations of the GNAS1 gene in fibrous dysplasia of the jaws, while ossifying fibromas are found lacking (Hasselblatt, Jundt et al. 2005; Eversole, Su et al. 2008; Nasser 2009; Noudel, Chauvet et al. 2009).

JPOF might be easily mistaken for psamomatous meningioma, and in JPOF with a neurocranial location the likelihood of a misdiagnosis is increased. Even though there is frequent immunohistochemical negativity for epithelial membrane antigen (EMA) in JPOF, there are reported cases with EMA positivity; it is also positive for vimentin, smooth muscle actin and CD10, with lack of expression of CD34, S100 protein and cytokeratins. The diagnosis should be based on morphological, clinical and radiographic findings (Hasselblatt, Jundt et al. 2005; Noudel, Chauvet et al. 2009; Sarode, Sarode et al. 2011).

8. Genomic alterations

Cytogenetic analysis was done in only a few cases of ossifying fibroma. In one case of COF of the mandible, deletions were detected in 2q31-32 q35-36 (Dal Cin, Sciot, et al. 1993).A study of 3 cases of JPOF of the orbit demonstrated non random chromosome break points at Xq26 and 2q33 resulting in (X;2) translocations (Sawyer, Tryka,et al.1995). Regarding OF NOS there are reports that identify mutations in HRPT2 a gene that encodes parafibromin protein. Psammomatoid ossifying fibroma has been associated to chromosomal breakpoints t(X;2)(q26;q33) and interstitial insertion of bands 2q24.2q33 into Xq26.

Hyperparathyroidism associated ossifying fibroma has been associated with mutations in tumor suppressor gene HRPT2.

The rare gigantiform cementoma is related to an autosomal dominant inheritance in some cases whereas others are "familial". Among the few cases that have been reported, the gene appears to have a high level of penetrance with variable expressivity (Young, Markowitz et al. 1989; Finical, Kane et al. 1999; Abdelsayed, Eversole et al. 2001; Rossbach, Letson et al. 2005).

9. Treatment and prognosis

Complete excision of a OF lesion is the treatment of choice and it can be curative. Despite its benign features, they can be locally invasive, causing significant morbidity, and fatal consequences may be induced by intracranial extension (Baumann, Zimmermann et al. 2005; Cruz, Alencar et al. 2008; Bohn, Kalmar et al. 2011; Linhares, Pires et al. 2011). However, a surgical approach is dictated more by anatomic location and tumor size than by histologic subtype (Shields, Peyster et al. 1985; Hartstein, Grove et al. 1998; Smith, Newman et al. 2009).

Radiotherapy is generally contraindicated because of the risk of malignant transformation and the potentially harmful late effects in children (Nakagawa, Takasato et al. 1995; Noudel, Chauvet et al. 2009).

The clinical course of JTOF is characterized by infrequent recurrence following conservative excision. One or more recurrences were observed in 3 of 10 patients reported by Slootweg et al (Slootweg, Panders et al. 1994). Eventual complete cure could be achieved in those cases without resorting to radical surgical intervention. Malignant transformation has not been reported. Regarding JPOF, surgical excision is the treatment of choice, although recurrence even after definitive surgery is not unusual. Recurrence rates of 30% have been reported. In some cases, multiple recurrences over a long follow-up period are reported. No malignant change has been observed. Treatment for gigantiform cementoma is resection with immediate or staged reconstruction (Finical, Kane et al. 1999).

Overall recurrence rates after resection is reported to range from 30 to 56% and this is likely to be due to incomplete excision resulting from the infiltrative nature of the tumor borders more than to any intrinsic biological properties (Brannon and Fowler 2001; MacDonald-Jankowski 2004; Noudel, Chauvet et al. 2009).

10. Conclusion

Ossifying fibromas comprises entities with different morphological features that can be mistaken for other benign fibro-osseous lesions; this similarity and overlapping microscopic characteristics turns the multidisciplinary approach, comprehending clinical, radiological and pathological aspects, more reliable for a correct diagnosis.

They have locally aggressive behavior, with high recurrence rate, particularly in partial and incomplete excisions, with complete removal being the gold standard treatment. Prognosis is good, without metastases in the reported cases.

Author details

Bruno Carvalho, Manuel Pontes, Helena Garcia, Paulo Linhares and Rui Vaz
Centro Hospitalar de São João, Faculdade de Medicina da Universidade do Porto;
Hospitais da Universidade de Coimbra – Centro Hospitalar Universitário de Coimbra, Portugal

Acknowledgement

The authors thank Dr. Manuel Jácome of Department of Pathology of the IPOFG-Oporto for the courtesy of the images provided. The authors thank Dr. Hélder Rodrigues of Department of Pathology of CHUC for his assistance.

11. References

Abdelsayed, R. A., L. R. Eversole, et al. (2001). "Gigantiform cementoma: clinicopathologic presentation of 3 cases." *Oral Surg Oral Med Oral Pathol Oral Radiol Endod* 91(4): 438-444.

Barnes L, E. J., Reichart P, Sidransky D, editors (2005). "World Health Organization Classification of Tumours. Pathology and Genetics of Head and Neck Tumours . Lyon." *IARC Press*: 283–328.

Baumann, I., R. Zimmermann, et al. (2005). "Ossifying fibroma of the ethmoid involving the orbit and the skull base." *Otolaryngol Head Neck Surg* 133(1): 158-159.

Bohn, O. L., J. R. Kalmar, et al. (2011). "Trabecular and psammomatoid juvenile ossifying fibroma of the skull base mimicking psammomatoid meningioma." *Head Neck Pathol* 5(1): 71-75.

Brannon, R. B. and C. B. Fowler (2001). "Benign fibro-osseous lesions: a review of current concepts." *Adv Anat Pathol* 8(3): 126-143.

Caylakli, F., F. Buyuklu, et al. (2004). "Ossifying fibroma of the middle turbinate: a case report." *Am J Otolaryngol* 25(5): 377-378.

Cruz, A. A., V. M. Alencar, et al. (2008). "Ossifying fibroma: a rare cause of orbital inflammation." *Ophthal Plast Reconstr Surg* 24(2): 107-112.

Dal Cin, P., R. Sciot, et al. (1993). "Chromosome abnormalities in cementifying fibroma." *Cancer Genet Cytogenet* 71(2): 170-172.

El-Mofty, S. (2002). "Psammomatoid and trabecular juvenile ossifying fibroma of the craniofacial skeleton: two distinct clinicopathologic entities." *Oral Surg Oral Med Oral Pathol Oral Radiol Endod* 93(3): 296-304.

Eversole, L. R., A. S. Leider, et al. (1985). "Ossifying fibroma: a clinicopathologic study of sixty-four cases." *Oral Surg Oral Med Oral Pathol* 60(5): 505-511.

Eversole, R., L. Su, et al. (2008). "Benign fibro-osseous lesions of the craniofacial complex. A review." *Head Neck Pathol* 2(3): 177-202.

Finical, S. J., W. J. Kane, et al. (1999). "Familial gigantiform cementoma." *Plast Reconstr Surg* 103(3): 949-954.

Gogl, H. (1949). "Das Psammo-osteoid-fibroma der Nase und ihrer Ne-benh \um[ohlen." *Monatsschr F Ohrenheilk Lar Rhin* 83: 1–10.

Hartstein, M. E., A. S. Grove, Jr., et al. (1998). "The multidisciplinary management of psammomatoid ossifying fibroma of the orbit." *Ophthalmology* 105(4): 591-595.

Hasselblatt, M., G. Jundt, et al. (2005). "Juvenile psammomatoid ossifying fibroma of the neurocranium. Report of four cases." *J Neurosurg* 102(6): 1151-1154.

Linhares, P., E. Pires, et al. (2011). "Juvenile psammomatoid ossifying fibroma of the orbit and paranasal sinuses. A case report." *Acta Neurochir (Wien)* 153(10): 1983-1988.

MacDonald-Jankowski, D. S. (2004). "Fibro-osseous lesions of the face and jaws." *Clin Radiol* 59(1): 11-25.

Margo, C. E., B. D. Ragsdale, et al. (1985). "Psammomatoid (juvenile) ossifying fibroma of the orbit." *Ophthalmology* 92(1): 150-159.

Mohsenifar, Z., S. Nouhi, et al. (2011). "Ossifying fibroma of the ethmoid sinus: Report of a rare case and review of literature." *J Res Med Sci* 16(6): 841-847.

Nakagawa, K., Y. Takasato, et al. (1995). "Ossifying fibroma involving the paranasal sinuses, orbit, and anterior cranial fossa: case report." *Neurosurgery* 36(6): 1192-1195.

Nasser, M. J. (2009). "Psammomatoid ossifying fibroma with secondary aneurysmal bone cyst of frontal sinus." *Childs Nerv Syst* 25(11): 1513-1516.

Noudel, R., E. Chauvet, et al. (2009). "Transcranial resection of a large sinonasal juvenile psammomatoid ossifying fibroma." *Childs Nerv Syst* 25(9): 1115-1120.

Rossbach, H. C., D. Letson, et al. (2005). "Familial gigantiform cementoma with brittle bone disease, pathologic fractures, and osteosarcoma: a possible explanation of an ancient mystery." *Pediatr Blood Cancer* 44(4): 390-396.

Sarode, S. C., G. S. Sarode, et al. (2011). "Juvenile psammomatoid ossifying fibroma: a review." *Oral Oncol* 47(12): 1110-1116.

Sawyer J. R., Tryka A.F., et al. (1995). "Nonrandom chromosome breakpoints at Xq26 and 2q33 characterize cementoossifying fibromas of the orbit." *Cancer* 76(10): 1853–1859.

Shields, J. A., R. G. Peyster, et al. (1985). "Massive juvenile ossifying fibroma of maxillary sinus with orbital involvement." *Br J Ophthalmol* 69(5): 392-395.

Slootweg, P. J. and H. Muller (1990). "Juvenile ossifying fibroma. Report of four cases." *J Craniomaxillofac Surg* 18(3): 125-129.

Slootweg, P. J., A. K. Panders, et al. (1994). "Juvenile ossifying fibroma. An analysis of 33 cases with emphasis on histopathological aspects." *J Oral Pathol Med* 23(9): 385-388.

Smith, S. F., L. Newman, et al. (2009). "Juvenile aggressive psammomatoid ossifying fibroma: an interesting, challenging, and unusual case report and review of the literature." *J Oral Maxillofac Surg* 67(1): 200-206.

Su, L., D. R. Weathers, et al. (1997). "Distinguishing features of focal cemento-osseous dysplasias and cemento-ossifying fibromas: I. A pathologic spectrum of 316 cases." *Oral Surg Oral Med Oral Pathol Oral Radiol Endod* 84(3): 301-309.

Young, S. K., N. R. Markowitz, et al. (1989). "Familial gigantiform cementoma: classification and presentation of a large pedigree." *Oral Surg Oral Med Oral Pathol* 68(6): 740-747.

Chapter 8

Morphology of the Intestinal Barrier in Different Physiological and Pathological Conditions

Jesmine Khan and Mohammed Nasimul Islam

Additional information is available at the end of the chapter

http://dx.doi.org/10.5772/50659

1. Introduction

Beside its main function of digestion and absorption, intestinal mucosa acts as an important barrier to toxic and harmful materials and protects an individual from different antigenic and inflammatory reactions. The intestinal barrier is composed of a mucin layer covering the cells, enterocytes and the apical junctional complex in between the cells [1].

The epithelium of the small intestine is characterized by villi & crypts. Villi are folds of the epithelium into the lumen with a core of lamina propria. Villi are tallest in the jejunum and shortest in ileum. The lamina propria core contains white blood cells, lacteals, a rich fenestrated capillary network, nerves; and scattered smooth muscle cells.

The villus epithelium is composed of enterocytes and goblet cells. Enterocytes are columnar absorptive cells and has an apical striated border of microvilli. Goblet cells secrete mucin to provide a protective coating. Only a few goblet cells are present in the the upper small intestine, more in the ileum.

The apical junctional complex consists of a network of tight junction proteins and the adherens junction [2]. They are anchored in the cell via the filamentous actin cytoskeleton [3]. Zonula occludens proteins (ZO-1, ZO-2 and ZO-3) are important intracellular tight junction proteins, linking the cell cytoskeleton to the transmembrane TJ proteins such as claudins, occludin and junctional adhesion molecules (JAM). Whereas occludin and JAM have a regulatory role, transmembrane protein claudins, abundantly present between adjacent healthy intestinal epithelial cells, are mainly responsible for the intestinal barrier function [4].

Crypts are folds of the epithelium that invaginate down into the lamina propria. Many of the cells in the crypt serve as precursors for enterocytes or goblet cells of the villi. Paneth cells are situated at the base of the crypts. Enteroendocrine cells are scattered through the small intestinal crypts.

Microvilli are folds of the apical plasma membrane of each enterocyte with a core of actin cytoskeleton. A thick glycoprotein coat, the glycocalyx covers the microvilli. The glycocalyx contains hydrolytic enzymes such as enteropeptidase, dipeptidases and disaccharidases.

Lymphoid cells are found throughout the GI tract lamina propria, submucosa and even the epithelium itself and are known as gut associated lymphoid tissue or GALT. Aggregated nodules are found in the jejunum and ileum, with more prominent ones in the ileum and known as Peyer's patches.

At the site of Peyer's patches, the overlying villi are frequently absent. The epithelium covering a patch is called the follicle associated epithelium (FAE). The FAE is composed of specialized cells called "M" cells. M cells pinocytose a representative sample of intraluminal antigens and transcytose them across to intraepithelial antigen presenter cells.

Recently, disruption of the above mentioned structures during several physiological or pathological conditions has been reported, which were associated with impaired intestinal barrier function and lead to the passage of intraluminal solutes into the systemic circulation [5,6,7].

Investigations showed that the changes of intestinal barrier function were mainly due to the relaxation of the tight-junction between intestinal epithelial cells [8]. Some studies proposed that factors causing alterations in gut microbiota, hormones secreted by the enterocytes and changes of related enzymatic system caused damage of intestinal barrier, and the enteric bacteria and endotoxin reinforced the damage [9].

Histopathological data of the gastrointestinal barrier of human being is scarce. This chapter mainly focuses on the research findings of the morphological changes of the gut during intestinal barrier dysfunction in laboratory animals. Contents of the chapter will help the researchers interested in gastrointestinal morphological changes.

Discussion about the factors and type of morphological changes of the gastrointestinal barrier is provided below. For easy understanding, discussion is done under several headings.

2. Gender and age

Recently, Milićević Z and his team analyzed the effects of gender and ageing on the histoquantitative parameters of healthy jejunal and ileal mucosa. Computer-aided morphometric analysis of 24 jejunal and 25 ileal biopsy samples collected during routine endoscopy of healthy individuals with family history of intestinal malignancy was done. Jejunal mucosal thickness was significantly reduced in elderly subjects above 60 years of age ($p<0.05$), especially in elderly females compared to the adults ($p<0.05$). Jejunal villi were significantly wider in adults than in the elderly subjects ($p<0.05$), whereas ileal villi were significantly wider in elderly compared to adult subjects ($p<0.01$) and in male compared to female subjects ($p<0.05$). Other histoquantitative parameters eg. mucosa epithelium height, crypt numerical density, villous height, crypts and villous perimeter, diameter and epithelium height of jejunal and ileal mucosa were not different significantly in their observation [10].

3. Undernutrition

Adequate nutrition is necessary for the normal cell division and cell migration from the crypt to the villi thus in maintaining the gastrointestinal barrier. Diet with protein and vitamin restriction (75% protein and 50% vitamin restrictions) but not food restriction to weanling, Wistar/NIN male rats for 20 weeks significantly increased intestinal cell apoptosis observed by morphometry, Annexin V binding, M30 CytoDeath assay, and DNA fragmentation [11].

Providing a diet moderately deficient in protein, fat, and minerals to C57BL/6 mice from the 10 day of their life for 6 weeks resulted in decreased villous height and crypt depth in the jejunum of the undernourished weanlings, stained by haematoxylin and eosin (H&E) and observed under light microscope, increased claudin-3 expression, decreased epithelial cell proliferation measured by immunohistochemistry eg. MTS and bromodeoxyuridine assays and increased epithelial cell apoptosis as measured by annexin and 7-amino-actinomycin D staining. All these changes were associated with decreased transmucosal resistance and increased permeability to FITC-dextran indicating intestinal barrier dysfunction [12].

Cancer cachexia is also reported to induce alterations to some of the morphological parameters of the small intestine. Light microscopic observation of the H&E stained intestinal specimen of tumor-bearing mice was reported to have lower villus height and contour length than in healthy mice ($P > 0.05$). Villus width and crypt depth showed substantial evidence of atrophy ($P < 0.05$). Wasting of smooth muscle in the muscularis layer as indicated by a reduction in muscularis width was present on days 2 and 11 of tumor production ($P < 0.05$). [Villus contour length was calculated using the following equation: villus contour length = (2 × villus height) + (0.3 × villus width)] [13].

4. Psychological stress

Various kinds of psychological stresses such as chronic water avoidance stress (WAS) in rats and mice which mimics chronic depression in human being has been reported to compromise small intestinal mucosal structure and hamper intestinal barrier function. H&E and Periodic acid schiff (PAS) stain of the microtome sections of the small intestinal segments of the Sprague Dawley rats subjected to water avoidance stress for 10 days showed that villus height ($p<.005$), crypt depth ($p<0.00$), number of goblet cells in villus ($p<.0.00$) and crypt ($p<.0.03$) decreased significantly in the jejunum as compared to the control. Ileum also had atrophy but villus height and the number of goblet cells in the villi did not differ significantly. Number of polymorphonuclear neutrophil infiltration was significantly higher in stress group as compared to control ($p<0.00$) [6].

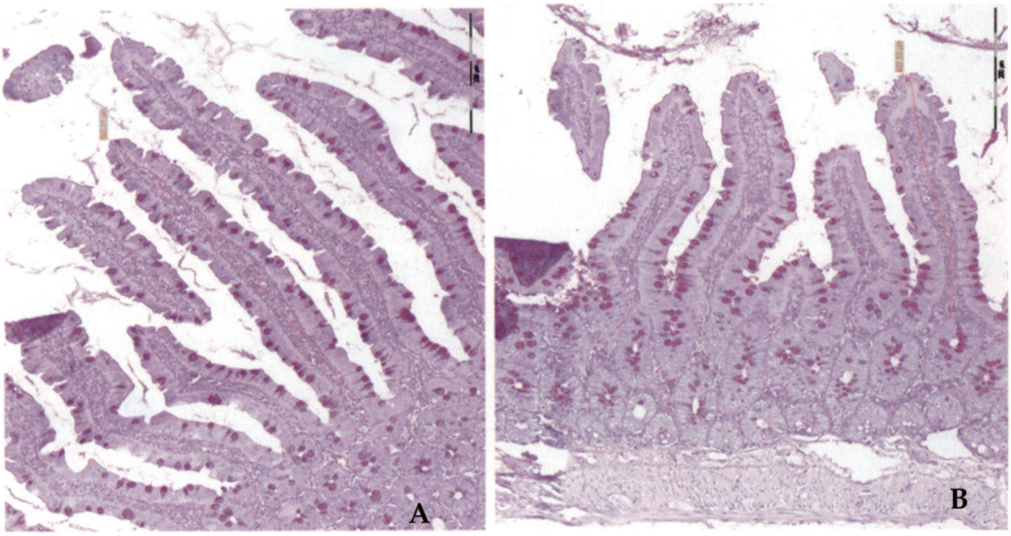

Figure 1. Light microscope findings of PAS stain of control (A) and WAS (B) rats of the mucosal layer of jejunum (× 100).

Microtome sections of the rat distal colon subjected to WAS stained with H&E showed inflammatory cell infiltration in the lamina propria of stressed rats fed with standard diet that was not observed in non-stressed rats [14].

Noise-induced stress (15 min of white noise at 90 dB daily for 3 wks) has been reported to disrupt the intestinal barrier of laboratory rats. Light microscopic observation of the ileum stained by H&E showed significantly more degranulated mast cells (mean+SE, 3.95+0.8 vs 0.35+ 0.29, respectively) and eosinophils (mean+SE 9.46+0.44 vs 4.58+0.38) per villus section adjacent to the Peyer patches in noise exposed rats than in quiet rats. The mean width of villus laminar propria was significantly greater in noise exposed rats than in quiet rats, suggesting edema. Mucosal epithelial cells of noise rats were often separated, sometimes detaching from the basement membrane, whereas those of quiet rats were intact. Recovery rats who were kept in quiet room for a further 3 weeks after the initial 3 weeks of noise exposure, showed no reduction in mast cell degranulation or mean width of villus lamina propria, but there were increased numbers of secreting goblet cells in the villi adjacent to Peyer patches and some recovery of epithelial integrity [15].

5. Nutrients

High fat diet consumption and obesity has recently been identified to be associated with compromised tight junction integrity of the enterocytes. An altered distribution such as substantial decreased staining of occludin and discontinuous signals for ZO-1, in the intestinal epithelium of leptin-deficient obese *ob/ob* mice was observed by immunocytochemistry of intestinal cryosections. Similar results were obtained in hyperleptinemic and functional leptin receptor deficient obese *db/db* mice. There was also a shift of intestinal junctional protein from the cytoskeleton of both these obese strains, causing a decrease in paracellular sealing [9].

Medium chain triglycerides (MCTs) enhance cell proliferation of the intestinal epithelium and mucous secretion from goblet cells in the small intestine. Number of goblet cells measured by periodic acid Schiff and alcian blue stain was significantly higher in rats given MCTs as compared to rats given corn oil (5 g/kg per day) or chow for 2 weeks. Proliferating cells on the villi and the crypts in the small intestine, detected by immunohistochemistry using monoclonal mouse anti rat Ki-67 antigen and the apoptotic cells detected by polyclonal rabbit anti single stranded DNA antibody were also significantly greater in rats given MCTs than rats given corn oil or normal rats. Both proliferative and apoptotic index were significantly increased in rats receiving MCTs.

These effects of MCTs might persuade further research on the role of MCTs on the histological changes of the gastrointestinal barrier in patients suffering from inflammatory bowel disease or enterogenous infections [16].

6. Parenteral nutrition

Observation of the Ileal segments of Sprague Dawley rats stained with H&E and PAS staining after seven days of standard total parenteral nutrition (TPN) under light microscope has been associated with villous atrophy, fewer goblet cells, atrophy of Peyer's patches. Decreased luminal mucus gel was observed by cryostat sections of frozen samples in liquid nitrogen followed by celloidin stabilization and PAS stain in rats receiving TPN [17]. Seven days of Alanyl glutamine supplemented TPN was able to attenuate the changes found in standard TPN observed under light microscope [18].

7. Infections

Enteroaggregative Escherichia coli strains have been associated with persistent diarrhea in several developing countries. Electron microscope observation showed that Enteroaggregative Escherichia coli strains caused total or partial villi destruction, vacuolization of basal cytoplasm of the enterocytes, epithelium detachment, derangement of the structure and epithelial cell extrusion in ileal mucosa. Bacterial aggregates associated with mucus and cellular debris was evident in the intestinal lumen and in the intercellular spaces of the destroyed epithelium, suggesting bacterial invasion which seemed to be secondary to the destruction of the tissue [19].

8. Inflammatory bowel disease

Duodenal biopsy of Celiac disease patients stained with H&E and studied under light microscope had a raised IEL count (> 20 per 100 enterocytes) and marked villous atrophy [20].

Expression of claudin-2 was distinctly different in active Chron's disease (CD) and ulcerative colitis (UC) in comparison to its expression pattern in controls. Claudin-2 expression was upregulated along the whole length of intercellular junction (ICJ) in biopsies from patients with active CD and UC in comparison to the biopsies from control patients, where its expression was limited to the uppermost part of ICJ. There was reduced expression of ZO-1 in UC and CD patients. On transmission electron microscopic examination, the pentalaminar structure of tight junction (TJs) was destroyed in patients with CD and UC but no significant change was seen in controls. The redistribution of claudin-2 expression was in accordance with the TJ ultrastructural changes in patients with UC and CD [21].

9. Diabetes mellitus

Endoscopic biopsy of eight insulin dependent diabetes mellitus patients without concomitant celiac disease was devoid of any sign of atrophy or inflammation under light microscope, whereas observation under transmission electron microscope showed remarkable ultra-structural changes in height and thickness of microvilli, space between microvilli and thickness of tight junctions in six out of the eight patients [22].

10. Surgery

Electron microscope observation of the samples of the laboratory animals underwent intestinal surgery reported lower expression of occludin. Administration of enteral nutrition (EN) after surgery induced greater expression of occludin in the intestine than in the animals receiving total parenteral nutrition (TPN). Intestinal epithelial tight junction and microvilli were more intact in the animals receiving post surgical EN as compared to those receiving post surgical TPN [23].

Destructive changes such as intense edema of the intestinal wall, mainly in the intestinal lamina propria, as well as blood vessel dilatation and congestion were observed in the intestinal obstruction model of mice. There was also a discrete increase in the cellularity of lamina propria. In addition to that, epithelial reactive changes, superficial erosions, edema, and enlargement of the intestinal villi were observed under light microscope [24].

11. Alcohol and drugs

Ethanol (0, 1, 2.5, 5, 7.5, and 10%) produced a progressive disruption of TJ protein (ZO-1) with separation of ZO-1 proteins from the cellular junctions and formation of large gaps between the adjacent cells of Caco-2 cell line as evidenced by immunofluorescent antibody labeling of ZO-1 proteins [25].

Immunofluorescence analysis of HT-29 cells showed a fragmented and granulous ZO-1 staining, after aspirin treatment. Treating both aspirin and heat-killed Lactobacillus acidophilus strain LB (LaLB) together with the culture supernatant, resulted in fine continuous linear web at cell-cell contacts similarly to control evaluated by immunofluorescence using an anti-ZO-1 antibody [26].

Prolonged subcutaneous injection of Methamphetamine (MA) for 12 weeks decreased the villi height and increased the number of goblet cells significantly as compared to the control group of rats as evidenced by light microscope observation of the H&E and PAS stained samples of the ileum. Withdrawal of MA was able to bring the morphology back to normal [27].

Quantitative analysis of ZO-1 expression in male Wistar rats receiving oral methotraxate (MTX, 15 mg/kg) for 3-5 days showed the absence of significant differences, whereas tyrosine dephosphorylation of ZO-1 was observed. An obvious reduction of ZO-1 immunostaining along the apical membrane of intestinal villi was also observed. These findings suggest that ZO-1 alterations may contribute to the disturbance of TJ barrier in MTX-treated rats, which leads to enhanced intestinal permeability [28].

Paclitaxel, a new chemotherapeutic agent induced apoptosis in 12.5% of jejunum villus cells observed under light microscope after Terminal deoxynucleotidyl transferase-mediated deoxyuridine triphosphate (dUTP)-biotin end labeling assay (TUNEL), which was reduced to 3.8% by granulocyte stimulating factor (G-CSF) treatment. Apoptosis in the control group was 0.6%. Paclitaxel treatment also resulted in villus atrophy observed under light microscope of H&E stained slides, which led to increased intestinal permeability. G-CSF treatment resulted in increased villus height and returned WBC counts to normal levels [29].

12. Radiation injury

Radiation exposure in cancer patients damages the intestinal epithelium and thus can hamper intestinal barrier function [30].

Disruption of the integrity of the intestinal barrier was observed in rat ileum following abdominal X-irradiation, depending on the post irradiation time and the delivered dose. The loss of barrier integrity was characterized by a disorganization of proteins of tight and adherent junctions as evidenced by immunohistochemical analyses of junctional proteins (ZO-1 and beta-catenin) observed by confocal microscope. A disorganization of the localization for ZO-1 and beta-catenin was also observed [31].

Epithelial cell damage was observed in the duodenum, jejunum, ileum and distal colon in paraffin and frozen section at 1, 6, 24, 96h, 1.5 and 3 months after a single dose of 25Gy administered percutaneously to the liver of rats. However, prolonged denudation of the villi together with destruction of the crypt lining was only observed in the ileum, resulting in deficient regeneration. In the colon, changes were minor. Radiation mucositis with granulocyte (MP0+) infiltration was seen from 1 to 24h in the duodenum and jejunum, when ED1+ macrophages, CD3+ T-lymphocytes, and CD34+ hematopoietic precursor cells were recruited, accompanied by an increase in the chemokines MCP-1, MIP-1α, MIP3α and Il-8. In the ileum, early granulocyte infiltration was delayed but continuous. Recruitment of macrophages and lymphocytes was deficient and induction of chemokines such as the adhesion molecules PECAM-1, ICAM-1 was lacking [32].

13. Others

Thirty percent total body surface area (TBSA) burn resulted in a significant increase in intestinal permeability. Burn injury resulted in a marked decrease in the levels of tight junction proteins occludin and ZO-1 at 6 and 24 h following burn analyzed by immunoblotting and immunohistochemistry and seen under confocal microscope [33].

Gut barrier dysfunction was evident in patients with multiple organ dysfunction (MODS). Breakdown and reorganization of occludin and ZO-1 away from tight junctions was found in all MODS patients analyzed by immunoblotting and immunofluorescence staining [34].

In animal model of cirrhosis of liver, ileal structure was altered by the presence of villous atrophy, lymphangiectasias and submucosal oedema as seen in H&E stained samples under light microscope [35].

Condition	Methods used	Findings	Author
Gender and age	Endoscopic biopsy, H&E stain, Computer-aided morphometric analysis.	Jejunal mucosal thickness was significantly reduced in elderly subjects above 60 years of age (p<0.05), especially in elderly females compared to the adults (p<0.05). ileal villi were significantly wider in elderly compared to adult subjects (p<0.01) and in male compared to female subjects (p<0.05).	Milićević Z
Under nutrition Diet with 75% protein and 50% vitamin restrictions to weanling, Wistar/NIN male rats for 20 weeks	Apoptosis observed by morphometry, Annexin V binding.	Significantly increased intestinal cell apoptosis.	Bodiga VL 2005
Diet moderately deficient in protein, fat, and minerals to C57BL/6 mice	H&E, immunohistochemistry eg. MTS and bromodeoxyuridine assays, annexin and 7-amino-actinomycin D staining.	Decreased villous height and crypt depth in the jejunum. Increased claudin-3 expression, decreased epithelial cell proliferation, increased epithelial cell apoptosis.	Ueno PM 2011
Cancer cachexia	Light microscopic observation of the H&E stained intestinal specimen of tumor-bearing mice.	Decreased villus height and contour length than in healthy mice ($P > 0.05$). Villus width and crypt depth showed substantial evidence of atrophy ($P < 0.05$).	Susan E 2000

Condition	Methods used	Findings	Author
Total parenteral nutrition	Ileal segments of rats stained with H&E and PAS staining and observed under light microscope.	Villous atrophy, fewer goblet cells, atrophy of Peyer's patches. Decreased luminal mucus gel.	Khan J 1999 Iiboshi Y 1994
High fat diet	Immunocytochemistry of intestinal cryosections of mice	Altered distribution such as substantial decreased staining of occludin and discontinuous signals for ZO-1	Suzuki T 2010
Medium chain triglycerides (MCTs)	Periodic acid Schiff and alcian blue stain.	Number of goblet cells measured was significantly higher in rats given MCTs as compared to rats given corn oil (5 g/kg per day) or chow for 2 weeks.	Iishi K 2009
	Immunohistochemistry using monoclonal mouse anti rat Ki-67 antigen, polyclonal rabbit anti single stranded DNA antibody.	Proliferating cells on the villi and the crypts in the small intestine, significantly greater in rats given MCTs than rats given corn oil or normal rats.	
Psychological stress	H&E and periodic acid Schiff stain of the microtome sections of the small intestinal segments of rats under light microscope.	Villus height (p<.005), crypt depth (p<0.00), number of goblet cells in villus (p<.0.00) and crypt (p<.0.03) decreased significantly in jejunum as compared to control. Number of polymorphonuclear neutrophil was significantly higher in stress group as compared to control (p<0.00).	Saudi WSW 2009
	Microtome sections of the rat distal colon stained by H&E.	Inflammatory cell infiltration in the lamina propria of stressed rats.	Larauche M 2012
	Light microscopic observation of the ileum stained by H&E.	Significantly more degranulated mast cells and eosinophils per villus section adjacent to the Peyer patches in noise exposed rats than in quiet rats. The mean width of villus laminar propria was significantly greater in noise rats than in quiet rats. Mucosal epithelial cells of noise rats were often separated, sometimes detaching from the basement membrane.	Baldwin AL 2006

Condition	Methods used	Findings	Author
Diabetes mellitus	Transmission electron microscope.	Remarkable ultra-structural changes in height and thickness of microvilli, space between microvilli and thickness of tight junctions.	Secondulfo M 2004
Surgery	Electron microscope.	Samples of the laboratory animals underwent intestinal surgery reported lower expression of occludin.	Zhang MM 2009
Infection	Electron microscope.	Enteroaggregative Escherichia coli strains caused total or partial villi destruction, vacuolization of basal cytoplasm of the enterocytes, epithelium detachment, derangement of the structure and epithelial cell extrusion in ileal mucosa of laboratory animals.	Andrade JA 2010
Inflammatory bowel disease	Hematoxylin-eosin and studied under light microscope. Immunohistochemistry. Electron microscope	Raised IEL count (> 20 per 100 enterocytes) and marked villous atrophy of duodenal biopsy. Reduced expression of ZO-1 in UC and CD patients. Pentalaminar structure of tight junction (TJs) was destroyed in patients with CD and UC	Dewar DH 2012 Das P 2012
Alcohol	Immunofluorescent antibody labeling of ZO-1 proteins.	Ethanol (0, 1, 2.5, 5, 7.5, and 10%) produced a progressive disruption of TJ protein (ZO-1) with separation of ZO-1 proteins from the cellular junctions and formation of large gaps between the adjacent cells of Caco-2 cell line.	Ma TY 1999
Drugs	Immunofluorescence analysis. H&E and PAS staining of ileum, observed under light microscope. Immunostaining.	HT-29 cell line showed a fragmented and granulous ZO-1 staining, after aspirin treatment. Prolonged Methamphatamine abuse in rats decreased the villi height and increased the number of goblet cells significantly as compared to the control group of rats. Reduction of ZO-1 along the apical membrane of intestinal villi was observed in methotraxate treatment in rats.	Montalto M 2004 Khan J 2008 Hamada K 2010

Condition	Methods used	Findings	Author
	Light microscope observation after Terminal deoxynucleotidyl transferase-mediated deoxyuridine triphosphate (dUTP)-biotin end labeling assay (TUNEL) and hematoxylin and eosin (H&E) staining.	Paclitaxel, a new chemotherapeutic agent induced apoptosis in 12.5% of jejunum villus cells. Apoptosis in the control group was 0.6%. also resulted in villus atrophy which led to increased intestinal permeability. Granulocyte colony-stimulating factor (G-CSF) treatment resulted in increased villus height and returned WBC counts to normal levels.	Zhang C 2011
Radiation injury	Immunohistochemical analyses of junctional proteins (ZO-1 and beta-catenin) and confocal microscopy. Light microscope observation.	Disorganization of the proteins of tight and adherent junctions. A disorganization of the localization for ZO-1 and beta-catenin was also observed. Prolonged denudation of the villi together with destruction of the crypt lining observed in the ileum. In the colon, changes were minor. Radiation mucositis with granulocyte (MP0+) infiltration was seen from 1 to 24h in the duodenum and jejunum, when ED1+ macrophages, CD3+ T-lymphocytes, and CD34+ hematopoietic precursor cells were recruited.	Dublineau I 2004 Cameron S 2011
Burn	Immunohistochemistry.	Marked decrease in the levels of tight junction proteins occludin and ZO-1 at 6 and 24 h.	Costantini TW 2009
Multiple organ dysfunction	Immunoblotting and immunofluorescence staining.	Breakdown and reorganization of occludin and ZO-1 away from tight junctions was found in all MODS patients.	Zhang JB 2010
Cirrhosis of liver	Light microscope.	In animal model of cirrhosis of liver, ileal structure was altered by the presence of villous atrophy, lymphangiectasias and submucosal oedema.	V Lorenzo Zúñiga 2006

Table 1. Summary of the morphological findings in different conditions affecting gastrointestinal barrier.

Although still at conceptual level, evidences are persuasive that use of the certain compounds, such as zinc, glutamine, probiotics etc has the potential to attenuate morphological changes by the above factors and might represent a simple device to prevent the occurrence or aggravation of chronic pathologies caused by intestinal barrier dysfunction.

14. Glutamine

Glutamine is an amino acid important for the growth of enterocytes. Electron microscopy of the intestine in a GLN-deprived infant rat model demonstrated intestinal intercellular junction breakdown [36].

Deprivation of GLN decreased claudin-1, occludin, and ZO-1 protein expression and caused a disappearance of perijunctional claudin-1 and a reduction of occludin but had no effect on ZO-1. Transmission electron microscopy revealed that methionine sulfoximine-treated cells in the absence of GLN formed irregular junctional complexes between the apical lateral margins of adjoining cells. These findings indicate that TJ protein expression and cellular localization in Caco-2 cell monolayers rely on GLN [37].

15. Zinc

Trace elements such as zinc may assist in the maintenance of intestinal barrier integrity. Caco-2 cells grown in zinc-deficient media had reduced TEER and altered expression of ZO-1 and occludin ie. localized away from the cell boundaries and less homogenicity as compared with the Caco-2 cells grown in zinc-replete media. This findings were accompanied by disorganization of F-actin filaments [38].

Electron microscopic studies showed that percentage of the disrupted (opened) tight junctions in experimental colitis were reduced by 50% with zinc supplementation [39].

16. Vitamin A

Retinoic acid (RA), the active form of vitamin A had significant trophic effects in resected and sham-resected rats. Exogenous RA stimulated the adaptive response of the intestine in 70% small bowel resection by 2 weeks, as manifested by a significant increase in crypt depth, villus height, and intestinal surface area of rats. The enlarged crypts and villi were due to adaptive hyperplasia and not to cellular hypertrophy. RA was also trophic in the intestine of control rats that were only subjected to transection and reanastomosis. Villus heights and crypt depths were measured in 20–50 well-oriented hematoxylin-eosin-stained crypt-villus units with the aid of a slide micrometer and Scion Image software. Apoptotic cells were identified by standard morphological changes, including nuclear condensation, perinuclear clearing, and cell shrinkage, and by staining for activated caspase-3 [40].

17. Arginine

Arginine is a dibasic amino acid with various metabolic and immunologic effects. Animal models of intestinal obstruction, treated with arginine presented preservation of the tissue structure. The villous epithelium was preserved and only discrete edema and enlargement were present at lamina propria [24].

18. Probiotic

Light microscope observation of Giemsa staining samples revealed that there was close interaction between luminal bacteria and the apical aspect of surface ileal enterocytes in rats subjected to WAS. Bacterial interactions with ileal enterocytes were not observed in sham stressed animals. Pretreatment with probiotics prevented the bacteria epithelial cell contacts induced by WAS.

TEM confirmed the findings demonstrated with light microscopy. While there were no bacteria adhering to the apical surface of enterocytes in sham stressed rats, multiple bacteria were observed closely adhering and internalised into ileal enterocytes in stressed rats. Electron dense condensation around the internalised bacteria consistent with polymerised actin was observed indicating that enterocytes underwent cytoskeletal rearrangements. Pretreatment with probiotics prevented WAS induced bacteria epithelial cell interactions [41].

19. Prebiotic

Prebiotic treated mice exhibited a decreased hepatic expression of inflammatory and oxidative stress markers. This decreased inflammatory tone was associated with a lower intestinal permeability and improved tight-junction ZO-1 and occludin integrity evidenced by qPCR and immunohistochemistry, compared to controls [9] .

Both fibre sources, wheat bran (rich in cellulose and hemicellulose) and pollen from Chinese Masson pine (Pinus massoniana) (rich in lignin) increased villus height of mucosa in jejunum (+10% on average) and ileum (+16% on average) in animal model of 48 weaned piglets [42].

Diet rich in arachidonic and docosahexaenoic acids, galacto- and fructo-oligosaccharides and Lactobacillus paracasei NCC2461 resulted in increased villus length in the small intestine to restore impaired intestinal barrier function and growth after neonatal stress in rats [43].

20. Flavonoid

Quercetin is the most common flavonoid in nature. High amounts of quercetin are found in onions, kale, and apples [44].

Flavonoids, quercetin and myricetin, enhanced barrier function in human intestinal Caco-2 cells. Suzuki and Hara recently reported that a 48-h exposure of quercetin enhanceds the intestinal barrier function through increasing claudin-4 expression in human intestinal Caco-2 monolayers. Quercetin promoted the assembly of TJ proteins, ZO-2, occludin, and claudin-1 and the expression of claudin-4 by inhibiting the PKCδ isoform [45].

Kaempferol, a natural flavonoid present in fruits, vegetables, and teas, provides beneficial effects for human health. Confocal microscopy showed kaempferol-induced assembly of occludin and claudin-3 occurred at the TJ of Caco -2 cells at 6 h postadministration [46].

Condition	Methods used	Findings	Author
Deprivation of Glutamine	Electron microscope observation	Decreased claudin-1, occludin, and ZO-1 protein expression and caused a disappearance of perijunctional claudin-1 and a reduction of occludin	Potsic B 2000
Zinc supplementation Zinc-deficient media	Electron microscope observation	Percentage of the disrupted (opened) tight junctions in experimental colitis were reduced by 50% with zinc. Caco-2 cells have reduced TEER and altered expression of ZO-1 and occludin ie. localized away from the cell boundaries and less homogenous compared with Caco-2 cells grown in zinc-replete media	Sturniolo GC, 2002 Finamore A 2008
Vitamin A	Light microscope, H&E and staining for activated caspase-3	Significant increase in crypt depth, villus height, and intestinal surface area of 70% bowel resection in rats.	Wang L 2007
Arginine	Light microscope	Animal models of intestinal obstruction treated with arginine presented preservation of the tissue structure. The villous epithelium was preserved and only	Viana ML 2010

Condition	Methods used	Findings	Author
		discrete edema and enlargement were present at lamina propria.	
Probiotics	Light microscope observation of Giemsa stained sample	Prevented WAS induced close interaction between luminal bacteria and the apical aspect of surface ileal enterocytes in rats.	M Zareie 2007
Prebiotics	qPCR and immunohistochemistry	Improved tight-junction ZO-1 and occludin	Cani PD 2009
Wheat bran and pollen from Chinese Masson pine	Light microscope observation of H&E stained samples	Increased villus height of mucosa in jejunum (+10% on average) and ileum (+16% on average) in animal model of 48 weaned piglets	Schedle K 2008
Diet containing arachidonic and docosahexaenoic acids, galacto- and fructo-oligosaccharides and Lactobacillus paracasei NCC2461	Light microscope observation	Increased villus length in small intestine after neonatal stress in rats.	García-Ródenas CL 2006
Quercetin	Confocal microscope observation	Promotes the assembly of TJ proteins, ZO-2, occludin, and claudin-1 and the expression of claudin-4	Suzuki T 2009
Kaempferol	Confocal microscope observation	Assembly of occludin and claudin-3 at the TJ of Caco -2 cells	Suzuki T 2011

Table 2. Summary of the histological findings of different modulating agents improving gastrointestinal barrier.

21. Conclusion

Emerging experimental evidences from animal models suggest that altered barrier function is a potential pathway for intestinal and extra intestinal inflammation. Although thousands of research findings are available dealing with gut barrier function during different physiological and pathological conditions, few articles focused on the histolological changes. In this chapter discussion was made in an attempt to provide a generalized idea of morphological changes during several conditions. Future researches are suggested to deal with the effect of different modulating agents on the histolological parameters of intestinal barrier. Therapeutic restoration of barrier function could improve pathophysiology and clinical outcomes of different diseases.

Author details

Jesmine Khan and Mohammed Nasimul Islam
Faculty of Medicine, Universiti Teknologi MARA (UiTM),
Shah Alam, Selangor, Malaysia

Acknowledgement

Authors are grateful to Dr. Shyamoli Mostoffa, pathologist and senior lecturer, School of Health Sciences, Universiti Sains Malaysia for her help in interpreting histological data of their research included in this chapter.

Histological images of rat jejunum were taken with permission from the International Medical Journal, Japan.

22. References

[1] Nusrat A, Turner JR, Madara JL (2000) Molecular physiology and pathophysiology of tight junctions. IV. Regulation of tight junctions by extracellular stimuli: nutrients, cytokines, and immune cells. Am J Physiol Gastrointest Liver Physiol 279(5):G851-7.

[2] Mitic LL, Anderson JM (1998) Molecular architecture of tight junctions. Annu Rev Physiol 60:121-42.

[3] Ivanov AI, McCall IC, Parkos CA, Nusrat A (2004) Role for actin filament turnover and a myosin II motor in cytoskeleton-driven disassembly of the epithelial apical junctional complex. Mol Biol Cell 15(6):2639-51. Epub 2004 Mar 26

[4] Turksen K, Troy TC (2004) Barriers built on claudins. J Cell Sci. 117:2435–2447

[5] Rahner C, Mitic LL, Anderson JM (2001) Heterogeneity in expression and subcellular localization of claudins 2, 3, 4, and 5 in the rat liver, pancreas, and gut. Gastroenterology 120(2):411-422

[6] Saudi WSW, Khan J, Islam MN (2009) Small intestinal morphology and permeability in chronic water avoidance stress in rats. IMJ16(2), 87-91

[7] Suzuki T, Hara H (2010) Dietary fat and bile juice, but not obesity, are responsible for the increase in small intestinal permeability induced through the suppression of tight junction protein expression in LETO and OLETF rats. Nutr Metab (Lond) 12;7-19

[8] Gasbarrini G, Montalto M. Structure and function of tight junctions. Role in intestinal barrier. Ital J Gastroenterol Hepatol.1999 Aug-Sep;31(6):481-8.

[9] P D Cani, S Possemiers, T Van de Wiele, Y Guiot, A Everard, O Rottier, L Geurts, D Naslain, A Neyrinck, D M Lambert, G G Muccioli, and N M Delzenne. (2009). Changes in gut microbiota control inflammation in obese mice through a mechanism involving GLP-2-driven improvement of gut permeability. Gut 58(8):1091-103. Epub 2009 Feb 24.

[10] Trbojević-Stanković JB, Milićević NM, Milosević DP, Despotović N, Davidović M, Erceg P, Bojić B, Bojić D, Svorcan P, Protić M, Dapcević B, Miljković MD, Milićević Z (2010) Morphometric study of healthy jejunal and ileal mucosa in adult and aged subjects. Histol Histopathol. Feb;25(2):153-8.

[11] Bodiga VL, Boindala S, Putcha U, Subramaniam K, Manchala R (2005) Chronic low intake of protein or vitamins increases the intestinal epithelial cell apoptosis in Wistar/NIN rats. Nutrition 21(9):949-60.

[12] Ueno PM, Oriá RB, Maier EA, Guedes M, de Azevedo OG, Wu D, Willson T, Hogan SP, Lima AA, Guerrant RL, Polk DB, Denson LA, Moore SR (2011) Alanyl-glutamine promotes intestinal epithelial cell homeostasis in vitro and in a murine model of weanling undernutrition. Am J Physiol Gastrointest Liver Physiol. 301(4):G612-22. doi: 10.1152/ajpgi.00531.2010. Epub 2011 Jul 28.

[13] Susan E. Samuels, Andrew L. Knowles, Thomas Tilignac, Eric Debiton, Jean Claude Madelmont, and Didier Attaix (2000) Protein Metabolism in the Small Intestine during Cancer Cachexia and Chemotherapy in Mice.Cancer Res 60,4968-4974.

[14] Baldwin AL, Primeau RL, Johnson W E (2006) Effect of noise on the morphology of the intestinal mucosa in laboratory rats. J Am Assoc Lab Anim Sci.45(1):74-82.

[15] De La Serre CB, Ellis CL, Lee J, Hartman AL, Rutledge JC, Raybould HE (2010) Propensity to high-fat diet-induced obesity in rats is associated with changes in the gut microbiota and gut inflammation. Am J Physiol Gastrointest Liver Physiol; 299(2):G440-8. Epub 2010 May 27.

[16] Ishii K, Kono H, Hosomura N, Tsuchiya M, Ohgiku M, Tanaka N, Fujii H (2009) Medium-chain triglycerides enhance mucous secretion and cell proliferation in the rat. J Gastroenterol. 44(3):204-11. Epub 2009 Feb 13.

[17] Iiboshi Y, Nezu R, Kennedy M, Fujii M, Wasa M, Fukuzawa M, Kamata S, Takagi Y, Okada A (1994) Total parenteral nutrition decreases luminal mucous gel and increases permeability of small intestine. JPEN J Parenter Enteral Nutr 18(4):346-50.

[18] Khan J, Iiboshi Y, Cui L, Wasa M, Sando K, Takagi Y, Okada A (1999) Alanyl-glutamine-supplemented parenteral nutrition increases luminal mucus gel and decreases permeability in the rat small intestine. JPEN J Parenter Enteral Nutr 23(1):24-31.

[19] Andrade JA, Freymüller E, Fagundes-Neto U (2010) Pathophysiology of enteroaggregative Escherichia coli infection: an experimental model utilizing transmission electron microscopy. Arq Gastroenterol. 47(3):306-12.

[20] Dewar DH, Donnelly SC, McLaughlin SD, Johnson MW, Ellis HJ, Ciclitira PJ (2012) Celiac disease: management of persistent symptoms in patients on a gluten-free diet. World J Gastroenterol. 28;18(12):1348-56.

[21] Das P, Goswami P, Das TK, Nag T, Sreenivas V, Ahuja V, Panda SK, Gupta SD, Makharia GK (2012) Comparative tight junction protein expressions in colonic Crohn's disease, ulcerative colitis, and tuberculosis: a new perspective. Virchows Arch.460(3):261-70.

[22] Secondulfo M, Iafusco D, Carratù R, deMagistris L, Sapone A, Generoso M, Mezzogiomo A, Sasso FC, Cartenì M, De Rosa R, Prisco F, Esposito V (2004) Ultrastructural mucosal alterations and increased intestinal permeability in non-celiac, type I diabetic patients. Dig Liver Dis. 36(1):35-45.

[23] Zhang MM, Cheng JQ, Lu YR, Zhai HJ, Chen YN, Wu XT (2009) Effects of enteral nutrition and parenteral nutrition on gut epithelial tight junction and barrier function in rats after surgical stress. Sichuan Da Xue Xue Bao Yi Xue Ban;40(4):615-8.

[24] Viana ML, Santos RG, Generoso SV, Arantes RM, Correia MI, Cardoso VN (2010) Pretreatment with arginine preserves intestinal barrier integrity and reduces bacterial translocation in mice. Nutrition 26(2):218-23. Epub 2009 Aug 5.

[25] Ma TY, Nguyen D, Bui V, Nguyen H, Hoa N (1999) Ethanol modulation of intestinal epithelial tight junction barrier. Am J Physiol. 276(4 Pt 1):G965-74.

[26] Montalto M, Maggiano N, Ricci R, Curigliano V, Santoro L, Di Nicuolo F, Vecchio FM, Gasbarrini A, Gasbarrini G (2004) Lactobacillus acidophilus protects tight junctions from aspirin damage in HT-29 cells. Digestion 69(4):225-8. Epub 2004 Jun 16.

[27] Jesmine Khan, Mohammed Nasimul Islam(2008) Effect of Methamphetamine on the small intestinal morphology of rats. IMJ 15(5), 385-388.

[28] Hamada K, Shitara Y, Sekine S, Horie T (2010) Zonula Occludens-1 alterations and enhanced intestinal permeability in methotrexate-treated rats. Cancer Chemother Pharmacol. 66(6):1031-8. Epub 2010 Jan 30.

[29] Zhang C, Xu YG, Duan XN, Liu YH, Zhao JX, Xu L, Ye JM (2011) Role of granulocyte colony-stimulating factor in paclitaxel-induced intestinal barrier breakdown and bacterial translocation in rats. Chin Med J (Engl). Jun;124(12):1870-5.

[30] Nejdfors P, Ekelund M, Weström BR, Willén R, Jeppsson B (2000) Intestinal permeability in humans is increased after radiation therapy. Dis Colon Rectum 43(11):1582-1587; discussion 1587-8.

[31] Dublineau I, Lebrun F, Grison S, Griffiths NM (2004) Functional and structural alterations of epithelial barrier properties of rat ileum following X-irradiation. Can J Physiol Pharmacol. 82(2):84-93.

[32] Cameron S, Schwartz A, Sultan S, Schaefer IM, Hermann R, Rave-Fränk M, Hess CF, Christiansen H, Ramadori G (2011) Radiation-induced damage in different segments of the rat intestine after external beam irradiation of the liver. Exp Mol Pathol. 29;92(2):243-258. [Epub ahead of print].

[33] Costantini TW, Loomis WH, Putnam JG, Drusinsky D, Deree J, Choi S, Wolf P, Baird A, Eliceiri B, Bansal V, Coimbra R (2009) Burn-induced gut barrier injury is attenuated by phosphodiesterase inhibition: effects on tight junction structural proteins. Shock. 31(4):416-22.

[34] Zhang JB, Du XG, Zhang H, Li ML, Xiao G, Wu J, Gan H (2010) Breakdown of the gut barrier in patients with multiple organ dysfunction syndrome is attenuated by continuous blood purification: effects on tight junction structural proteins. Int J Artif Organs. 33(1):5-14.

[35] V Lorenzo Zúñiga, C M Rodríguez Ortigosa, R Bartolí, ML Martínez Chantar, L Martínez Peralta, A Pardo, I Ojanguren, J Quiroga, R Planas, and J Prieto (2006) Insulin like growth factor I improves intestinal barrier function in cirrhotic rats. Gut 55(9): 1306–1312. doi: 10.1136/gut.2005.079988.

[36] Potsic B, Holliday N, Lewis P, Samuelson D, DeMarco V, and Neu J (2002) Glutamine supplementation and deprivation: effect on artificially reared rat small intestinal morphology. *Pediatr Res* 52: 430–436.

[37] Nan Li, Lewis P, Samuelson D, Liboni K, Neu J (2004) Glutamine regulates Caco-2 cell tight junction proteins. AJP-GI, 287(3). G726-33.

[38] Finamore A, Massimi M, Conti Devirgiliis L, Mengheri E (2008) Zinc deficiency induces membrane barrier damage and increases neutrophil transmigration in Caco-2 cells. J Nutr 138:1664–70.

[39] Sturniolo GC, Fries W, Mazzon E, Di Leo V, Barollo M, D'inca R (2002) Effect of zinc supplementation on intestinal permeability in experimental colitis. J Lab Clin Med 139: 311–315.

[40] Lihua Wang, Yuzhu Tang, Deborah C. Rubin, and Marc S. Levin (2007) Chronically administered retinoic acid has trophic effects in the rat small intestine and promotes adaptation in a resection model of short bowel syndrome. Am J Physiol Gastrointest Liver Physiol. 292(6):G1559-69. Epub 2007 Feb 15.

[41] M Zareie, K Johnson Henry, J Jury, PC Yang, BY Ngan, D M McKay, J D Soderholm, M H Perdue, and P M Sherman (2006) Probiotics prevent bacterial translocation and improve intestinal barrier function in rats following chronic psychological stress. Gut: 55(11): 1553–1560.

[42] Schedle K, Pfaffl MW, Plitzner C, Meyer HH, Windisch W (2008) Effect of insoluble fibre on intestinal morphology and mRNA expression pattern of inflammatory, cell cycle and growth marker genes in a piglet model. Arch Anim Nutr. 62(6):427-38.

[43] García-Ródenas CL, Bergonzelli GE, Nutten S, Schumann A, Cherbut C, Turini M, Ornstein K, Rochat F, Corthésy-Theulaz I (2006) Nutritional approach to restore impaired intestinal barrier function and growth after neonatal stress in rats. J Pediatr Gastroenterol Nutr.43(1):16-24.

[44] Hertog MGL, Hollman PCH, Katan MB (1992) Content of potentially anticarcinogenic flavonoids of 28 vegetables and 9 fruits commonly consumed in the Netherlands. J Agric Food Chem 40:2379–83).

[45] Suzuki T, Hara H (2009) Quercetin Enhances Intestinal Barrier Function through the Assembly of Zonnula Occludens-2, Occludin, and Claudin-1 and the Expression of Claudin-4 in Caco-2 Cells. J Nutr: 139(5), 965-974

[46] Takuya Suzuki, Soichi Tanabe and Hiroshi Hara (2011) Kaempferol Enhances Intestinal Barrier Function through the Cytoskeletal Association and Expression of Tight Junction Proteins in Caco-2 Cells. J Nutr: 141(1), 187-94

Chapter 9

Histological Change of Aquatic Animals by Parasitic Infection

Watchariya Purivirojkul

Additional information is available at the end of the chapter

http://dx.doi.org/10.5772/52769

1. Introduction

The aquatic parasite usually classified in six groups include Protozoa (Phylum Rhizopoda, Phylum Mastigophora, Phylum Ciliophora, Phylum Myxozoa, Phylum Microspora, Phylum Apicomplexa), Phylum Platyhelminthes (Turbellaria, Monogene, Digenia, Cestoda), Phylum Nematoda, Phylum Acanthocephala, Phylum Annelida and Phylum Arthropoda (Branchiura, Copepoda, Malacostraca (order Isopoda)). Because of their size are vary from microscopic size (1 μm) to macroscopic type (more than 1 meter in some species), more techniques will need to help scientist to classified them. Histological methods are becoming quite common in diagnostic methodology in aquatic animals for a long time (Klontz, 1985). From 1999 to 2012, the author collected more than 120 species of parasites from wild and cultured fish from freshwater and marine fish in many parts of Thailand; North of Thailand (Chiang Rai province, Payao province), North-east of Thailand (Nakornratchasima province, Kalasin province, Sakonnakorn province), East of Thailand (Chachoengsao province, Chonburi province, Rayong province, Trat province), Middle of Thailand (Suphan Buri province, Ratchaburi province, Phra Nakhon Si Ayutthaya province). The specimens from this study were fixed by fixative, dehydrated through a graded ethanol series and embedded in paraffin. Five micrometer thick sections were prepared and stained with Harris' hematoxylin and eosin (H&E). This method advantage to classify the disease because in some situation parasites hide deep in the organ that can not observe by the simple diagnosis such as brain, vertebrae and heart etc.. Moreover, histological study can explain the effect of parasite in the host and predict for chemical and drug therapy for aquatic animals more precisely.

All groups of aquatic parasite are explained at below:

2. Protozoa

The protozoa is a vast assemblage of essentially single celled eukaryotic organisms [2]. Protozoans can be ectoparasites or endoparasites depending on their species. Protozoan ectoparasites are the most common parasites encountered in cultured fish [3]. They are also frequently found in wild fish [4]. Ciliates and flagellates feed on the most superficial skin layer [4]. Parasites cause a reactive hyperplasia of the epithelium and increased mucus production. Hyperplasia appears as a cloundiness to the skin and leads to hypoxia if occur on the gills [4]. Microspora are intracellular and affect a wide variety of vertebrates and invertebrates, Myxosporea are largely intercellular and infect mainly fish [5].

2.1. Phylum Rhizopoda (amoeba)

Amoeba can infect on the external surface such as gill, skin and internal organ as intestine. *Paramoeba pemaquidensis* has caused chronic mortality [4]. This parasite causes proliferative gill lesions. Histopathological change includes focal lamellar hypertrophy with epithelial hyperplasia and metaplasia [4]. *Neoparamoeba perurans* causes amoebic gill disease (AGD) [6]. This parasite affects some species of fish farmed in the marine environment such as Atlantic salmon [7]. The gills of infected fish are pale, multifocal with diffused white AGD-like lesions. Histological changes in the gills are characterized by hyperplasia of epithelial like cells across the gill filaments. This resulted in the fusion of lamellae and the development of round to oval interlamellar vesicles. Hyperplasia of mucous cells are also observed in the gills [6].

2.2. Phylum Mastigophora (flagellated protozoa)

Aquatic parasites in this subphylum separated in two classes; Phytomastigophora and Zoomastigophora

Phytomastigophora contain chloroplasts in their cytoplasm [2]. Common type of this group was dinoflagellate parasites *Amyloodinium* sp. and *Piscinoodinium* sp. [2]. *Amyloodinium* sp. and *Piscinoodinium* sp. cause necrotic dermatitis to their host. *Amyloodinium ocellatum* is marine fish parasites that can infect both elasmobranchs and teleosts [4]. They attach to the host's epithelium by rhizoids (root-like structures) and feed on the host [4]. The gills are the primary site of infection. Heavy infestations can cause gill hyperplasia which include epithelium to severe hyperplasia of the entire gill filament, inflammation, hemorrhage and necrosis. In freshwater, *Piscinoodinium* is reported, histopathological changes are similar to *Amyloodinium* sp. Filament degeneration and necrosis may also occur [4].

Zoomastigophora do not contain chloroplasts in their cytoplasm [2]. Three orders; Kinetoplastida, Retortamonodida and Diplomonadida are usually reported as fish parasites [2].

Parasites of order Kinetoplastida have one or two flagella such as *Cryptobia* sp. [2]. *Cryptobia* spp. are reported to invade the gastric epithelium of European cyprinids and flounders, they may cause gastric dilation, lesions include submucosal granuloma, gastric perforation, peritonitis and full thickness necrosis of the body wall musculature (Ferguson, 1989).

Parasites of order Retortamonodida are possessing two to four flagella, one turned posteriorly such as genus *Ichthyobodo* [2]. *Ichthyobodo* is especially dangerous to young fish and can attack healthy fry and even eggs [4]. *Ichthyobodo necatrix* induces severe erosion and ulcerative dermatitis following epithelial hyperplasia and increased mucus production [4].

Parasites of order Diplomonadida have one to four flagella and two-fold rotational or bilateral symmetry such as *Hexamita* spp. and *Spironucleus* spp. [2]. *Hexamita* spp. are reported in the intestine of many fish such as siamese fighting fish, oscar, discus fish and rainbow trout, cause hexamitiasis [5]. This parasites are associated with a full-thickness gastritis and may penetrate blood vessels leading to dissemination [5]. *Spironucleus* sp. cause of hole-in-the-head disease of oscars, discus and other aquarium cichlids. This parasite ia associated with large erosions in the cranial cartilages, may ulcerate, resulting often in bilaterally symmetrical lesions [5].

2.3. Phylum Ciliophora

Members of this phylum have cilia in at least one stage of the life cycle. They always have two types of nucleus; micronucleus and macronucleus. Most of fish parasites can separate in three classes; Kinetofragminophorea, Oligohymenophorea and Prostomatea [2].

Members of class Kinetofragminophorea have oral ciliature slightly distinct from body ciliature such as *Chilodonella* spp. [2]. Only two species *C. piscicola* and *C. hexasticha* are pathogenic for fish [4]. *Chilodonella* spp. attach on fish skin and gills, this parasite causes infection in fish especially in ornamental fish (Koi, goldfish). *Chilodonella* sp. may feed directly on epithelium, appears to feed by penetrating the host cells with its cytostome and sucking their the contents [4, 8]. After infection, fish secrete excessive mucus, with acute to subacute dermatitis with hyperplasia [4].

Oral apparatus of the members of class Oligohymenophorea usually well defined and oral ciliature is distinct from somatic ciliature such as *Ichthyophthirius multifilis, Trichodina* sp. *Tetrahymena* sp. and *Epistylis* sp. *I. multifilis* parasitizing many species of wide and culture freshwater fish, cause Ich or white spot disease. This parasite is large in size (about 0.1-1.0 mm) contains a horseshoe-shaped macronucleus. Infected fish have the presence of small white spots on the skin or gills. *I. multifilis* cause acute to sub acute dermatitis with hyperplasia, they present within epidermis [5]. The epithelial erosion and ulceration that result from the parasites' entrance into and exit from the host are probably as damaging as its feeding activity. Lesions produced by the parasites may also lead to secondary microbial infections [4].

Trichodinid species (*Trichodina, Trichodinella, Tripartiella, Paratrichodina, Hemitrichodina* and *Vauchomia* sp.) especilly *Trichodina* sp. (Figure 1) are reported from infected skin and gills of freshwater and marine fish. They inhabit the surface of fish, adhere through the suction on the epithelium may cause damage [4,9]. They cause subacute dermatitis with hyperplasia [5]. Mortalities can be much higher, especially in young fish [4]. In incidental case, some species of Trichodina may infect the urinary bladder, oviducts or gastrointestinal tract [4]. In this case, unilateral aplasia of a ureter or chronic inflammation may result in cystic dilation of that portion proximal to the obstruction [5].

Tetrahymena sp. (Figure 1) is the parasite of freshwater fish, cause erosion of the cranium in Atlantic salmon [5]. Tetrahymena pyriformis are usually reported in the parasite of guppy, capable of disseminated infections with dermal ulceration. In some cases, this parasite may invade various internal organs, kidney or brain [4].

The peritrichous ciliate, *Epistylis* sp. and *Scyphidia* sp. are widely spread on fresh water fish such as cichlid and cyprinid. They may infect skin, fins, oral cavity and gills. *Epistylis* sp. is the most common and pathogenic type of sessile, colonial ectocommensal ciliate [4]. Host response for this infection occur by hemorrhagic lesions, necrotic dermatitis with ulceration [5]. In some case, *Vorticella* sp. was found on the thoracic appendages and the cercopods of fairy shrimps [10] (Figure 2). Although in much literature, *Vorticella* sp. is reported as a free-living organism, in some case, when aquatic animals are stressed by adverse environmental conditions and they are completely debilitated and moribund, these free-living ciliophorans become facultative parasites externally [11].

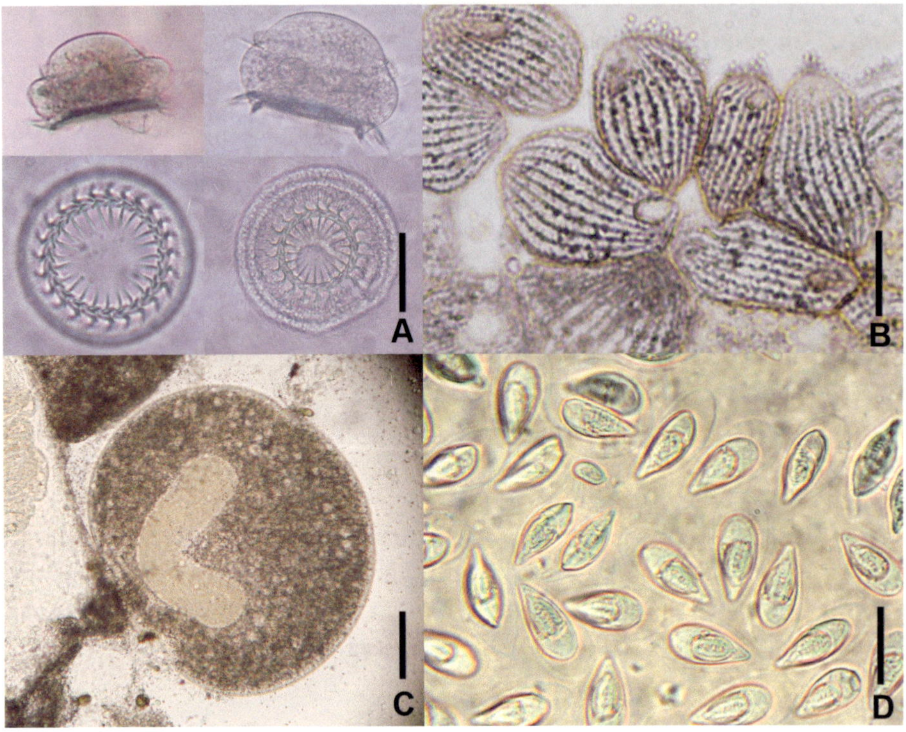

Figure 1. Some parasitic protozoa from aquatic animals.
(A) *Trichodina* spp. from *Pangasianodon gigas*. (scale bar = 50 μm) (source: Purivirojkul W, Areechon N, Purukkiate C. Parasites and bacteria of giant catfishes (*Pangasianodon gigas* Chevey) larva. Thai science and technology journal 2004; 12(3) 1-11.)
(B) *Tetrahymena* sp. from *Poecilia reticulata*. (scale bar = 50 μm)
(C) *Ichthyophthirius multifilis* from *Pangasianodon gigas*. (scale bar = 100 μm)
(D) Myxozoa (*Thelohanellus* sp.) from *Barbonymus gonionotus*. (scale bar = 20 μm)

Cryptocaryon irritans was the member of class Prostomatea, which cause marine white spot disease also present within epidermis as *I. multifilis*. This parasite cause acute to subacute dermatitis with hyperplasia [4].

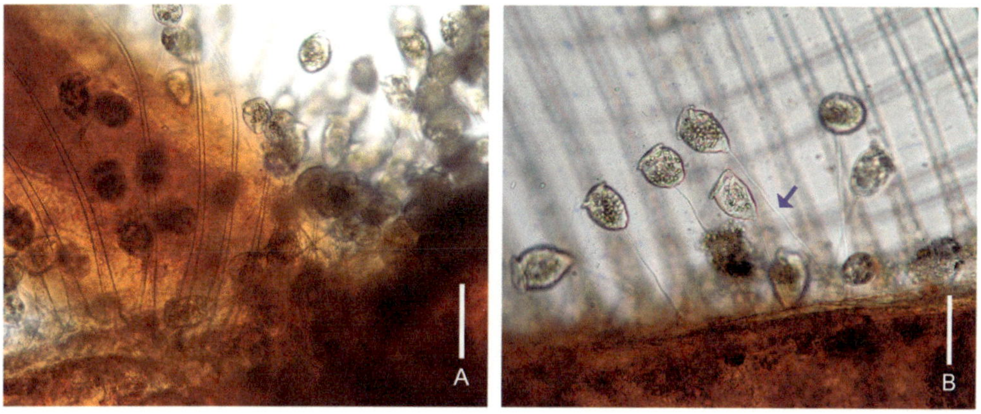

Figure 2. *Vorticella* sp.
(A) Clusters of *Vorticella* sp. infected on the cercopod of fairy shrimp.
(B) Myoneme of *Vorticella* sp. (arrow). (scale bar = 50 μm)

2.4. Phylum Myxozoa

Members of this phylum have spores of multicellular origin, with one or more polar capsules and valves [2]. Classification is based on spore morphology [5]. They are divided into two orders; Bivalvulida and Multivalvulida [2]. Spore of members of order Bivalvulida have two valves such as *Myxidium* sp., *Sphaerospora* sp., *Ceratomyxa* sp., *Thelohanellus* sp. (Figure 1) and *Myxobolus* sp. While spore of members of order Multivalvulida have three or more valves such as *Kudoa* sp. [2].

Parasites in this group settle in muscles and bones of fish hosts lead to fibroplasia and vertebral deformities. In muscle, dermal or sub-dermal cysts are reported [5]. A few myxosporean genera develop intracellularly in skeletal muscle, while others have some development stages that are intracellular [5]. *Myxobolus* spp., infect bone causes vertebral deformities especially *M. cerebralis*, causes whirling disease in farmed salmon and trout. This parasite develops within cartilage, causing lysis and may lead to skeletal abnormalities [5]. The parasite may distort the vertebrae and cause compression lesions [5].

Myxobolus sp. occurred as intact plasmodia between muscle fibers, often adjacent to vertebral spines. The inflammatory response consisted of melanin-laden macrophages and associated with fibroplasia [12]. Many species of *Myxobolus* spp. are reported in fish such as *M. hakyi* in *Pangasianodon hypophthalmus* [13]. *M. hendricksoni* is found in the optic lobes, cerebellum, ventricles and meninges of the fathead minnow. Host response is minimal even though large areas of the brain may be occupied by the parasites [5]. In minnows, *Myxobolus* are found in dorsal root ganglia and spinal canal [5].

The pathology of *Henneguya* spp. is related to the site of infection in the gill (lamellae, filaments or arch) [14]. *H. tunisiensis* infecting the gill arches of *Symphodus tinca*, the parasites develop plasmodia in the connective tissue elements of the gill arch, under the mucosal epithelium. Large plasmodia are usually situated at the ends of the gill arch and induce the compression of the capillaries and retraction of the neighbouring tissue [14]. *H. creplini* infecting the gills of *Stizostedion lucioperca*. The plasmodia located in gill lamellae cause epithelial hyperplasia, and the formation of a thick layer of granular tissue [15]. *H. salminicola* infect pacific salmon muscle cause grossly visible opaque milky white blotches or streaks [5].

Myxosporidiosis associated with the genera *Mitrospora* sp. and *Sphaerospora* sp. found in the kidney caused degenerative changes within tubular epithelium and cast. *Ceratomyxa shasta* is parasite of salmonids that induces granulomatous lesions throughout the viscera, including the kidney [5]. This parasite causes granulomatous peritonitis and sometime total loss of the gall bladder [5]. *Myxidium oviformis* in Atlantic salmon causes severe cholangiohepatitis and inflammation of the gall bladder with emaciation of the host [5]. *Kudoa* sp. release myolytic enzymes after the death of the fish thereby resulting in rapid liquefaction [5].

2.5. Phylum microspora

The phylum Microspora is comprised of unicellular organisms living as intracellular parasites in a variety of invertebrates and in all five classes of vertebrate hosts [16]. Their extrusion apparatus, always with a polar tube and cap [2]. Microsporidia are currently classified on the basis of their ultrastructural features, including size and morphology of the spores, number of coils of the polar tube, developmental life cycle and host-parasite relationship [17].

Some species infect the muscle, dermal or subdermal cysts are seen and often rupture through the skin [5]. Some species form cysts within the intestinal wall such as *Thelohanellus kitauei*, cause intestinal giant cystic disease of carp [5]. The intracellular parasite, *Ichthyosporidium, Glugea* and *Spraguea* replicate and cause cytomegaly, leads to atrophy and encapsulating fibroplasia. A large xenoma with a refractile wall and filled with refractile spores may elicit the formation of granulation tissue [5]. Moreover, *Glugea* spp. cause serious pathological changes in a variety of tissues. It infects macrophages and other mesenchymal cells that subsequently undergo massive hypertrophy, causing space-occupying compression and deformations [5].

Many species of microsporidians do not induce hypertrophy of the myocyte but rather replicates within the sarcoplasm, eventually occupying and destroying it such as *Pleistophora* [5]. *P. macrozorcidis* infect the ocean pouts *Macrozoarces americanus*, their cyst within the muscle give the gross appearance of neoplasms [5]. These may cause pressure necrosis of the overlying skin with release of spores into the water as a consequence [5]. *P. longifilis* is recorded from the testis of *Barbus flaviatilis* in Germany [5]. In some species such as *P. ovariae*, ovaries are the prime target of this parasite in golden shiner *Notemigonus crysoleucas*. The large cysts are considered to reduce fecundity, cause pressure atrophy of adjacent uninfected ova and parenchyma and lead to sterility [5].

The genera *Heterosporis, Kabatana, Microsporidium, Pleistophora* and *Thelohania* have been found to infect muscle tissue [16]. Some microsporidian may infect brain and heart for example, *Spraguea lophii* is found in the cerebrospinal ganglia of angle fish, *Lophius* spp.

where it evokes grossly visible xenoma formation [5]. *Loma* sp. cause endarteritis of epizootic proportions in juvenile Chinook salmon [5].

The aquatic parasite microsporideans, such as *Pleistophora* sp. infect muscle of fairy shrimp *Branchinella thailandensis* [10]. In host' muscle, white tubular masses are seen which are indicative of microsporidian infection. Close contact between the sporophorous vesicle and degenerating muscle fibers are observed, but there is no evidence of xenoma or a host response to the parasite (Figure 3). In another case, *Thelohania* (*Agmasoma*) infect both the hepatopancreas and abdominal muscle of Pacific white shrimp (*Litopenaeus vannamei*). Affected shrimp show a whitish or milky appearance in various parts of the body. As the shrimp grow larger, this clinical signs are more easily observed especially dorsally from the hepatopancreas to the middle of the body. Histological changes found in microsporidian infection of most of the hepatopancreas. Hepatopancreatic tubules of the heavily infected shrimp are dilated and necrotic. Gills and striated abdominal muscle are mostly infected by microsporidia [18] (Figure 4).

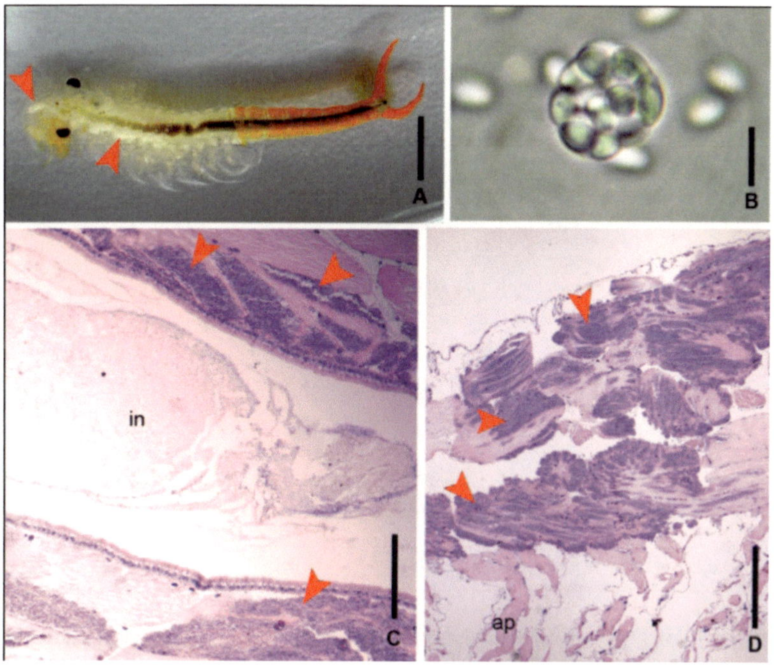

Figure 3. Fairy shrimp *Branchinella thailandensis* infected with microsporidia.
(A) *B. thailandensis* infected with microsporidia, white tubular masses (arrow) indicative of microsporidia infection. (scale bar = 3 mm)
(B) Fresh spores of *Pleistophora* sp. showing one group of spores in a sporophorous vesicle. (scale bar = 6 μm) (source: Purivirojkul W., Khidprasert S. First report of microsporidiosis in fairy shrimp *Branchinella thailandensis* (Sanoamuang, Saengphan and Murugan, 2002). Aquaculture 2009; 289 (1-2) 185-190)
(C) Longitudinal section of *B. thailandensis* at intestine region, the muscle fibers were damaged by microsporidia (arrow). (scale bar = 100 μm) (in = intestine)
(D) Longitudinal section of muscle at the dorsal part of *B. thailandensis* shows degenerating muscle fibers (H&E). (scale bar = 500 μm) (ap = appendage of fairy shrimp)

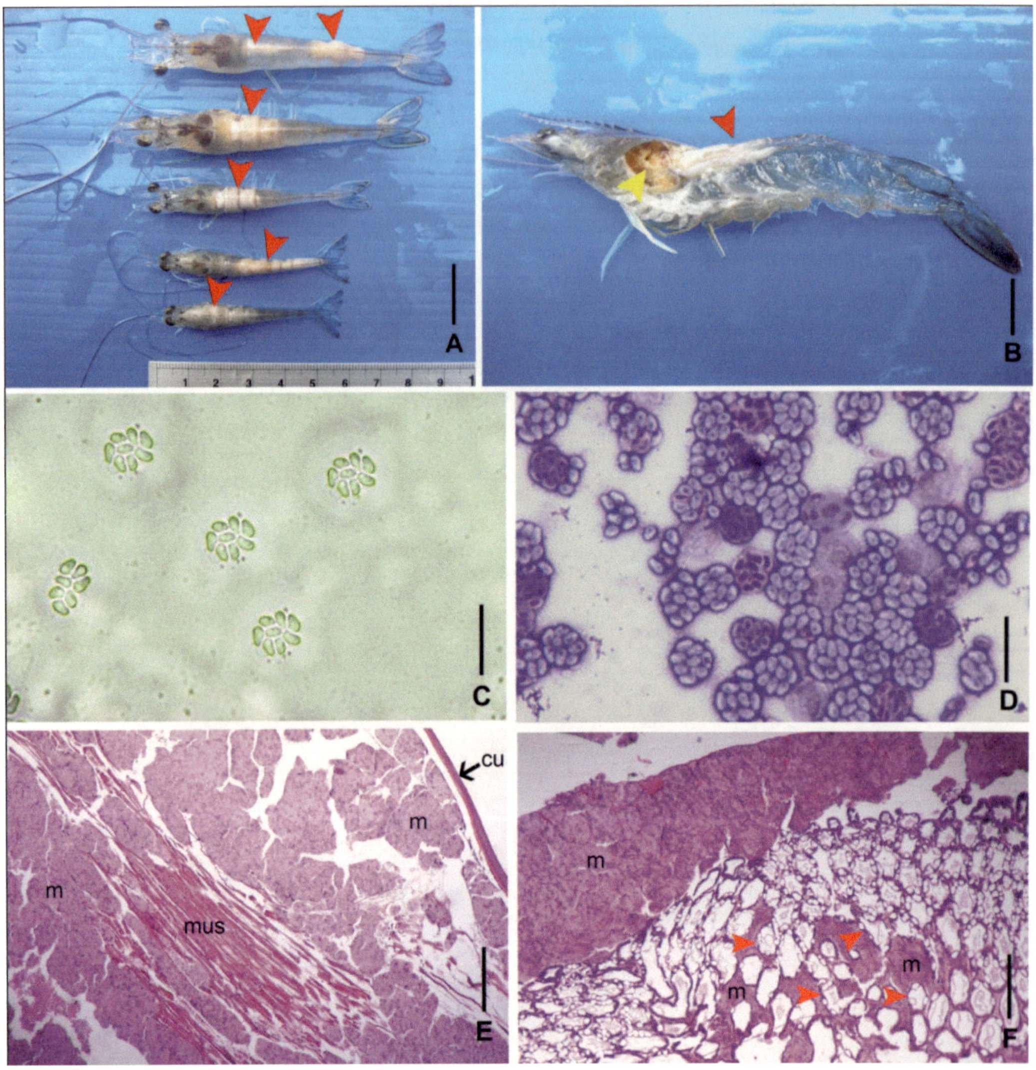

Figure 4. Microsporidian (*Thelohania*) infection in Pacific white shrimp (*Litopenaeus vannamei*) (Photo from Associated Professor Dr. Chalor Limsuwan).
(A) Various size Pacific white shrimp were infected by microsporidia (arrow). (scale bar = 1.5 cm)
(B) Long section of Pacific white shrimp, showed white masses of microsporidian in infested striated muscle (red arrow) and hepatopancreas (yellow arrow). (scale bar = 1 cm)
(C) Fresh spores of *Thelohania* sp. showing 8 spores in a sporophorous vesicle.
(D) Giemsa's strain of *Thelohania* sp. (C,D scale bar = 15 μm)
(E) Striated muscles of infected shrimp, the muscle fibers were damaged and replaced by microsporidia. (scale bar = 200 μm)
(F) Hepatopancreatic tubule epithelium of heavily microsporidian-infected shrimp were dilated and necrotic (arrows). (scale bar = 200 μm)
(cu = cuticle, m = microspore, mus = striated muscles)

2.6. Phylum Apicomplexa

Members of this phylum have a unique organelle, the apical complex, visible only with the electron microscope [2]. They are intracellular parasites, the apical complex serves to assist in penetrating the host cell [2]. The genus *Eimeria* is often reported as fish parasite both marine and freshwater fish. *Eimeria subepithelialis* is the cause of nodular coccidiosis in European carp, the mucosa is damaged when the parasites are released [5]. *Eimeria brevoortiana* are present in the testis of menhaden and get shedded with the milt [5]. In some case, this group of parasite can destroy host tissue such as *Calyptospora* (*Eimeria*) *fundulil* can damage 85% of the liver and pancreas of killifish *Fundalus grandis* when infect in large number [5].

3. Phylum platyhelminthes

Members of phylum Platyhelminthes have a dorsoventrally flattened, bilaterally symmetrical body. This phylum is the first phylum which exhibit three primary germ layers; ectoderm, mesoderm and endoderm. Aquatic parasitology in this phylum includes four classes; Turbellaria, Monogene, Digenia and Cestoda.

3.1. Turbellaria

Although, most of turbellarian are free-living worms but *Ichthyophaga* and *Paravortex* are reported as fish parasites. *Paravortex* spp. infest a wide variety of fishes and molluscs [19-20]. They induce a hypermelanization reaction, resulting in dark foci on the skin, there may be acute, focal dermatitis and hemorrhage [4]. *Piscinquilinus* (*Ichthyophaga*) sp. is reported in marine fish such as a parrotfish (*Scarus ribulatus*). This parasite induces a proliferative epithelial response [4].

3.2. Monogenea

Monogenes are common parasites of the skin and gills of both marine and freshwater fish [4]. Monogenes feed on the superficial layers of the skin and gills, causes skin cloudiness or focal reddening resulting from excess mucus production [4]. Large numbers of monogenes can kill small fish [4]. Taxonomic identification of monogenes is based on the morphology of opishaptor (posterior attachment organ), mode of reproduction and presence of eye spot, etc. [4]. However, *Dactylogyrus* spp. (gill flukes) usually attaches to the gills of freshwater fish (Figure 5). *Gyrodactylus* spp. (skin flukes) usually attached to the skin of freshwater fish. Monogenes have the simple life cycle without having intermediate hosts.

In skin area, epithelial hyperplasia or hemorrhage are found in monogene infected area [21]. Heavy monogenean infections by their attachment and feeding can induce a range of histopathological changes to the epithelium [22], sometimes severe dermatitis with hyperplasia [5]. *Gyrodactylus* sp. parasite on fish skin may cause superficial lesions of the epidermis. This parasite attaches to and feeds on the epidermis, causes an increase in production of mucus. The excess mucus disturbs the respiratory function of the skin [5].

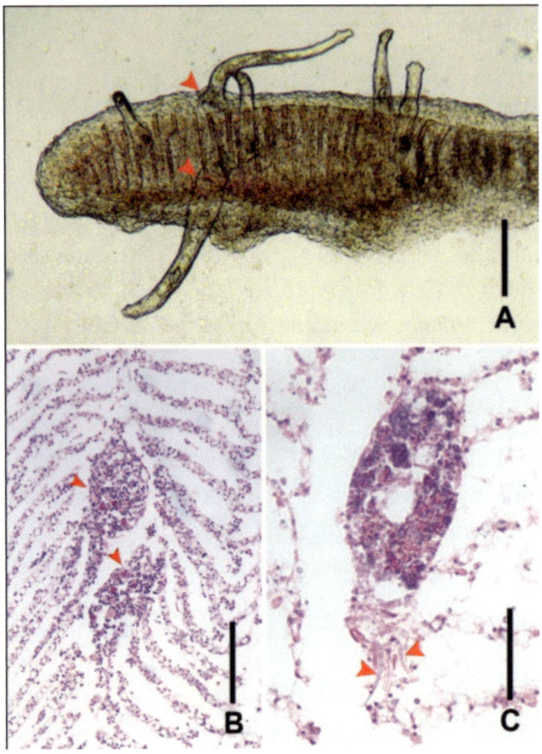

Figure 5. Monogene infested on gill of fish.
(A) Fresh sample, opishaptor (arrows) attach to gill filament of fish. (scale bar = 70 μm)
(B) *Dactylogyrus* sp. infested on gill filaments of *Barbonymus gonionotus*. Hyperplasia of gill filament were observed (arrows). (scale bar = 70 μm)
(C) Anchor of *Dactylogyrus* sp. (arrows) attached to the gill filaments of *Barbonymus gonionotus*. (scale bar = 50 μm) (Photo by Ms.Tanawan Leeboonngam).

Most of monogene infect the gill area (Figure 5), a proliferation of epithelial tissue resulting in the fusion of the secondary lamellae by the attach of the opisthaptor. In some gills, this latter pathology was accompanied by the presence of blood vessel aneurysms (telangiectasis) [22]. Histopathological change by monogene on fish gill was also studied by [22]. In the histological sections of cultured European sea bass, *Dicentrarchus labrax*, the opisthaptors of the parasites *Diplectanum aequans* were observed to penetrate in the basal membrane of primary lamella where they induced a hyperplastic response. Disruption and fusion of the secondary lamellae are common in all infected specimens where several individuals are with erosion and inflammation of the epithelium of the primary and secondary lamellae. The infection of monogenes in fish gills have an impact on the host's ability to regulate its ion balance. This parasite can reduce the number of chloride cells which are the main site of ion absorption and secretion [23].

Another site of infection are reported in *Neobenedenia melleni* which causes serious skin damage and has a predilection for the eye [4]. The hooks of parasite cause ophthalmic lesions leading to blindness [24].

3.3. Digenea

Digeneans have two suckers to attach their host; oral sucker surrounding the mouth and ventral sucker (acetabulum) on the ventral surface. The life cycle of this group consists of intermediate hosts (one or two types) and final host. They form seven different developmental stages; egg, miracidium, sporocyst, rediae, cercariae, metacercariae and adult. In Aquatic animals, sporocyst stage usually found in infected gastropod (Mollusca: Gastropoda) (Figure 6A). Metacercariae (Figure 6B) and adult may be found as parasites of fish. Metacercariae encyst Metacercariae are found in many sites throughout the host such as gill, fin, bone, muscle, eyeballs, brain, spinal cord, nervous system, intestinal peritoneum, liver, gall bladder, heart ventricle and kidney [4]. Adult trematodes are found in skin, gill, intestine, stomach, pyloric caeca. Sometime other larval stages are reported to effect the aquatic animals such as *Sanguinicola klamathensis* miracidium cause acute hemorrhage of the gills accompanies the mass exodus of this parasite [5].

Many species of freshwater fishes serve as second intermediate host of digenetic trematode [25]. Five families of digenetic trematodes metacercariae are reported from fresh water fish namely, Clinostomidae, Diplostomidae, Isoparorchiidae, Strigeidae and Heterophyidae [26-27]. Trematodes metacercariae encyst in different organs of fish such as fin, skin, gill, branchial chamber, body cavity and other internal organs (intestinal peritoneum, liver, gall bladder, heart ventricle, on the bulbus arteriosus, kidney) [28-30]. Invasions of metacercariae of numerous trematode species result in pathogenic changes occurring in different organs of the intermediate hosts affected [31].

Metacercariae of *Apophallus* sp. are encapsulated by new bone or present within vertebral spines. The metacercariae are associated with prominent dysplastic and cartilage proliferation, often resulting in complete encapsulation of the parasite [12]. Proliferation of branchial cartilage can occur in response to encysted digenetic metacercariae [5]. Some metacercariae encyst within filamental cartilage of goldfish gill. The hyperplastic response has distorted the normal architecture [5]. Metacercariae of heterophyid digeneans cause prominent dysplastic and proliferative changes in the gill cartilage of freshwater fishes [32-33]. Histopathological examination of the infected fish gills reveals the cartilage proliferation around metacercarial cysts, hyperplasia, hypertrophy and fusion in the affected gill filaments [34]. Lesions of the gills associated with parasitic infection vary with the agent, host and density of infection [2]. Metacercariae of *Centrocestus* sp. located in gill cartilage cause similar respiratory stress in cichlids and carp and mortality in farmed Japanese elvers [35].

Digeneans metacercariae are frequently found in the skin. Metacercaria may or may not evoke a melanin response, if they do, the parasites become a grossly visible as black spot such as *Cryptocotyle lingua* which cause black spot disease [5]. Also in other species, *Diplostomulum* sp. cause of black spot disease, they invade in the epidermis. The black spots are due to melanophore infiltration of the dermis in response to the presence of the metacercariae [5]. Muscle infections by *Bucephalus polymorphus* causes vertebral deformities in cyprinid fishes [36]. *Euclinostomum heterostomum* is very widespread in many regions in Europe, Asia and Africa [37]. Metacercariae of this parasite infect in the muscular tissues of freshwater fish.

Histopathological section has shown metacercariae invaded into the muscular tissue and was encapsulated by a sheet of connective tissue in host musculature (Figure 7).

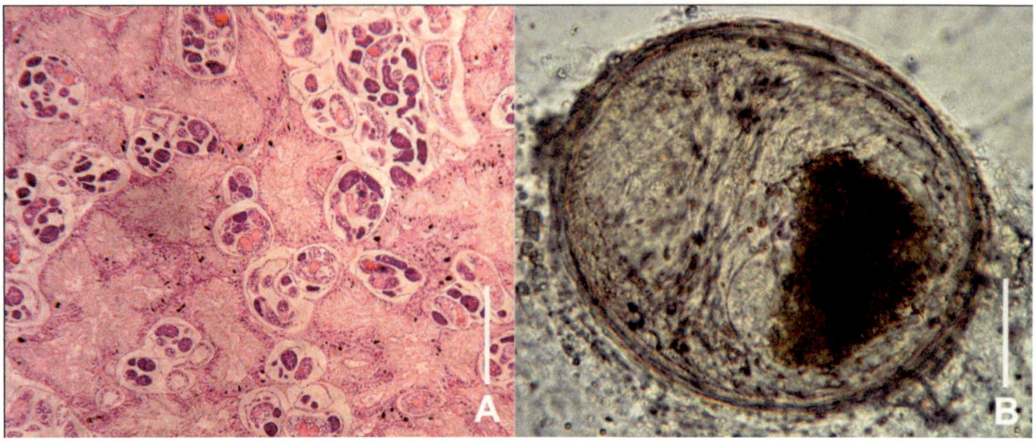

Figure 6. Some larval stage of digeneans.
(A) Sporocyst stage infected gastropod. (scale bar = 200 µm)
(B) Metacercaria infected fish muscle. (scale bar = 40 µm)

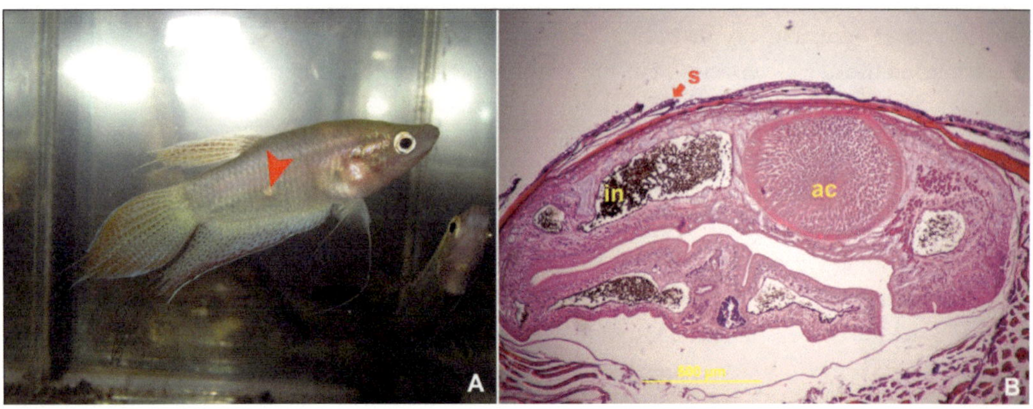

Figure 7. *Euclinostomum* sp. metacercariae infected in the muscle of *Trichopsis vittata*.
(A) *Trichopsis vittata* infested with metacercaria of *Euclinostomum* sp. (arrow) (Photo from Mr. Montri Sumontha)
(B) Histopathological section of fish muscle infected by *Euclinostomum* sp. metacercariae showed metacercariae invaded into the muscular tissue and was encapsulated by sheet of connective tissue in host musculature. (ac = acetabulum, in = intestine, s = scale)

Examples of some metacercariae such as *Diplostomum spathaceum*, *Cotylurus erraticus* parasite in eyeballs and brain of numerous cyprinids, destroy the structure of the eye and cause disappearance of rods following blindness [31, 38-39]. *Bucephalus polymorphus* and *Rhipidocotyle illense* are occurred in eyeballs, brain, spinal cord and nervous system coats. Histopathological changes are found as cornea delamination and retina damage leading to blindness [40-41]. Metacecariae of *Apophallus brevis* (sand-grain grub) found in yellow perch causing bony cysts within the lumen of the peripheral vasculature, especially in the axial musculature, but also of the extrinsic muscles of the eye [5]. Some metacercariae are occasionally found within extralenticular sites such as cornea and retina, usually with minimal inflammatory reaction [5]. Immature *Diplostomum* can be found in many host fish tissues including all portions of the eye, often causing very little host reaction [5].

In kidney, vast necrosis of the endoparenchymal tissue and hemorrhage from the main kidney vein near metacercaria cyst are found [31]. In kidney parenchyma, complex granulation of connective tissue cells and blood morphotic elements are seen. Metacercaria cyst wall with connective tissue fiber layer results in congested and necrotically changed kidney parenchyma . Degeneration necrosis of the kidney tissue are reported. [31].

In pericardium, inflammational infiltration, destroyed structure and fragmentation of muscle fibers, necrotic lesion, extravasation of erythrocytes, cytolysis of muscle fibers and karyolysis or heteropyknosis of nuclei were found in pericardium when fish are infected by metacercariae this also include losses of muscle tissue [31]. The degenerative and inflammational processes are associated with disturbed circulation [31]. For more cases, metacercariae of digenean *Stephanostomum baccatum* infected rainbow trout pericardium. A constrictive pericarditis is occasionally seen in severe fibrogranulomatous responses [5].

In some case, adult *Sanguinicola inermis* infected in the branchial and other vessels of fish, released eggs that hatched in the gill capillaries. These then migrated out of the vessels, causing hemorrhage and possibly death [5].

3.4. Cestoda

Cestode (tapeworms) body consists of three regions; scolex, neck and strobila. Cestodes do not have a digestive system, for this reason adult forms are usually found in host intestine to absorb host nutrients through the integument. The attachment of cestode in fish intestine cause necrosis, hemorrhage and inflammation at attachment points, space occupying distension of the intestine and possible perforation for example pseudophylliidean tapeworm, *Bothriocephalus gowkongensis* found to infect the cyprinids [5].

Larval stage of cestodes are also reported as parasite in fish. The larval cestode *Diphyllobothrium dentriticum* can cause severe granulomatous enteritis in trout and lead to peritonitis with visceral adhesions and death [5]. Larval tapeworm, *Ligula* is found in the peritoneal cavity, will cause pressure atrophy of ovaries [5].

4. Phylum Nematoda

Nematodes are invertebrate round worms, they are elongated, cylindrical form with unsegmented body. The diseases occur due to the adult and larval nematodes which are very common in marine fishes. The nematode parasites infect various tissues and organs of fish such as stomach, intestine, liver, gonads, visceral mesenteries, peritoneum body cavity, blood vessels, swim bladder, and connective tissues, fin, orbits of the eye and brain [42]. Most species of nematodes in adult stage live in the alimentary canal except the family Philometridae which are found in body cavity, liver and gonads [42]. *Philometra* spp. and

Philometroides spp. cause chronic active ulcerative dermatitis [5]. *Philometra* sp. may encyst within the testes cause trauma from migrating of this parasite [5]. Moreover, *Philometra* is found in the ovaries (Figure 8A) as well as testis and although there may be little effect on egg production, in some cases there is hemorrhage, fibrosis, and increased number of melanomacrophages [5].

Nematode larvae are more harmful than adults and can penetrate into the tissues of various organs, causing severe tissue damage and destruction of the cells of the organ [42]. Ascarididans (Order Ascaridida) are reported to parasitize fish and cephalopods [43]. Their larval stage occurs in the internal organ or maybe digestive tracts of marine fish (Figure 8B). Pathogenesis is a result of their mode of feeding, attachment and movement or migration within the host [42]. Ascarididans genera *Phocanema* (*Pseudoterranova*) and *Contracaecum* are found within the muscle, the effect on the fish is usually minimal [5]. Another genus of Ascarididans, *Anisakis simplex* causes infection of cod, where gastritis, craterous granulomatous lesions can be found [5]. Larval stage of *Anisakis* can be present in number which is large enough to represent a space occupying threat to normal functioning [5]. The infected intestine by the nematode parasites causes destruction, atrophy of intestinal mucosa, necrosis and degeneration of the intestinal tissue, causing damage to the whole thickness of the bowel wall due to nematode larvae [42]. *Capillaria* spp. may cause hepatic destruction if the infection is massive, either by virtue of the parasites themselves or their eggs [5].

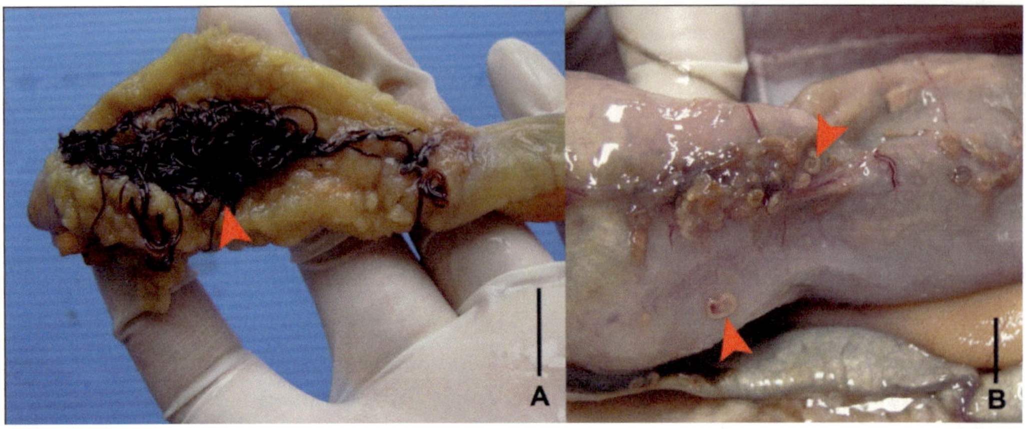

Figure 8. Nematode infest marine fish.
(A) *Philometra* sp. (arrow) is found in the ovary of marine fish *Lutianus johni*.
(B) Larval stage of ascarididans (arrow) occur in the internal wall of marine fish *Trichiurus haumela*.
(scale bar = 1 cm)

In reference [42] reported the histological change of the intestinal wall of *Pomadasys maculatum* with nematode where erosion of intestinal wall with loss of villous epithelial lining was usually seen. If the fish get infected with nematode, all the intestinal morphology become lost. Villious structures are not differentiated and appear as string of tissues. The mucosa of infected intestine appeared congested and edematous. The deformation of mucosa and submucosa results in separation of muscle fibers. The shape of villi are changed as compared with the normal shapes [42].

5. Phylum Acanthocephala

Acanthocephala is a phylum of parasitic worms which have the presence of an evertable proboscis (Figure 9). Body of acanthocephalan consist of two part presoma (proboscis, anterior neck, and posterior neck) and metasoma (trunk). The proboscis extend through the host epithelium into the submucosa with limited hemorrhaging at the point of attachment. The lumen of the host intestine was obstructed, and compressed villi were present [44]. Attachment point of acanthocephalans may be necrotic and can be even perforated, leading to peritonitis [5]. In reference [45] reported the histopathological changes when the presoma and the anterior part of the metasoma of *Longicollum pagrosomi* passed through the intestinal wall and infect the intestinal tissue, perforating the loose connective tissue. In the inflammatory connective tissue, collagen and muscle fibers were fragmented and revealed partial necrosis. Lipid drops and eosinophilic granular cells aggregated in the connective tissue of the tissue capsule.

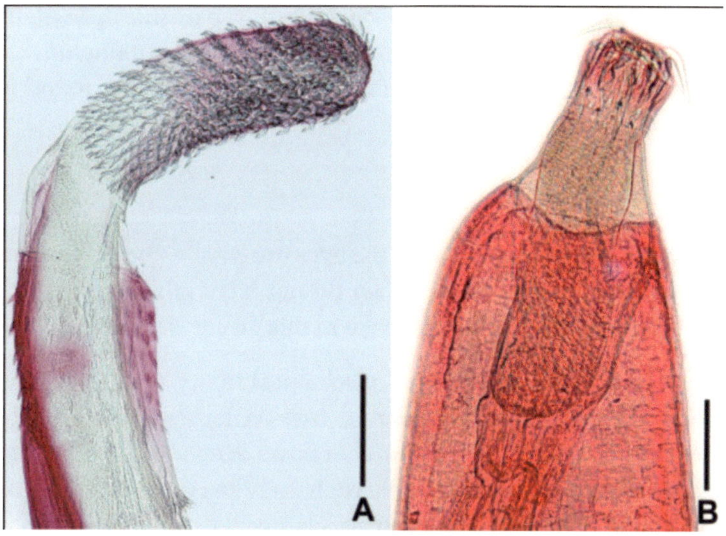

Figure 9. Anterior part of some acanthocephalans from marine fish.
(A) *Serrasentis* sp.
(B) *Neoechinorhynchus* sp. (scale bar = 130 μm)

In reference [46] observed heavy infections of acanthocephalan parasite, *Tenuiproboscis* sp. in the mangrove red snapper (*Lutjanus argentimaculatus*). They found that the large number of acanthocephalans in the posterior region of the intestine, almost blocking the lumen. At the site of parasite attachment, the surface of the intestine appeared thickened and the mucosal epithelium showed compression and abrasion. Intestinal folds were eroded along with the thickening of lamina propria. The presoma of the parasites pierced the mucosal epithelium, lamina propria, muscle layers and serosa, reaching the peritoneal cavity, surrounded by a tunnel with collagenous fibers and granulocytes. Inflammation, granular tissue formation, connective tissue proliferation and associated host immune reactions were evident.

6. Phylum Annelida

Annelids are eucoelomate, exhibit metamerism. They are known as segmented worms. The phylum is divided into three classes; Polychaeta, Oligochaeta and Hirudinea. Only class Hirudinea (leeches) are parasites, with a fixed number of body segments 34. They have anterior and posterior suckers, leeches can attach to hosts by using this sucker. Leeches are rare in cultured fish but are occasionally seen in wild or pond-raised fish [4]. Heavily infected fish often have a chronic anaemia [4]. This group of parasite cause skin lesions of fish. They damages the skin and small round wounds are found. In other site of infections, destruction of the fins and erosion of epithelium of the isthmus region of fish are also reported. *Piscicola* spp. cause ulcerative dermatitis with hyperemia, hemorrhage and epidermal hyperplasia [5].

7. Phylum Arthropoda

The body of arthropods consists of head, thorax and abdomen. They have exoskeleton and have jointed appendages, one pair to each somite, but in parasitic species, the appendages usually reduce or lost. All aquatic parasites are the members of Subphylum Crustacea. Class Branchiura, Copepoda and Malacostraca (order Isopoda) are usually found as parasites in aquatic animals.

7.1. Class Branchiura

The branchiurans are flattened crustaceans. the eyes are sessile, the antennae are very small, the abdomen is small and unsegmented. They do not have gills, most of branchiurans are parasites of fish. A known genus of fish parasite in this group is *Argulus* (Figure 10).

Argulus sp. has a preoral stylet causes local mechanical injury and especially the release of digestive enzymes, giving rise to systemic as well as local effects [5]. They scrape the epithelium while feeding, causing erosions and at times deep ulcers extending to bone. They attach to the host by pressing their shield-like cephalothorax onto the skin like a sucker. The second antennae and maxillipeds are used as clamps [4]. It may cause small petechial hemorrhages at feeding sites and also necrotizing and ulcerative dermatitis [4, 47].

The copepod body is short and cylindrical. The head and thorax are fused to form a cephalothorax. Parasitic copepods are increasingly serious problems in cultured fish and can also impact wild populations. Most parasites affect marine fish [4]. Parasitic copepods attached to the host by frontal filament of chalimus larvae [4]. Most sites of infections are gill, fin or skin but sometimes they can attach to oral cavity or eye. Such as Greenland sharks had copepods embedded in both corneas [5]. Histopathological change of fish infected by copepod are epithelial erosions, ulceration around the site of attachment of the parasite's mouth organs, hemorrhages and around the penetration sites of the claws there occur tissue necrosis, proliferation happens around the site of penetration of antennae [4]. Some copepods may be deeply embedded within the skin and elicit host response, mainly localized in mild dermal fibrosis and epidermal hyperplasia [5].

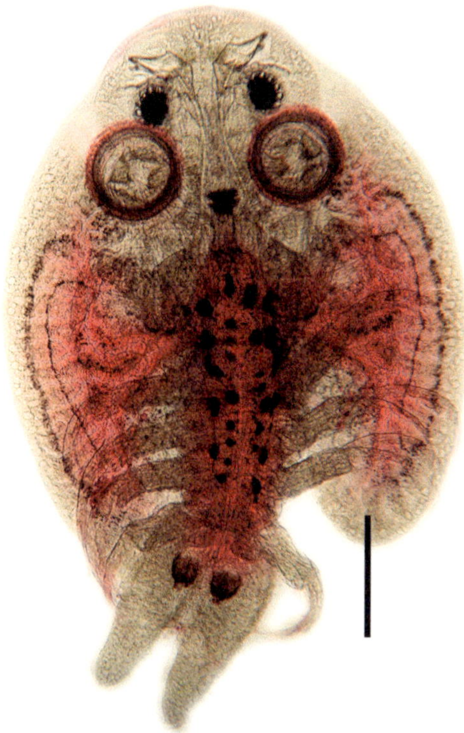

Figure 10. *Argulus* sp. (scale bar = 1 mm)

7.2. Copepoda

Lernaea spp. (anchor worms) insert part of their body, burrow deeply into tissues and evokes severe acute inflammation [4, 47]. Necrotizing and ulcerative dermatitis are seen [5]. Hemorrhage at the site of attachment, or hyperplasia or fibroblast may develop at the attachment site [4]. Heavy infections can lead to debilitation, secondary infection by bacterial or fungal infection will follow [48].

Ergasilus spp. have antennae modified for gasping the host and large trunk for reproductive products [49] mostly infected the gills of freshwater fish and marine fish [4]. Ergasilid copepods have extrabuccal digestion that leads to lysis of tissue and hyperplasia at the point of attachment [5]. In reference [50] study the host (*Abramis brama*) response when attach by *E. sieboldi* on their gill. The parasite elicits an intense host cellular reaction at the site of attachment with a high number of inflammatory cells, eosinophilic granular cells and neutrophilic granular cells.

Lepeophtheirus causes severe ulcerative dematitis with loss of substantial areas of the skin [5]. In some case, this copepod only superficially attach to the skin such as in *L. pectoralis*, the slight penetration of this parasite elicits massive dermal fibroplasia with hemorrhage in severe cases and a chronic inflammatory infiltrate [5].

In elasmobranch, *Eudactylina* sp. found from gill of shark *Chiloscyllium punctatum*. Histological examination of gill tissue has shown hyperplasia of the gill filaments and fusion of secondary lamellae and finally loss of respiratory surface area (Figure 11).

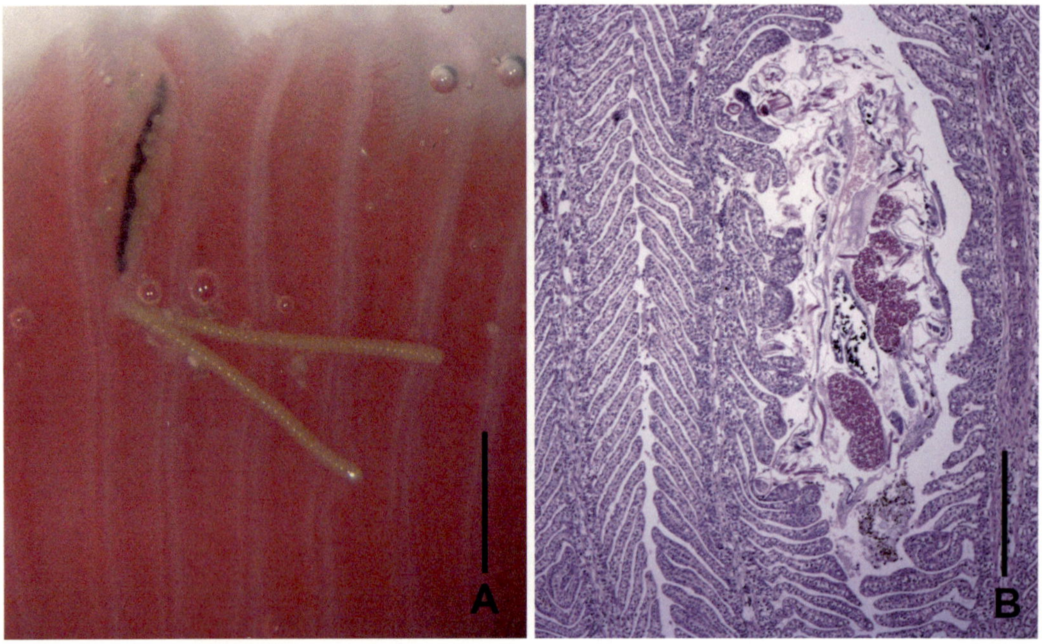

Figure 11. *Eudactylina* sp. from gill of *Chiloscyllium punctatum*.
(A) Fresh sample.
(B) Gill filament, sagittal section. The histological structures of the secondary lamellae pathology, gill lamellae were damaged at attach site. (scale bar = 1 mm)

7.3. Order Isopoda

Isopod predominantly attach to the body or fins of the fish, although some have been discovered inside gill chambers, buccal cavities and body pouches [51-53]. They occur in marine, estuarine and freshwater habitats, especially in the near shore coastal environment [52,54]. Single isopod can cause damage with their biting and sucking mouth parts. Heavy infestations of parasitic juveniles can kill small fish when they first attach [4].

Many genera of isopods are reported as parasite of fish both teleost and elasmobranch such as *Livoneca*, *Alitropus*, *Nerocila*, *Gnathia*, *Cirolana*, *Rocinela* and *Aega*. Recently, *Nerocila depressa* is found to attach to the bodies of *Sardinella albella* [55]. The hooks of the pereopods penetrate into the skin and anchor the isopod to the fish host. At the mouth part or pereopod site of attachment, the skin (epidermis and dermis) are eroded and exposed to the underlying tissue (Figure 12).

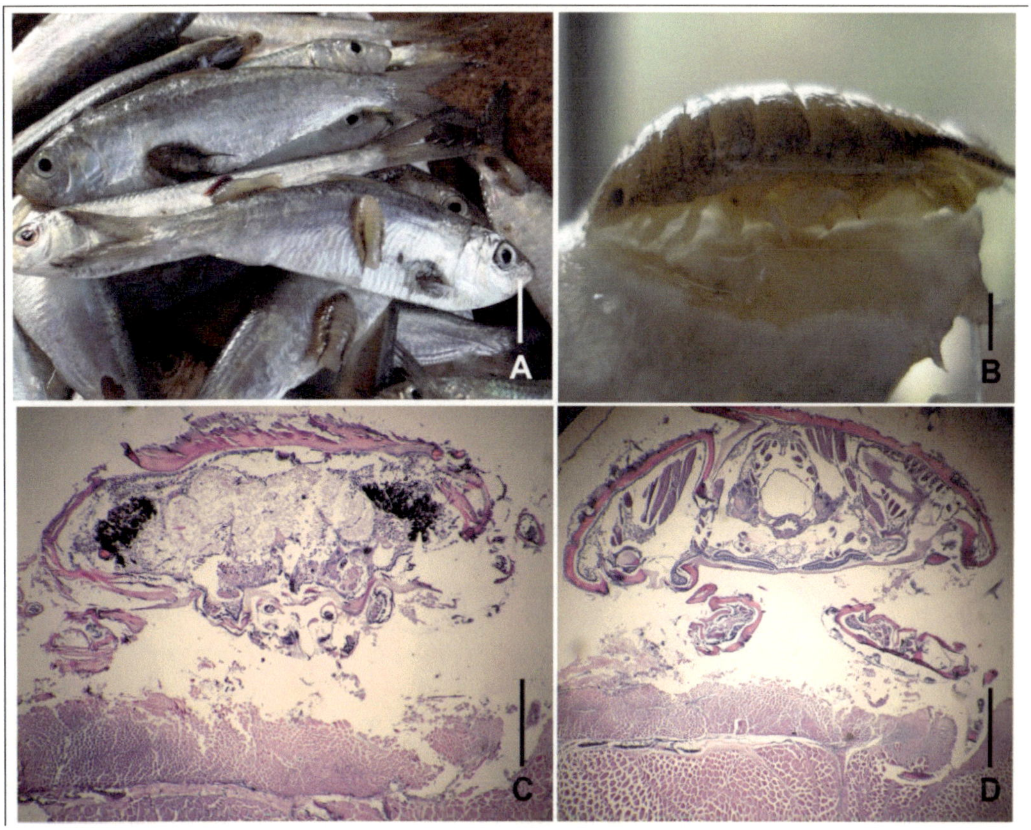

Figure 12. *Nerocila depressa* attached to the bodies of *Sardinella albella*.
(source: Printrakoon C, Purivirojkul W. Prevalence of *Nerocila depressa* (Isopoda, Cymothoidae) on *Sardinella albella* from a Thai estuary. Journal of Sea Research 2011; 65(2) 322–326.)
(A) *Nerocila depressa* attached *Sardinela albella*. (scale bar = 2 cm)
(B) *N. depressa* using hook-like legs penetrated in the skin of *S. albella*.
(scale bar = 250 μm)
(C) Pathology at the skin caused by biting mouthparts (arrow) of *N. depressa*.
(scale bar = 300 μm)
(D) Pathology of the skin caused by piercing of the pereopods (arrow). (scale bar = 300 μm)

8. Phylum Mollusca

The larvae of fresh water bivalve molluscs (Bivalvia: Unionoida) are often found attached to the gills and outer surfaces of fish. The larvae have thin bivalve shells often with little hooks on their inner edge [2]. This larva stage call "glochidia", usually found from gill both wide and cultured freshwater fish. Histopathology change of host by glochidia infection found hyperplasia of the epithelium, granulomatous dermatitis [5]. After glochidia attached the gills or outer surfaces of fish, epidermal or branchial epithelial cells of the host ultimately encapsulate the larva, completely enveloping it to form a cyst [56] (Figure 13). However, the glochidia must attach to a suitable host fish, if a glochidium attaches to a fish that is unsuitable as a host, an "abnormal" cyst may form and finally glochidium may death [57-58].

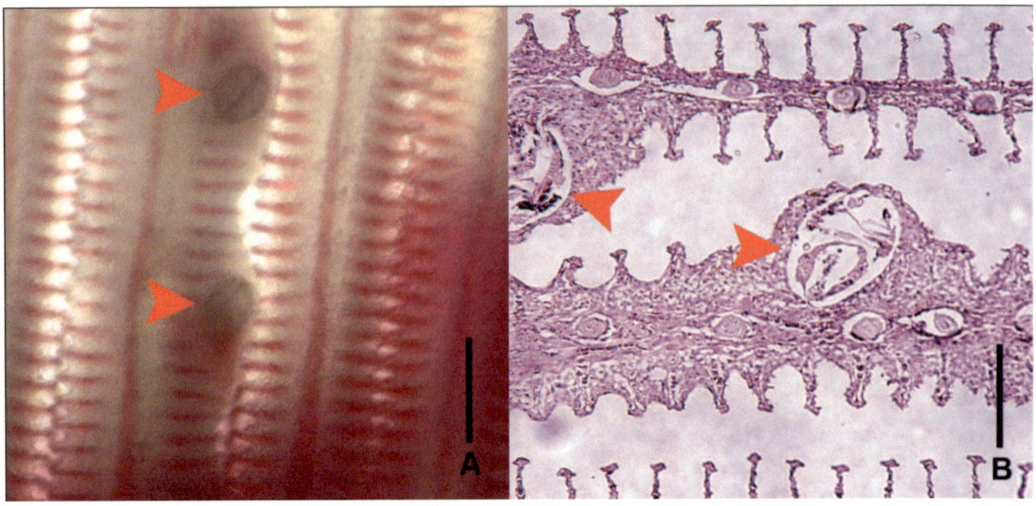

Figure 13. Glochidia of freshwater mollusc from the gill of *Pangasianodon gigas*.
(source: Purivirojkul W, Areechon N, Purukkiate C. Parasites and bacteria of giant catfishes (*Pangasianodon gigas* Chevey) larva. Thai science and technology journal 2004; 12(3) 1-11.)
(A) glochidia attached to the gills of a giant catfish (arrows). (scale bar = 400 μm)
(B) Host tissue has completely surrounded the glochidia (arrow). (scale bar = 250 μm)

9. Conclusion

Although the first step of identifying parasitic specimen is the direct wet mount but in some case the parasites are difficult to distinguish grossly, histology has a role in helping to identify intracellular parasite. Tissue stains not only use for the identification of the parasite but also in the visualization of cellular morphology [59]. Moreover, histopathology can use for examining each organ system for tells tale changes due to pathogenic agents and confirm the diagnosis [60].

Author details

Watchariya Purivirojkul
Department of Zoology, Faculty of Science, Kasetsart University, Thailand

Acknowledgement

The author would like to thank Associated Professor Dr. Chalor Limsuwan, Mr. Montri Sumontha and Dr. Cheewarut Printrakool for provide their own picture for this chapter and also thanks to Assistant Professor Siriwan Khidprasert for provide fairy shrimp specimens.

10. References

[1] Klontz GW. Diagnostic methods in fish diseases: Present status and needs. In: Ellis AE. (ed.) Fish and shellfish pathology. London: Academic press; 1985. p1-10.

[2] Roberts RJ. Fish pathology, 3rd edition. London: W.B. Saunders publishing; 2001.

[3] MacMillan JR. 1991 Biological factors impinging upon control of external protozoan fishparasites. Annual Review of Fish Disease 1 119-131.

[4] Noga EJ. Fish disease: diagnosis and treatment. Iowa: Iowa state university press; 2000.

[5] Ferguson H. Systemic pathology of fish: a text and atlas of comparative tissue responses in diseases of teleosts. Ames: Iowa state university Press; 1989.

[6] Bustos PA, Young ND, Rozas MA, Bohle HM, Ildefonso RS, Morrison RN, Nowak BF. Amoebic gill disease (AGD) in Atlantic salmon (Salmo salar) farmed in Chile. Aquaculture 2011; 310 281–288.

[7] Young ND, Crosbie PBB, Adams MB, Nowak BF, Morrison RN. *Neoparamoeba perurans* n. sp., an agent of amoebic gill disease of Atlantic salmon (*Salmo salar* L.). International Journal for Parasitology 2007; 37 1469–1481.

[8] Wiles M, Cone D, Odense PH. Studies on Chilodonella cyprinid and C. hexasticha (Protozoa: Ciliata) by scanning electron microscope. Canadian Journal of Zoology-Revue Canadienne de Zoologie 1985; 63 2483-2487.

[9] Lom J. Adhesive disc of Trichodinella epizootica – ultrastructure and injury to the host tissue. Folia Parasitologica 1973; 20 193-202.

[10] Purivirojkul W., Khidprasert S. First report of microsporidiosis in fairy shrimp *Branchinella thailandensis* (Sanoamuang, Saengphan and Murugan, 2002). Aquaculture 2009; 289 (1-2) 185-190.

[11] Basson L, Van As J. Trichodinidae and other Ciliophorans (Phylum Ciliophora). In: Woo PTK. (ed.) Fish diseases and disorders Volume 1: protozoan and metazoan infections 2nd edition. London: CAB international; 2006. p154-182.

[12] Kent ML, Watral VG, Whipps CM, Cunningham ME, Criscione CD, Heidel JR., Curtis L R, Spitsbergen J, Markle DF. A Digenean Metacercaria (*Apophallus* sp.) and a Myxozoan (*Myxobolus* sp.). Associated with Vertebral Deformities in Cyprinid Fishes from the Willamette River, Oregon. Journal of Aquatic Animal Health 2004; 16 116–129.

[13] Baska F, Voronin VN, Eszterbauer E, Müller L, Marton S, Molnár K. Occurrence of two myxosporean species, *Myxobolus hakyi* sp. n. and *Hoferellus pulvinatus* sp. n., in *Pangasianodon hypophthalmus* fry imported from Thailand to Europe as ornamental fish. Parasitology Research 2009; 105 1391–1398.

[14] Bahri S, Marton S, Marques A, Eszterbauer E. *Henneguya tunisiensis* n. sp. (Myxosporea: Bivalvulida), a new gill parasite of *Symphodus tinca* (L.) (Teleostei: Labridae) off Tunisia. Systematic Parasitology 2010; 76 93–101.

[15] Molnár K. Taxonomic problems, seasonality and histopathology of *Henneguya creplini* (Myxosporea) infection of the pikeperch *Stizostedion lucioperca* in Lake Balaton. Folia Parasitologica 1998; 45 261–269.

[16] Lom J, Dyková I, Myxozoan genera: definition and notes on taxonomy, life-cycle terminology and pathogenic species. Folia Parasitologica 2006; 53 1-36.

[17] Sprague VV, Becnel JJ, Hazard EI. Taxonomy of phylum Microspora. Critical Reviews in Microbiology 1992; 18 285–395.

[18] Prasertsri S, *Limsuwan C*, Chuchird N. The Effects of Microsporidian (*Thelohania*) Infection on the growth and histopathological changes in pond-reared pacific white shrimp (*Litopenaeus vannamei*). Kasetsart Journal Natural Science 2009; 43 680 - 688.
[19] Cannon LRG. Turbellaria of the world. Brisbane: Queensland Museum; 1986.
[20] Kent ML, Olson AC. Interrelationships of a parasitic turbellarian (*Paravortex* sp.) (Graffillidae, Rhabdocoela) and its marine fish hosts. Fish Pathology 1986; 21 65–72.
[21] Kabata Z. Parasites and diseases of fish cultured in the tropics. London: Taylor and Francis Ltd.; *1985*.
[22] Dezfuli BS, Giari L, Simoni E, Menegatti R, Shinn AP, Manera M. Gill histopathology of cultured European sea bass, *Dicentrarchus labrax* (L.), infected with *Diplectanum aequans* (Wagener 1857) Diesing 1958 (Diplectanidae: Monogenea). Parasitology Research 2007; 100 707–713.
[23] Pritchard JB. The gill and homeostasis: transport under stress. The American Journal of Physiology-Regulatory, Integrative and Comparative Physiology 2003; 285 1269–1271.
[24] Nigrelli RF. Mortality statistics for specimen in New York Aquarium 1939 1940; Zoologica, scientific contributions of the New York Zoological Society 25 525-552.
[25] Purivirojkul W. A survey of fish species infected with trematode metacercariae from some areas in northeast Thailand. Journal of Fisheries Technology Research 2011; 5(2) 75-86.
[26] Han ET, Shin EH, Phommakorn S, Sengvilaykham B, Kim JP, Rim HJ, Chai JY. *Centrocestus formosanus* (Digenea: Heterophyidae) Encysted in the Freshwater Fish, *Puntius brevis*, from Lao PDR. Korean Journal of Parasitology 2008; 46 49–53.
[27] Vankara AP, Mani G, Vijayalakshmi C. A report on various digenetic metacercariae from the freshwater fishes of River Godavari, Rajahmundry. Journal of Parasitic Diseases 2011; 35 177-185.
[28] Odening K, Mattheis T, Bockhardt I. 1970. The life cycle of *Cotylurus c. cucullus* (Thoss) (Trematoda, Strigeida) in the Berlin area. Zoological yearbooks, Department of Systematics, 97 125-198. (In German)
[29] Scholz T, Aguirre-Macedo ML, Salgado-Maldonado G. Trematodes of the family Heterophyidae (Digenea) in Mexico: a review of species and new host and geographical records. Journal of Natural History 2001; 35 1733-1772.
[30] Steele E, Hicks T. Histological effect of *Ascocotyle tenuicollis* (Digenea: Heterophyidae) metacercarial infection on the heart of *Fundulus heteroclitus* (Teleostei: Cyprinodontidae). Journal of the South Carolina Academy of Science 2003; 1 10-18.
[31] Orecka-Grabda T. Hemato-and histopathological changes in the whitefish (*Coregonus albula* (L.) invaded by metacercariae of *Cotylurus erraticus* (Syn. Ichthyocotylurus) (Rudolphi, 1809). Acta Ichthyologica et Piscatorial 1991; 21 3-19.
[32] Blazer VS, Gratzek JB. Cartilage proliferation in response to metacercarial infections of fish gills. Journal of Comparative Pathology 1985; 95(2) 273-280.
[33] Olson RE, Pierce JR. A Trematode metacercaria causing gill cartilage proliferation in steelhead trout from Oregon. Journal of Wildlife Diseases 1997; 33(4) 886-890.

[34] Shoaibi Omrani B, Ebrahimzadeh Mousavi HA, Sharifpour I. Occurrence and histopathology of *Ascocotyle tenuicollis* metacercaria in gill of platyfish (*Xiphophorus maculatus*) imported to Iran. Iranian Journal of Fisheries Sciences 2010; 9(3) 472-477.
[35] Paperna I. Diseases caused by parasites in the aquaculture of warm water fish. Annual Review of Fish Disease 1991; 1 155–194.
[36] Baturo B. Pathological changes in cyprinid fry infected by *Bucephalus polymorphos* Baer, 1827 and *Rhipidocotyle illensis* (Ziegler, 1883) metacercariae (Trematoda, Bucephalidae). Acta Parasitologica Polonica 1980; 27 241–246.
[37] Yamaguti S. Systema Helminthum Vol 1. The digenetic trematodes of vertebrates. Part I & II. New York: Interscience Pub Inc; 1958.
[38] Kozicka J. Diseases of fishes Drużno lake (Parasitofauna of the biocoenosis of Drużno lake. Part VIII). Acta Parasitologica Polonica 1958; 6(20) 393-432.
[39] Kozicka J. Diseases of fishes Drużno lake (Parasitofauna of the biocoenosis of Drużno lake. Part VIII) Acta Parasitologica Polonica 1959; 7(1) 1-72.
[40] Grabda E, Grabda J. Mass invasion of metacercariae of *Bucephalus polymorphus* Bear, 1827, in the eye of bream, *Abramis brama* (L.). Wiadomości parazytologiczne 1967; 13(6) 733-735. (in Polish)
[41] Baturo-Warszawska B. Pathological changes in cyprinid fry infected by Bucephalus polymorphus Bear, 1827 and Rhipidocotyle illensis (Ziegler, 1883) metacercariae (Trematoda, Bucephalidae). Acta Parasitologica Polonica 1980; 27 241-246.
[42] Akhtar Y. Feeding habits and nematode parasites of some fishes of Karachi coast. PhD thesis. Jinnah university for women for fulfillment; 2008.
[43] Purivirojkul W. An investigation of larval Ascaridoid nematodes in some marine fish from the Gulf of Thailand. Kasetsart Journal Natural Science 2009; 43(5) 85-92.
[44] Amin OM, Heckmann RA. Description and pathology of *Neoechinorhynchus idahoensis* n. sp. (Acanthocephala: Neoechinorhynchidae) in *Catostomus columbianus* from Idaho. Journal of Parasitology 1992; 78(1) 34-39.
[45] Kim SR, Lee JS, Kim JH, Oh MJ, Kim CS, Park MA, Park JJ. Fine structure of *Longicollum pagrosomi* (Acanthocephala: Pomphorhynchidae) and intestinal histopathology of the red sea bream, *Pagrus major*, infected with acanthocephalans. Parasitology Research 2011; 109(1) 175-84.
[46] Sanil NK, Asokan PK, John L, Vijayan KK. Pathological manifestations of the acanthocephalan parasite, *Tenuiproboscis* sp. in the mangrove red snapper (*Lutjanus argentimaculatus*) (Forsskål, 1775), a candidate species for aquaculture from Southern India. Aquaculture 2011; 310(3-4) 259–266.
[47] Ferguson HW. Systemic Pathology of Fish. Ames: Iowa State University Press; 1989.
[48] Noga EJ. The importance of *Lernaea cruciata* (Le Sueur) in the initiation of skin lesions in largemouth bass, *Micropterus salmoides* (Lacepede), in the Chowan River, North Carolina, USA. Journal of Fish Disease 1986; 9 295-302.
[49] Kabata Z. Parasites and diseases of fish cultured in tropics. London: Taylor and Francis; 1985.

[50] Dezfuli BS, Giari L, Konecny R, Jaeger P, Manera M. Immunohistochemistry, ultrastructure and pathology of gills of *Abramis brama* from Lake Mondsee, Austria, infected with *Ergasilus sieboldi* (Copepoda). Disease of Aquatic Organism 2003; 53 257–262.

[51] Brusca RC. A monograph on the Isopoda: Cymothoidae (Crustacea) of the eastern Pacific. Zoological Journal of the Linnean Society 1981; 73 117–199.

[52] Lester RJG, Hayward CJ. Phylum Arthropoda. In: Woo PTK. (ed.) Fish Diseases and Disorders Vol 1: Protozoan and Metazoan Infections. 2nd edition. London: CAB international; 2006. p466-565.

[53] Alas A, Öktener A, Iscimen A, Trilles JP. New host record, *Parablennius sanguinolentus* (Teleostei, Perciformes, Blenniidae) for *Nerocila bivittata* (Crustacea, Isopoda, Cymothoidae). Parasitology Research 2008; 102 645–646.

[54] Sullivan M, Stimmelmayr R. Cymothoid isopods on coral reef fishes in the near shore marine environment of St.Kitts, Lesser Autilles: Proceedings of the 11th International Coal Reef Symposium, July 7–11, 2008, Ft. Lauderdale, Florida; 2008.

[55] Printrakoon C, Purivirojkul W. Prevalence of *Nerocila depressa* (Isopoda, Cymothoidae) on *Sardinella albella* from a Thai estuary. Journal of Sea Research 2011; 65(2) 322–326.

[56] Rogers-Lowery CL, Dimock Jr RV. Encapsulation of Attached Ectoparasitic Glochidia Larvae of Freshwater Mussels by Epithelial Tissue on Fins of Naïve and Resistant Host Fish. Biological Bulletin 2006; 210 51–63.

[57] Meyers TR, Millemann RE, Fustish CA. Glochidiosis of salmonid fishes. IV. Humoral and tissue responses of coho and Chinook salmon to experimental infection with *Margaritifera margaritifera* (L.) (Pelecypoda: Margaritanidae). Journal of Parasitology 1980; 66 274–281

[58] Waller DL, Mitchell LG. Gill tissue reactions in walleye *Stizostedion vitreum vitreum* and common carp *Cyprinus carpio* to glochidia of the freshwater mussel *Lampsilis radiata siliquoidea*. Diseases of Aquatic Organisms 1989; 6 81–87.

[59] Woods GL, Walker DH. Detection of infection or infectious agents by the use of cytologic and histologic stains. Clinical Microbiology Reviews 1996; 9 382-404.

[60] Gupta E, Bhalla P, Khurana N, Singh T. Histopathology for the diagnosis of infectious diseases. Indian Journal of Medical Microbiology 2009; 27(2) 100-106.

Toxicology of the Bioinsecticides Used in Agricultural Food Production

Neiva Knaak, Diouneia Lisiane Berlitz and Lidia Mariana Fiuza

Additional information is available at the end of the chapter

http://dx.doi.org/10.5772/52070

1. Introduction

As populations grow in numbers, the demands for food production increase and are generally met by the intensification of livestock breeding and the increase of agricultural activities. This in turn increases the quantity of chemical pesticides required to control the losses in production caused by insect pests preying on the food plants and disturbing the animals. Once applied these pesticides may cause resistance to the synthetic molecules, contaminate biotic and abiotic components like plants, soil, water and/or the local water network and can also effect non-targeted organisms, such as fish, small mammals, birds and so on.

Contamination of rivers with chemical pesticides is almost always due to excess material being carried away by rain or irrigation waters or by erosion of contaminated soil particles (1, 2). Therefore, as this generalized contamination of the environment increases, researchers are seeking alternative methods for controlling the pests but which cause less damage than the chemical products (3).

In the biological control system, the bacteria of the *Bacillus* genus have considerable potential for use as control agents, because, as well as being lethal to the insect pests, they remain viable for long periods in storage (4). Amongst these bacteria, *Bacillus thuringiensis* has achieved commercial-scale success in controlling various insect pests, plant pathogens, nematodes and mites, mainly because this micro-organism has a high specificity to the pest-targets (5).

In addition to the use of microorganisms, various botanical pesticides are being studied and can be associated with Integrated Pest Management (IPM). The products originating in plants refer to plant species that, over a long time developed defense mechanisms against herbivores, pathogens and other stress agents. Among the toxins produced by these plants are found nitrogenous substances such as non-protein amino acids, cyanogenic glycosides, certain peptides and proteins, and several alkaloids. The toxicity of a substance is related to the dose taken by the insect, its age, the absorption mechanism and the manner of excretion (6).

In this chapter we address the toxicological aspects of microbial and botanical biopesticides that act by ingestion, with emphasis on histopathological analysis of tissues and cells in the alimentary channel of the Lepidoptera as well as the specificity of the *B. thuringiensis* bacteria, aqueous extracts and oil essential of medicinal and forest.

2. Histology of lepidoptera

The alimentary channel of insects is composed of three main regions with different embryological origins: stomodeum or foregut, middle or midgut and hindgut or proctodeu. This canal represents a contact area between the insect and the environment and is the focus of much of the applied research concerning pest control (7, 8), especially the midgut region where the epithelial cells are involved in the processes of absorption and secretion of enzymes (columnar cells), ion homeostasis (goblet cells), endocrine function (endocrine cells) and the renovation of the epithelia (regenerative cells) (9, 10, 11). A defense mechanism in this region is the peritrophic membrane, which plays a fundamental role in the biology of the midgut, being positioned between the food contents and epithelial layer, performing the function of protecting the epithelium from mechanical damage, and in addition acts as a barrier against toxins and chemicals harmful to the insects (12, 13).

In Lepidoptera, the midgut epithelium is composed of four cell types (Figure 1) which are involved in the processes of absorption and secretion of enzymes (columnar cells), ion homeostasis (goblet cells), endocrine function (endocrine cells) and the renewal of the epithelium (regenerative cells) (14, 15). The regenerative cells are undifferentiated and are responsible for the renovation of the midgut epithelium, substituting the cells that wear out and are lost during the digestive process – they also make it possible for the alimentary channel to grow larger at each ecdysis. They are found at the base of the midgut, alone or in groups, and there are no differences in their abundance along the midgut (16, 17, 18).

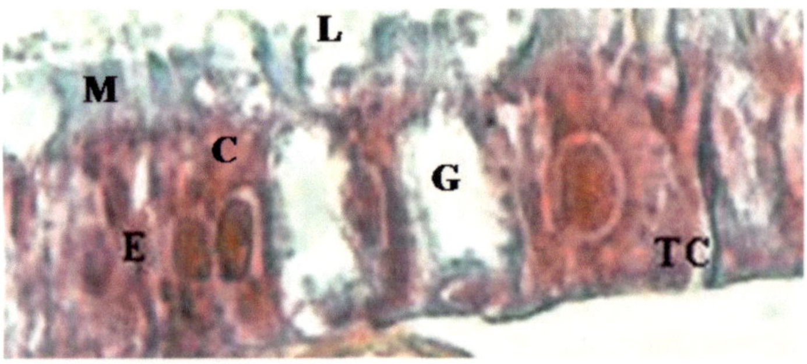

Figure 1. Types of cells found in Lepidoptera. L=lumen; TC=connective tissue; E=epithelium, C=columnar cells; G=globet cells;

Changes in the alimentary canal, especially in the region of the midgut, can affect the growth and development of insects, as well as all the physiological events, because these processes depend on adequate food, on its absorption and transformation in the alimentary canal (9, 11).

Among the insects, the Lepidoptera order causes the greatest economic losses in crops – in maize and rice which are attacked principally by *Spodoptera frugiperda,* in sugar-cane attacked by the stem-borer *Diatraea saccharallis* and in soybeans mainly by the Lepidoptera pest *Anticarsia gemmatalis*.

All regions of the epithelial layer of the alimentary canal of *S. frugiperda* caterpillars are coated with a single layer of cells, with a flat morphology in the stomodeum region and cubic morphology in the proctodeus (19). The muscles are arranged along the channel in a uniform manner (7). According to Cavalcante & Cruz-Landim (20) and Pinheiro et al. (16), in the midgut epithelium four cell types predominate: columnar, goblet, regenerative, and endocrine cells. These cells predominate along the *S. frugiperda* midgut epithelium and are considered responsible for the absorption of digested food, and demonstrate morphology similar to that of other Lepidoptera (8, 21). Studies by Harper & Hopkins (22) and Harper & Granados (23), indicate that these epithelial cells are also responsible for secretion of a micro fiber net soaked in a matrix of proteins and glycoproteins -denominated a peritrophic membrane – which performs various functions such as: the protection of the epithelium against chemical and mechanical damage caused by the alimentation, the creation of a physical barrier against micro-organisms and digestion division (18).

Pinto & Fiuza (24), analyzing the histology of the midgut of *A. gemmatalis* caterpillars with an optical microscope, observed that the alimentary canal is divided basically into three portions, which are: the anterior intestine or stomodeum, the middle intestine or mesentero, and the posterior intestine or proctodeus. The cells do not have a cuticle coating, the intestinal wall being constituted by an epithelium of approximately 40μm in height, which is separated from the haemolymph only by a thin layer of loose connective tissue. The cylindrical and goblet cells are evenly distributed along the intestine section. In the intestinal lumen is a thin membrane, called the peritrophic membrane, which surrounds the bolus of food, separating it from the epithelial cells of the midgut. The apical surface of the cylindrical cells has dense microvilli measuring 3μm in height. The goblet cells show invaginations of the intestinal lumen as far as the nucleus.

3. Microbial biopesticides

Among the microbial insecticides, the *Bacillus thuringiensis* bacterium is highlighted because it shows great promise for development in the line of organic products and in the area of genetically modified plants. Besides being a sporulent bacteria found naturally in the soil, it is distinguished by its production of protein inclusions with insecticidal activity against several orders of insects and phytonematodes (25, 26). According to Shelton et al. (27), the first biopesticide containing subspecies of *B. thuringiensis* were sold in France in 1930. In 1995 more than 180 products based on this bacterial species were recorded by the Environmental Protection Agency (EPA) in the United States of America. In a study by

Fiuza & Berlitz (28) they stated that *B. thuringiensis* formulas were then being marketed in Brazil. These are described in Table 1.

Products	Companies	*B. thuringiensis* (Bt)	Target insects
Dipel	Abbott	*Bt kurstaki*	Lepidoptera
Thuricide	Sandoz	*Bt kurstaki*	Lepidoptera
Agree	Mitsui	*Bt aizawai*	Lepidoptera
Bactur	Milenia Agrociências	*Bt kurstaki*	Lepidoptera
Ecotech Pro	Bayer	*Bt kurstaki*	Lepidoptera
Bactospeine	Solvay	*Bt kurstaki*	Lepidoptera
Javelin	Sandoz	*Bt kurstaki*	Lepidoptera
Foray	Novo-Nordisk	*Bt kurstaki*	Lepidoptera
Biobit	Novo-Nodisk	*Bt kurstaki*	Lepidoptera
Foil/Condor	Ecogen	*Bt kurstaki*	Lepidoptera
Delfin	Sandoz	*Bt kurstaki*	Lepidoptera
Cutlass	Ecogen	*Bt kurstaki*	Lepidoptera
LarvoBt	Fermone	*Bt kurstaki*	Lepidoptera
Nubilacid	Radonja	*Bt kurstaki*	Lepidoptera
MVP	Mycogen	*Bt kurstaki*	Lepidoptera
Bac-control	Agricontrol	*Bt kurstaki*	Lepidoptera
XenTari	Abbott	*Bt aizawai*	Lepidoptera
M-One	Mycogen	*Bt san diego* *Bt tenebrionis*	Coleoptera
Di-Terra	Abbott	*Bt san diego* *Bt tenebrionis*	Coleoptera
Trident	Sandoz	*Bt san diego* *Bt tenebrionis*	Coleoptera
Novodor	Novo Nordisk	*Bt san diego* *Bt tenebrionis*	Coleoptera
M-One Plus	Mycogen	*Bt san diego* *Bt tenebrionis*	Coleoptera
Foil	Ecogen	*Bt* (recombinant)	Coleoptera

*Table adapted by Fiuza & Berlitz (28)

Table 1. Products made from *Bacillus thuringiensis* for controlling agricultural pest*

3.1. Case studies

A study by Berlitz & Fiuza (29) evaluated the toxicity of *B. thuringiensis aizawai* on *S. frugiperda* and demonstrated that, 6 hours after the application of the treatments, an increase in the cell volume occurred and the intestinal microvilli ruptured. Significant differences in the cell volume of the treatment as compared with that of the control caterpillars were observed 12 hours after the application.

In the histopathological analysis of the midgut of *S. frugiperda* caterpillars treated with the *B. thuringiensis thuringiensis* 407 (pH 408) strain, structural changes were observed six hours after application of the treatment (HAT), where there were cells in the intestinal lumen and elongation of the microvilli, as compared to the control. After nine applications of the treatment (HAT) the action was intensified with vacuolization of the cytoplasm, and the beginning of the degradation of the peritrophic membrane – this was entirely absent after 12 HAT.

Treatment with *B. thuringiensis kurstaki* HD-73 strain was similar, except that rupture of the microvilli (BBMV's) and vacuolization of the cytoplasm began at 12 HAT. The results of the histopathological analysis of the midget of *S. frugiperda* caterpillars demonstrate that treatment with the *B. thuringiensis thuringiensis* strain was more efficient, because the degradations of the microvilosities started 9 hours after treatment application (HAT), while in the *B. thuringiensis kurstaki* the same effect was noticed only after 12 HAT (30).

Knaak and Fiuza (31) tested the nuclear polyhedrosis virus of *Anticarsia gemmatalis* (VPN*Ag*) and *B. thuringiensis kurstaki* HD-1 (Dipel®) in 2_{nd} instar caterpillars of *A. gemmatalis* (Lepidoptera, Noctuidae), and observed that when both entomopathogens are utilized simultaneously they are more efficient, because they caused alterations in the intestinal cells after 6 HAT while when used separately they produced the alteration only after 12 HAT.

If the dose of toxin administered does not cause the death of the insect, its cells are substituted permitting normal alimentation and the recuperation of the insect (32). Several studies report on the cell changes produced in the middle intestine of caterpillars intoxicated with Cry proteins from *B. thuringiensis* - for example: the increase in the volume of the epithelium cells, the rupture of the microvilli, cytoplasmic vacuolization, the changes in cytoplasmic organelles and cell hypertrophy (30, 33-35).

Studies of the mode action of the *B. thuringiensis* Cry proteins seek to clarify the mechanisms by which these proteins produce their entomopathogenic effects and to elucidate the specificity of the various toxins.

3.2. Mode action of the *Bacillus thuringiensis* Cry proteins

When the crystals of *B. thuringiensis* are ingested by susceptible insects they are solublized under alkaline conditions in the middle intestine and then broken into smaller fragments by proteases (5, 36, 37). Binding occurs because of the association of the activated toxin with specific proteins located in the microvilli of the epithelial cells of the middle intestine (38) and is followed by the formation of the pore (39) – the ion flux from this pore leads to cell lyses and consequently, to the death of the susceptible insect (5).

The solubility of the protein and crystals in liquids with alkaline pH values such as those in the middle intestine of the insects liberates the protoxins of 130-140kDa for Cry1 and 70kDa for Cry2. This phase determines the specificity of the *B. thuringiensis* isolate to the target species, both because of the alkalinity of the digestive system and because of the composition of the *B. thuringiensis* crystals.

1. The protoxins are activated by the digestive enzymes, forming toxic fragments of 60-65kDa. At this stage both the photolytic composition and the structure of the crystal protein are important. The toxins recognize specific receptors in the microvilli of the epithelial cells of the middle intestine of susceptible larvae to which they bind. Studies made with BBMV (*Brush Border Membrane Vesicles*) isolated from the larvae of Lepidoptera show that the strong binding affinity between the toxin and the receiver is considered an important factor in determining the insecticidal spectrum of the Cry proteins (40). Research data demonstrates that there is a positive correlation between binding, in vitro, of the toxin in the intestinal receptor and the toxicity, in vivo. On the other hand, other studies describe that while the recognition of the receptor is necessary it is not sufficient in itself to provoke the toxicity, which suggests the existence of other factors related to the mode of action of the Cry proteins. In 1994, Knight et al. (41) isolated from the BBMV of *Manduca sexta* (Lep., Sphingidae) larvae an aminopeptidase N implicated in the interaction of the toxin Cry1Ac. The receptor models now described demonstrate that an insect may present, in variable quantities, various kinds of receptors which could be recognized by different toxins. Research data show that these models may explain the specificity of the *B. thuringiensis* toxins.
2. After recognition of the receptor, the toxins induce the formation of pores in the cellular membrane of the intestinal epithelia.
3. The formation of pores in the cellular membrane provokes an ionic imbalance between the cytoplasm and the cell´s external environment. Histopathological analysis performed after the intoxication of insects reveal destruction of the microvilli, epithelial cell hypertrophy, cytoplasmic vacuolization and cellular lyses which cause paralysis and death of the insect.

When selecting insecticidal proteins, synthesized by this bacteria, a preliminary in vitro analyzes of membrane receptors can facilitate a rapid determination of the range of action of Cry proteins against the target species. The evaluation of the toxicity in vivo can then be limited to those isolates which were pre-selected as active in vitro.

3.3. Detection of receptors in tissues of insects

3.3.1. Preparation of the tissues of insects

The insect´s digestive tubes are dissected and fixed for 24h in *Bouin Hollande Sublimé* 10%, washed in distilled water for 12 hours and dehydrated in an ethanol mixture increasing in strength gradually from 70 to 100% (42). The tissues are then impregnated in mixed baths (ethanol/toluene/Paraplast) and embedded in 100% Paraplast at 58°C. The longitudinal or transverse sections, 7-10 mm thick, prepared using LKB microtome are mounted on glass slides, tanadas with poly-l-lysine at 10% and stored at 4°C for subsequent analysis of the histology of the receptors.

3.3.2. Labeling of Cry proteins with biotin

Cry proteins can be biotinylated, according to the method described in Bayer & Wilcheck (43), where the incorporation of biotin at the N-terminal of the protein is done using BNHS (biotinyl-N-hydroxysuccinimide) in a buffer of sodium bicarbonate, pH 9.

The reaction product should be purified with Sephadex G-25 (Sigma), and the fractions biotinylated and identified by dot-blot, which uses a nitrocellulose membrane, the conjugate of streptavidin alkaline phosphatase diluted in TST buffer (Tris-Triton-Saline, pH 7.6) and the revelation substrate (BCIP and NBT in a Tris buffer, pH 9.5).

The concentration of biotinylated Cry proteins can be determined by the Bradford method (44) using BSA as the protein standard. The purity and integrity of the labeled proteins can be evaluated by western blot using a nitrocellulose membrane (Sigma) and Towbin buffer, pH 8.3 with 10% ethanol. The membranes can be developed using the same technique described in the dot-blot.

3.3.3. In vitro detection of membrane receptors

3.3.3.1. Pre-treatment of tissues

The in vitro analyses of the receptors of Cry proteins of *B. thuringiensis* are performed with histological sections of the digestive systems of larvae being studied. The actual detection results from incubation with the tissue proteins, wich have been previously dew axed and rehydrated as shown in the drawing.

3.3.3.2. Reactions with biotinylated proteins (45)

In the analyses with biotinylated Cry proteins, histological sections are incubated at room temperature for 1 hour with the biotinylated proteins. Proteins not bound to the receptor sites are removed with TST, pH 7.6.

At the next step, the tissues are treated with streptavidin conjugated to an enzyme (peroxidase or alkaline phosphatase) or fluorochrome (fluorescein or phycoerythrin), diluted in a TST buffer. The resulting "protein-receptor" complex reaction, using the enzyme conjugate, can be developed with the DAB substrate for peroxidase (Figure 2A) and with BCIP/NBT for alkaline phosphatase (Figure 2B). The sections are fixed with Pertex mounting medium between the slide and the glass cover slip.

To develop tissues treated with fluorescein the histological sections are mounted with *Mowiol* and stored at 4°C for analysis by optical microscopy (OM - Figure 3A) or by laser scanning microscopy (LSM – Figure 3B).

3.3.3.3. Immune detection reactions of protein receptors

In immunohistochemical analyzes with unlabeled proteins (native preoteins), the receptors are developed with the primary antibody (AC_1 specifically against the Cry protein) and secondary antibody (AC_2, directed against the AC_1) conjugated to an enzyme or fluorochrome, which are developed and assembled according to the method described above.

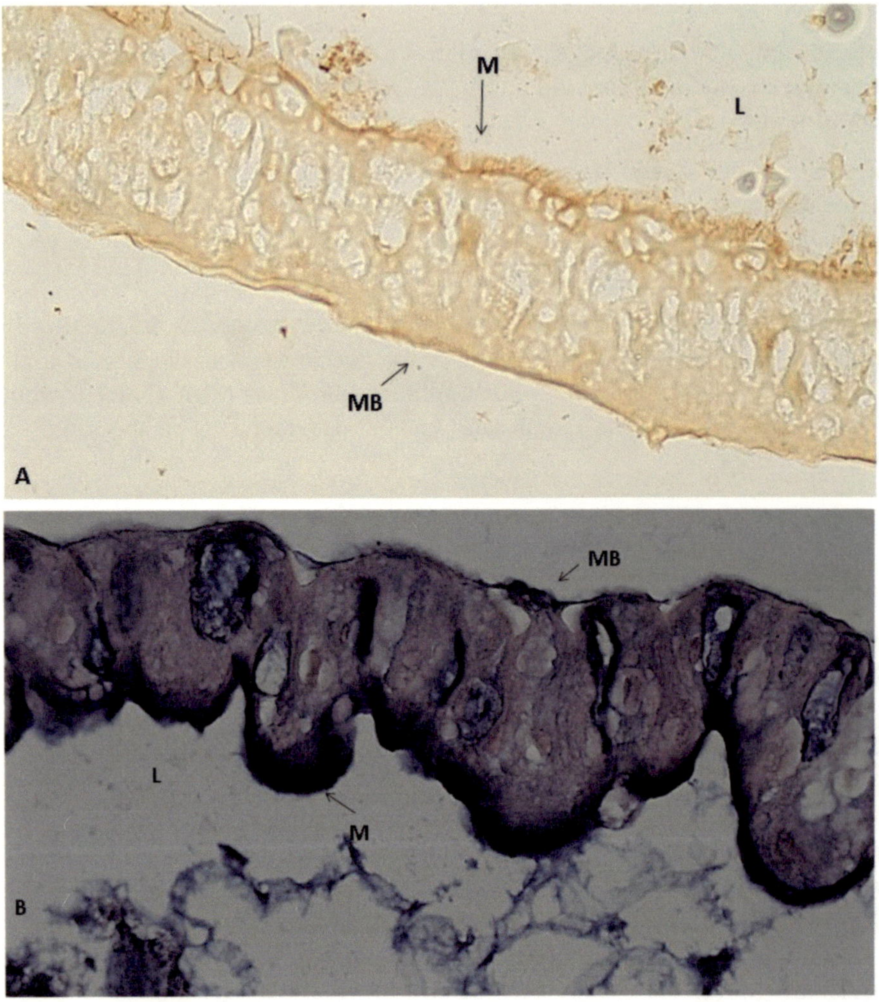

Figure 2. Cry proteins biotinylated receptor, in Lepidoptera insect tissue revealed with peroxidase (A) and alkaline phosphatase (B). (MB) Basal Membrane; (L) Lumen; (M) microvilli.

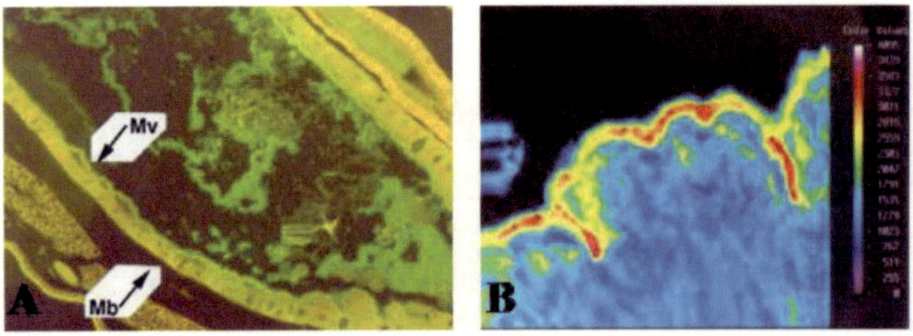

Figure 3. Receivers biotinylated Cry proteins, detected in the tissues of insects with fluorescein and observed in MO (A) and MVL (B) (45).

In immuno localization, the caterpillars are previously treated in vivo with the Cry proteins and after wards the tissues and the immunohistochemical reactions are prepared.

In both methods, the controls are prepared by alternative omission of each step of the reaction, to eliminate the possibility of false-positive reactions. The samples developed with enzymes like peroxidase and alkaline phosphatase can be evaluated by optical microscopy.

4. Plant bioinsecticides

Until quite recently the use of chemical insecticide has been the most widely used method of controlling insect pests. However, the products are expensive and in some cases inefficient and hazardous if used intensively and/or incorrectly. However, some success has been achieved in programs of Integrated Pest Management (IPM) with an alternative to chemicals extracted from various secondary metabolites present in roots, leaves and seeds of plants as an alternative to chemicals called "plant pesticides" (46-48).

The natural products obtained from vegetable raw materials present a wide variety of molecules, with great diversity in structure and biological activity (49). This wide range of new sites of action on target organisms can be considered another reason for the growing interest in phytotoxins, because, even if not commercially available able, they may suggest lines for the synthesis of entirely new products (50). This is important if we consider the speed with which the insects and micro-organisms have developed resistance to chemicals commonly used as biological control agents of target species.

According to Mello & Silva-Filho (51), the components of insecticides can be divided into the following groups: (i) derivatives of chemical compounds (tannins, terpenoids, flavonoids, alkaloids, quinones, linomoides, phenols), (ii) molecules produced from the processing proteins (chitinase, lectins, inhibitors alpha-amylase and proteinase inhibitors) and (iii) volatile compounds of plants such as essential oil. In this case, the chemical components can be divided into two classes. The first, based on biosynthesis, in which are found the derivates of the terpenoids, is formed via the mevalonic acetate, and the second, by derivatives which are located in the phenylpropanoid, aromatic compounds formed by way of shikimic acid (52).

Normally, the oily essential in the leaves and resins contain some constituents in high concentration, and about 30-40 minor compounds at concentrations less than 1% (53). These substances are found in plants in the form of complexes, whose components are integrated and reinforce its action on the organism. Even when the plant has only one active principle, this has a beneficial effect superior to that produced by the same substance produced by chemical synthesis. However, the use of botanical insecticides depends on identification of the active compounds, their mode of action, production, formulation, stability, dose, action on natural enemies, field persistence, toxicity tests for record, among others (54).

The Laboratory of Microbiology and Toxicology at the UNISINOS University uses two models for histopathologic analysis:

1. Following treatment with plant extracts or oily essences 10 larvae of the insect target are collected in periods of 1, 3, 6, 9, 12, 24 and 48 hours after treatment (HAT).The specimens are fixed in aqueous paraformaldehyde and then dehydrated in ethanol solutions of increasing strength (50, 70, 90 and 100%). After dehydration, the larvae are embedded in resin (Leica Historesin) for 12 h. After that the specimens are put into molds of solid polypropylene using the same resin with a polymerize. The resin blocks are mounted on supports after polymerization, and cut into 3mm thick sections in a microtome with a glass blade. The histological sections are stretched out onto glass slides and stained with Schiff-Naphtol Blue Black periodic acid, dehydrated, and mounted between the glass slides and the cover slips with *Entellan*.
2. After application of the treatments with plant extracts or essential oil, 10 target insect larvae in each treatment, are collected in periods of 3, 6, 9, 12, 24 and 27HAT. After fixation in *Bouin Hollande Sublime-BHS* for 24 hours (38), the larvae are subjected to dehydration in increasingly strong ethanol solutions, followed by rapid baths of xylene and impregnation in paraffin. Longitudinal histological sections of the midgut are realized at a thickness of 5µm. Coloration is applied with *Azul de Heidenhain* (41), which differentiates the microvilli of the middle intestine by the presence of glycoproteins which can be observed by the system of comparative histology in an optical microscopy.

Knaak et al. (55) found that the toxicity of the extracts of *Petivesia alliacea, Zingiber officinale, Ruta graveolens, Malva silvestris, Baccharis genistelloides* and *Cymbopogon citratus* caused damage such as: vacuolization of the cytoplasm, disruption of microvilli, peritrophic membrane destruction and cell changes in the midgut of *S. frugiperda* (Figure 4). This study the changes mentioned in the previous work were not observed until 48HAT, which was the maximum time rated.

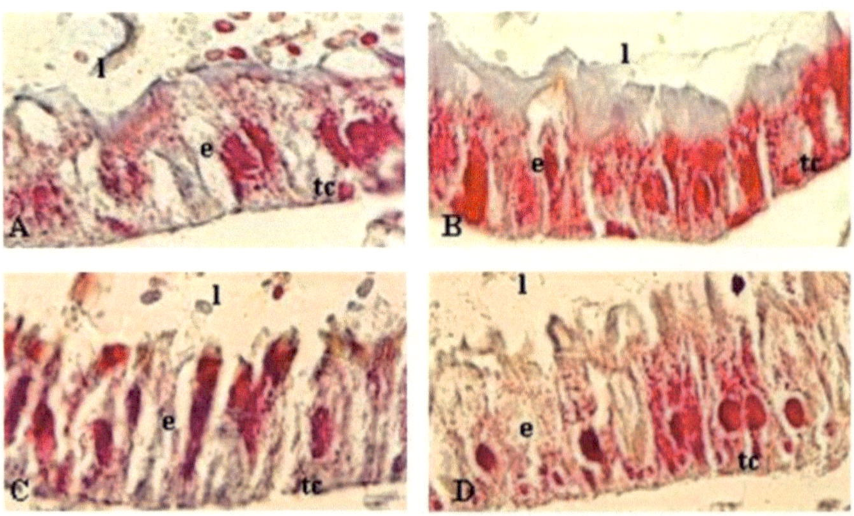

Figure 4. Longitudinal sections of the midgut of *Spodoptera frugiperda* caterpillars treated with plants extrats, (A) *Petivesia aliacea* (24 HAT), (B) *Petivesia aliacea* (24 HAT); (C) *Zingiber officinale* (6 HAT); (D) *Zingiber officinale* (27 HAT); (E) *Z. officinale* (6 HAT); (F) *Z. officinale* (24 HAT); (G) Controle. Increase 400X; bar=2.44µm; →=changes; TC=connective tissue; M=microvilli; E=epithelium; L= lumen.

The chemical compounds (tannins, terpenoids, flavonoids, alkaloids, quinones, linomoides, phenols), molecules produced from the processing of proteins (chitinase, lectins, alfa-amylase inhibitor and proteinase inhibitors) and volatile compounds from the plant [56, 57], present in plant extracts, undergo different changes according to the physico-chemical conditions along the digestive tract of insects.

In treatments with the essential oil of *R. graveolens* and *Malva* sp., cellular projections were observed in the intestinal lumen at 9 HAT, and the oil of *R. graveolens* caused cell elongation at 12 HAT. Thus, it appears that changes in the structure of the midgut of *S. frugiperda* may increase during the treatment with essential oils. The intensity of the pathological effects is dependent on time period and the concentration used (58).

In the treatments with essential oil of *Z. officinale* and *C. citratus*, was observed projections of epithelial cells in the lumen, at 3 and 6HAT respectively (Figure 5A, D and E). After 24 hours treatment with *C. citratus* (Figure 5B), we observed elongation of the microvilli, while in the treatment with *Z. officinale* cell elongation occurred (Figure 5G). At 24HAT with the *Z. officinale* oil several morphological changes occurred, such as: cellular disorganization, destruction of the epithelium, of the microvilli and the peritrophic membrane. It can still be observed that the changes are dependent on the time period and the concentrations used (56).

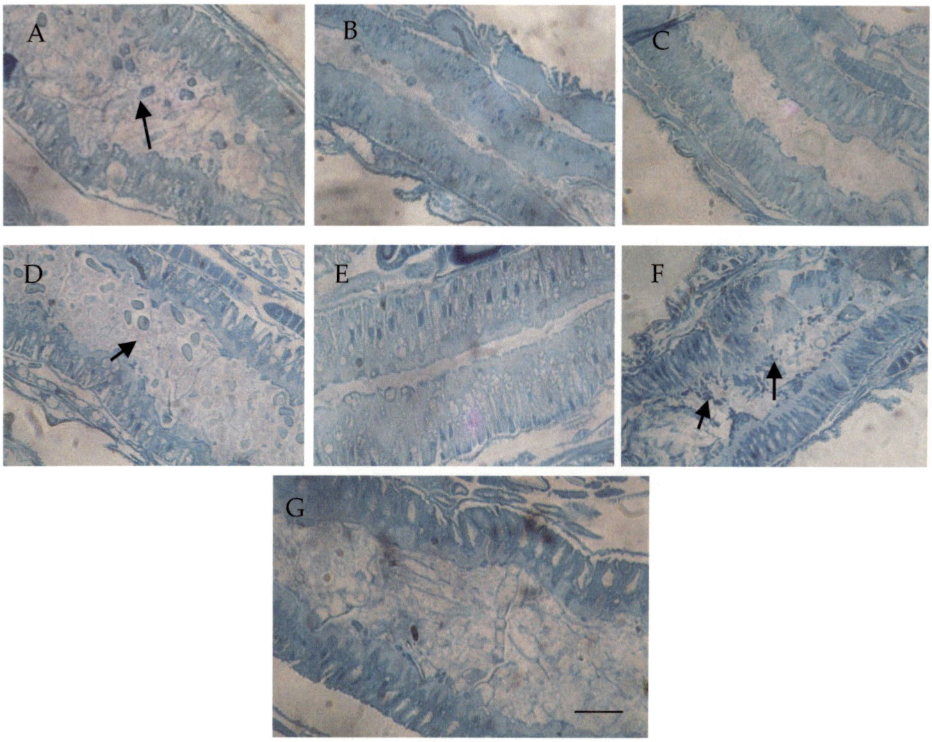

Figure 5. Longitudinal sections of the midgut of *Spodoptera frugiperda* caterpillars treated with essential oils, (A) *Cymbopogon citratus* (6 HAT) (B) *C. citratus* (24 HAT); (C) *C. citratus* (48 HAT); (D) *Zingiber officinale* (3 HAT); (E) *Z. officinale* (6 HAT); (F) *Z. officinale* (24 HAT); (G) Controle. Increase 400X; bar=2.44μm; →=changes; TC=connective tissue; M=microvilli; E=epithelium; L= lumen.

Knaak et al. (55) evaluated the effect of the interaction of various plant extracts with Xentari®, *B. thuringiensis aizawai,* in the midgut of *S. frugiperda,* demonstrating that the histopathological effects of *Z. officinale, M. silvestris, R. graveolens* and *B. genistelloides,* in the midgut of *S. frugiperda* were more intense when compared to extracts of *P. alliacea and C.citratus,* which showed a positive interaction with Xentari®, accelerating the process of destruction of intestinal cells, which represents a reduction in the lethal time of the target species, *S. frugiperda.*

Some plants are outstanding, for instance, *Melia azedarach,* a plant similar to *Azadirachtina indica* which produces azadirachtine efficiently for more than 400 species of insects (58), its active ingredient is already a commercial product called Neemix 4.5®. This causes different reactions in insects, acting as an alimentary inhibitor retarding growth, reduces fertility, and causes morphogenetic and behavioral changes (59).

The toxicity of cinnamon is related to the presence of different compounds, such as salanalina, meliaterina and meliacarpinina E, from which additionally other derivatives can be obtained which show insecticidal action against the Coleopteran orders (Curculionidae, Tenebrionidae and Chrysomelidae) and Lepidoptera (60-62), amongst others.

Correia et al. (63) evaluated the histology of the alimentary canal of larvae of *S. frugiperda* treated with neem (Neemseto®) at concentrations 0.5 and 1.0%, on non-treated leaves. They found that regions of the stomodeum and proctodeus showed no morphological changes. However, the middle intestinal region, showed morphological changes that varied in intensity according to the exposure time and concentration (0.5 and 1.0%). After 48h and 96h of treatment, tissue changes were observed in the larvae treated with neem – the cells of the epithelial lamina became slender and elongated. It was not possible to distinguish cell types beyond reducing significantly reducing the secretion activity of the two concentrations studied, in comparison with the control.

5. Conclusion

In toxicological analysis of microbial biopesticides, with *Bacillus thuringiensis* as the object of analysis, the labeling detected in the region of the microvilli of the cells of the intestinal epithelial cells revealed the presence of membrane receptors of Cry proteins in the midgut of the larvae of the insects when compared to the controls representing the alternative omission of different components of the reactions, as can be seen by the absence of staining on the microvilli of intestinal epithelial cells of the insects used here as a model of this approach to the study. The imunedetections and the detection of biotinylated Cry proteins were used by various authors, for identifying the intestinal membrane receptors, in larvae of different species of Lepidoptera (33, 45, 64-65), Diptera (66) and Coleoptera (33, 67). These authors proved that the binding of the Cry proteins to the microvilli of the insect´s midgut indicate the existence of a receptor specific to the cited protein in the target insect.

Considering therefore, the studies of receptors in vitro and the toxicological analyses in vivo, it can be confirmed that the methods for detection of membrane receptors can be applied in selecting the toxins of *B. thuringiensis* that are active against insects, and that there is a positive correlation between the in vitro and the in vivo analysis. However, to determine the median lethal concentration (LC_{50}) of a Cry protein a bioassay is necessary since the binding of proteins to the receptors may vary in concentration and affinity, as previously described by several authors for different insect species (64, 68, 69, 70). Other studies show that the Cry proteins that are toxic to insects correspond to those which bind irreversibly to the epithelial cell receptors of the target insects (71).

In the case of plant insecticides, chemical compounds, (tannins, terpenoids, flavonoids, alkaloids, quinones, phenols and linomoides), the molecules produced from the processing of proteins (chitinase, lectins, inhibitors alpha-amylase and proteinase inhibitors) and volatile compounds from plants, such as the oily essences present in plants (57) undergo different changes according to the physical and chemical conditions along the digestive tract of the insects.

In recent years, in the search for alternative methods to control agricultural pests without using artificial chemical substances, research was expanded to obtain greater knowledge on the mode action of microbial toxins and plant insecticides. Studies realized in vitro on the cells and tissues of the alimentary canal of insects, especially of Lepidoptera, have identified and located the receptors in the target species. Thus, for the application of plant and microbial toxins as biopesticides, it is fundamental to evaluate the range of action and the specificity of the active ingredient. In this context, Fiuza (72) mentions that the analysis in vitro of membrane receptors can be considered an indispensable tool due to the large number of botanical compounds plus the isolates, the strains and proteins of *B. thuringiensis* that have been identified, and which have considerable potential for pest management.

Author details

Neiva Knaak, Diouneia Lisiane Berlitz and Lidia Mariana Fiuza
University of Vale do Rio dos Sinos, Laboratory of Microbiology and Toxicology, São Leopoldo, RS, Brazil

6. References

[1] Cáceres, O. et al. (1981). Resíduos de pesticidas clorados em água das cidades de São Carlos e Araraquara. *Ciência e Cultura*, São Paulo, Vol. (33): 1622-1626.

[2] Aguiar, L.H. & Moraes, G. (1999). Hepatic alanine and aspartic amino transferases of the freshwater teleost. *Bryconcephalus* (Matrinchã) exposed to the organophosphorous methyl parathion (folidol 600 registred), *Fish response totoxic-environments,* Kennedy, Canadá. pp. 145-152.

[3] Carlini, C.R. & Grossi-de-Sá, M.F. (2002). Plant toxic proteins with insecticidal properties. A review on their potentialities as bioinsecticides. *Toxicon,* Vol. 40: 1515-1539.

[4] Alves, S. B. (1998). *Controle microbiano de insetos*. 2.ed. Piracicaba: FEALQ, 1163p.

[5] Schnepf, E., Crickmore, N., Van Rie, J., Lereclus, D., Baum, J., Feitelson, J., Zeigler, D.R. & Dean, D.H. (1998). *Bacillus thuringiensis* and its pesticide crystal proteins. *Microbiology Molecular Biology Reviews*, Vol. (62): 775-806.

[6] Saito, M.L. & Lucchini, F. (1998). Substâncias obtidas de plantas e a procura por praguicidas eficientes e seguros ao meio ambiente. Jaguariúna: EMBRAPA-CNPMA. 46p.

[7] Chapman, R.F. (1998). *The insects: structure and function*, 4th ed., Cambridge, Cambridge University Press, 788p.

[8] Levy, S.M., A.M.F. Falleiros, E.A. Gregório, N.R. Arrebola & L.A. Toledo. (2004). The larval midgut of *Anticarsia gemmatalis* (Hübner) (Lepidoptera: Noctuidae): light and electron microscopy studies of the epithelial cells. *Brazilian Journal of Biology*, Vol. (64): 633-638.

[9] Mordue (Luntz), A.J. & Blackwell A. (1993). Azadirachtin: an update. *Journal of Insect Physiol*ogy, Vol. (39): 903-924.

[10] Chiang, A.S., Yen, D.F. & Peng, W.K. (1986). Defense reaction of midgut epithelial cells in the rice moth larva (*Corcyra cephalonica*) infected with *Bacillus thuringiensis*. *Journal of Invertebrate Pathology*, Vol. (47): 333-339.

[11] Mordue (Luntz), A.J. & Nisbet A.J. (2000). Azadirachtin from the neem tree *Azadirachta indica:* its action against insects. *An. Soc. Entomol. Brasil*, Vol. (29): 615-632.

[12] Lehane, M.J. (1997). Peritrophic matrix structure and function. *Ann Ver.Entomol*, Vol. (42): 525-550.

[13] Terra, W.R. (2001). The origin and functions of the insect peritrophic membrane and peritrophic gel. *Arch. Insect Biochem. Physiol.*, Vol. (47): 47-61.

[14] Terra, W.R. & Ferreira, C. (2005) Biochemistry of digestion. In Comprehensive Molecular Insect Science (Gilbert LI, Iatrou K & Gill SS, eds), Vol. 4, pp. 171–224. Elsevier, Oxford.

[15] Pinheiro, D.O., Quagio-Grassiotto, I. & Gregório, E.A. (2008). Morphological regional differences of epithelial cells along the midgut in *Diatraea saccharalis* Fabricius (Lepidoptera: Crambidae) larvae. *Neotropical Entomology*, Vol. (37): 413-419.

[16] Pinheiro, D.O., Silva, R.J., Quagio-Grassiotto, I. & Gregório, E.A. (2003). Morphometric study of the midgut epithelium in larvae Of *Diatraea saccharalis* Fabricius (Lepidoptera: Pyralidae). *Neotropical Entomology*, Vol. (32): 453-459.

[17] Wanderley-Teixeira, V., Teixeira, A.A.C., Cunha, F.M., Costa, M.K.C.M., Veiga, A.F.S.L. & Oliveira, J.V. (2006). Histological description of the midgut and thepy loric valve of *Tropida criscollaris* (Stoll, 1813) (Orthopetera: Romaleidae). *Brazilian Journal of Biology*, Vol. (66): 104.

[18] Martins, G.F., Neves, L.A.O. & Serrão, J.E. (2006). The regenerative cells during the metamorphosis in the midgut of bees. *Micron*, Vol. (37): 161-168.

[19] Correia, A.A., Wanderley-Teixeira, V., Teixeira, A.A.C., Oliveira, J.V. & Torres, J.B. (2009). Morfologia do canal alimentar de lagartas de *Spodoptera frugiperda* (J.E. Smith) (Lepidoptera:Noctuidae) alimentadas com folhas tratadas com Nim. Neotropical Entomology, Vol. (38): 1-9

[20] Cavalcante, V.M. & Cruz-Landim, C. (1999). Types of cells present in the midgut of the insects: a review. *Naturalia*, Vol. (24): 19-39.

[21] Levy, S.M., Falleiros, A.M.F., Gregório, E.A., Arrebola, N.R. & Toledo, L.A. (2004). The larval midgut of *Anticarsia gemmatalis* (Hübner) (Lepidoptera: Noctuidae): light and electron microscopy studies of the epithelial cells. Braz J Biol, Vol. (64): 633-638.

[22] Harper, M.S. & Hopkins, T.L. (1997). Peritrophic membrane structure and secretion in European corn borer larvae (*Ostrinia nubilalis*). *Tissue Cell*, Vol. (29): 463-475.

[23] Harper, M.S. & Granados, R.R. (1999). Peritrophic membrane structure and formation of larval *Trichoplusia ni* with an investigation on the secretion patterns of a PM mucin. *Tissue Cell*, Vol. (31): 202-211.

[24] Pinto, L.M.N.P. Histologia do intestino médio de lagartas de *Anticarsia gemmatalis* Hübner 1818 (Lepidoptera, Noctuidae). *Acta Biologica Leopoldensia*, Vol. (22): 89-95.

[25] Crickmore, N., Zeigler, D.R., Schnepf, E., Van Rie, J., Lereclus, D., Baum, J., Bravo, A. & Dean, D.H. (2005). *Bacillus thuringiensis* toxin nomenclature. [Online.] http://www.lifesci.su

[26] Marroquin, L.D.; Elyasnia, D.; Griffitts, J.S.; Feitelson, J.S. & Aroian, R.V. (2000). *Bacillus thuringiensis*: toxin susceptibility and isolation of resistance mutants in the nematode Caenorhabditis elegans. *Genetics*, Vol. (155): 1693-1699.

[27] Shelton, A. M., Ahao, J.Z. & Roush, R.T. (2002). Economic, ecologycal, food safety and social consequences of the deployment of Bt trangenic plants. *Annual Review of Entomology*, Vol. (47): 845-881.

[28] Fiuza, L.M. & Berlitz, D.L. (2009). Produtos de *Bacillus thuringiensis*: registro e comercialização. *Biotecnologia Ciência & Desenvolvimento*, Vol. (38): 58-60.

[29] Berlitz, D.L. & Fiuza, L.M. (2004). Avaliação toxicological de *Bacillus thuringiensis aizawai* para *Spodoptera frugiperda* (Lepidoptera: Noctuidae), em laboratório. *Biociências*, Vol. (12): 115-119.

[30] Knaak, N., Franz, A.R., Santos, G.F. & Fiuza, L.M. (2010). Histopathology and the lethal effect of Cry proteins and strains of *Bacillus thuringiensis* Berliner in *Spodoptera frugiperda*J.E. Smith Caterpillars (Lepidoptera, Noctuidae). *Brazilian Journal Biology*, Vol. (70): 677-684

[31] Knaak, N. and Fiuza, LM., 2005. Histopathology of A*nticarsia gemmatalis* Hübner (Lepidoptera; Noctuidae) treated with *Nucleopolyhedrovirus* and *Bacillus thuringiensis* serovar *kurstaki*. *Brazilian Journal of Microbiology*, vol. 36, no. 2, p. 195-199.

[32] Spies, A.F. & Spence, K.D. (1995). Effect sublethal *Bacillus thuringiensis* crystal endotoxin treatment on the larval midgut of a moth, *Manduca sexta*. *Tissue and Cell*, Vol. (17): 394-397.

[33] Bravo, A., Hendrickx, K., Jansens, S. & Peferoen, M. (1992). Immunocytochemical analysis of specific binding of *Bacillus thuringiensis* insecticidal crystal proteins to lepidopteran and coleopteran midgut membranes. *Journal of Invertebrate Pathology*, Vol. (60): 247-253.

[34] Griego, V.M., Fancher, L.J. & Spence, K.D. (1980). Scanning electron microscopy of the disruption of tobacco horn worm, *Manduca sexta*, midgut by *Bacillus thuringiensis* endotoxin. *Journal of Invertebrate Pathology*, Vol. (350): 186–189.

[35] Mathavan, S., Sudha, P.M. & Pechimuthu, S.M. (1989) Effect of *Bacillus thuringiensis* on the midgut cells of *Bombyxmori* larvae: A histopathological and histochemical study. *Journal of Invertebrate Pathology,* Vol. (53):217–227.

[36] Shao, Z., Cui, Y., Yi, H., Ji, J. & Yu, Z. (1998). Processing of Δ-endotoxin of *Bacillus thuringiensis* subsp. *Kurstaki* HD-1 in *Heliothis armigera* midgut juice and the effect of proteases inhibitors. *Journal of Invertebrate Pathology*, Vol. (72): 73-81.

[37] Tojo, A. & Aizawa, K. (1983). Dissolution and degradation of *Bacillus thuringiensis* δ endotoxin by gut juice protease of the silkworm *Bombyx mori. Appl. Environ. Microbiology*, Vol. (45): 576-580.

[38] Schwartz, J.L., Juteau, M., Grochulski, P., Cygler, M., Prefontaine, G., Brousseau, R. & Masson, L. (1997). Restriction of intramolecular movements within the Cry1Aa toxin molecule of *Bacillus thuringiensis* through disulfide bond engineering. *FEBS Lett.*, Vol. (410): 397-402.

[39] Masson, L., Tabashnik, B.E., Liu, Y.B. & Schwartz, J.L. (1999). Helix 4 of the *Bacillus thuringiensis* Cry1Aa toxin lines the lumen of the ion channel. *Journal of Biology Chemical,* Vol. (274): 31996-32000.

[40] Fiuza, L. M., Nielsen-Leroux, C., Goze, E., Frutos, R. & Charles, J.F. (1996). Binding of *Bacillus thuringiensis* Cry1 toxins to the midgut brush border membrane vesicles of *Chilosuppressalis* (Lepidoptera, Pyralidae): evidence of shared binding sites. *Applied Environmental Microbiollogy,* Vol. (62): 1544-1549.

[41] Knight, P., Crickmore, N. & Ellar, D. (1994). The receptor for *Bacillus thuringiensis*CryIAc delta-endotoxin in the brush border membrane of the lepidopteran *Manduca sexta* is aminopeptidase N. *Molecular Microbiology,* Vol. (11): 429-436.

[42] Brandtzaeg, P. (1982). Tissue preparation methods for imunocytochemistry. In: Bullock, G. & Petruz, P., *Techniques in imunocytochemistry*. Academic Press, London. pp. 49-51.

[43] Bayer, E. & Wilcheck, M. (1990). Protein biotinylation. *Methods in Enzymology,* Vol. (184): 138-159.

[44] Bradford, M. (1976). A rapid and sensitive method for the quantitation of microgram quantities of protein utilizing the principle of protein-dye binding. *Analytical Biochemistry,* Vol. (72): 248-254.

[45] Fiuza, L.M. (1995). Etude des sites récepteurs et de la toxicité des delta-endotoxines de *Bacillus thuringiensis* Berliner chez les larves de la Pyrale du riz, *Chilo suppressalis* Walker. *Thèse de doctorat en Sciences Agronomiques,* ENSA-M, Montpellier, France. 180p.

[46] Schmutterer, H. (1990). Properties and potential of natural pesticides from the neem tree, *Azadirachta indica. Annu. Rev. Entomology,* Vol. (35): 271-297.

[47] Roel, A.R., Vendramim, J. D., Frighetto, R.T.S. & Frighetto, N. (2000) Atividade tóxica de extratos orgânicos de *Trichilia pallida* Swartz (Meliaceae) sobre *Spodoptera frugiperda* (J.E. Smith). *An. Soc. Entomol. Brasil,* Vol. (29): 799-808.

[48] Roel, A.R. (2001). Utilização de plantas com propriedades inseticidas: uma contribuição para o desenvolvimento rural sustentável. Ver Int Desenv Local Vol. (1): 43-50.

[49] Reigosa, M. & Pedrol, N. (2002). *Allelopathy from molecules to ecosystems.* Plymouth: Science Publishers, 316p.

[50] Duke, S.O., Dayan, F.E. & Rimando, A.M. (2000). Natural products and herbicide discovery. IN: Cobb, A.H.; Kirkwood, R.C. (Ed.). *Herbicides and their mechanisms of action*. Sheffield: Academic Press, pp.105-133.

[51] Mello, M.O. & Silva-Filho, M.C. (2002). Plant-insect intections: na evolutionary arms race between two distinct defense mechanisms. *Brazilian Journal of Plant Physio*logy, Vol. (14): 71-81

[52] Strapazzon, J.O. (2004). Composição química e análise antimicrobiana do óleo volátil de *Annona squamosa* L. (Ariticum.) Chapecó, SC. Monografia de graduação. Universidade Comunitária Regional de Chapecó, 53 p.

[53] Takabayashi, J., Dicke, M. & Posthumus, M. A. (1994). Volatile herbivore-induced terpenoids in plant-mite interactions: variation caused bybiotic and abiotic factors. *Journal of Chemical Ecology*, Vol. (20): 1329-1354. http://dx.doi.org/10.1007/BF02059811

[54] Martinez, S.S. & Emdem, H.F. (2001). Redução do crescimento, deformidades e mortalidade de *Spodoptera littoralis* (Boisduval) (Lepidoptera: Noctuidae) causadas por Azadiractina. *Neotropical Entomology*, Vol. (30): 113-125.

[55] Knaak, N., Tagliari, M.S. & Fiuza, L.M. (2010). Histopatologia da interação de *Bacillus thuringiensis* e extratos vegetais no intestino médio de *Spodoptera frugiperda* (Lepidoptera: Noctuidae). *Arquivos do Instituto Biológico*, São Paulo, Vol. (77): 83-89.

[56] Knaak, N. 2011. Potencial dos óleos essenciais e proteínas vegetais, obtidos de plantas medicinais, no controle de pragas da cultura do arroz irrigado.Tese de Doutorado, Programa de Pós-Graduação em Biologia da Universidade do Vale do Rio dos Sinos. 107p.

[57] Simões, C.M.O., Schenkel, E.P., Gosmam, G., Mello, J.C.P., Mentz, L.A. & Petrovick, P.R. (2003). Farmacognosia da Planta ao medicamento. 5ª ed., Porto Alegre, Universidade, 1102 p.

[58] Martinez, S.S. (2002). O nim – *Azadirachta indica*: natureza, usos múltiplos, produção. Londrina, Instituto Agronômico do Paraná, 142p.

[59] Breuer, M.; Hoste, B.; De Loof, A. & Naqvi, S.N.H. (2003). Effect of *Melia azedarach* extract on the activity of NADPH-cytochrome c reductase and cholinesterase in insects. *Pestic. Bioch. Physiology*, Vol. (76): 99-103.

[60] Huang, Y., Tan, J.M.W.L., Kini, R.M. & Ho, S.H. (1997). Toxic and antifeedant action of nutmeg oil against *Tribolium castaneum* (Herbst) and *Sitophilus zeamais* Motsch. Journal of Stored Products Research, Vol. (4): 289-298.

[61] Bohnenstengel, F.I.; Wray, V.; Witte, L.; Srivastava, R.P. & Proksch, P. (1999). Inseticidal meliacarpins (C-seco limnoids) from *Melia azedarach*. *Phytochemistry*, Vol. (50): 977-982.

[62] Carpinella, M.C.; Defago, M.T.; Valladares, G. & Palacios, S.M. (2003). Antifeedant and inseticide proprieties of a limnoid from *Melia azedarach* (Meliaceae) with potential use for pest management. *J. Agric. Food Chemistry*, Vol. (51): 369-374.

[63] Correia, A.A., Wanderley-Teixeira, V., Teixeira, A.A.C., Oliveira, J.V. & Torres, J.B. (2009). Morfologia do Canal Alimentar de Lagartas de Spodoptera frugiperda (J.E. Smith) (Lepidoptera: Noctuidae) Alimentadas com Folhas Tratadas com Nim. *Neotropical Entomology*, Vol. (38): 083-091.

[64] Denolf, P., Jansens, S., Peferoen, M., Degheele, D. & Van Rie, J. (1993). Two different delta-endotoxin receptors in the midgut brush border membrane of the European corn borer, *Ostrinia nubilalis*. *Applied Environmental Microbiollogy*, Vol. (59): 1828-1837.

[65] Estada, U. & Ferre, J. (1994). Binding of insecticidal crystals proteins of *Bacillus thuringiensis* to the midgut brush border of the Cabbage Looper, *Trichoplusiani* and selection for resistance to one of the crystal proteins *Applied Environmental Microbiollogy*, Vol. (60): 3840-3846.

[66] Ravoahangimalala, O., Charles, J-F. & Schoeller-Raccaud, J. (1993). Immunological localization of *Bacillus thuringiensis* serovar *israelensis* toxins in midgut cells of intoxicated *Anopheles gambie* larvae (Diptera: Culicidae). *Research of Microbiology*, Vol. (144): 271-278.

[67] Boets, A., Jansens, S., Denolf, P., Peferoen, M. Degheele, D. & Van Rie, J. (1994). Sequential observations of toxin distribution and histopathological effects of CryIIIA in the gut of intoxicated *Leptinotarsa decemlineata* larvae. *XXVIIth Annual Meeting of the Society for Invertebrate Pathology*, pp. 377.

[68] Van Rie, J., Jansen, S., Höfte, H., Degheeled, D. & VanMellaert, H. (1990). Receptors on the brush border membrane of the insect midgut as determinants of the specificity of *Bacillus thuringiensis* δ-endotoxins. *Applied Environ. Microbiology*, Vol. (56): 1378-1385.

[69] Lee, M.K., You, T.H., Young, B.A., Cotrill, J.A., Valatis, A.P. & Dean, D.H. (1996). Aminopeptidase N purified from Gypsy moth brush border membrane vesicles is a specific receptor for *Bacillus thuringiensis* Cry1Ac toxin. *Applied Environmental Microbiollogy*, Vol. (62): 2845-2849.

[70] Hua, G., Masson, L., Jurat-Fuentes, J.L., Schwab, G. & Adang, M.J. (2001). Binding Analyses of *Bacillus thuringiensis* Cry delta-endotoxins using brush border membrane vesicles of *Ostrinia nubilalis Applied Environmental Microbiollogy*, Vol. (67): 872-879.

[71] Liang, Y., Patel, S.S. & Dean, D.H. (1995). Irreversible binding kinetics of *Bacillus thuringiensis* Cry1A delta-endotoxins to Gypsy moth brush border membrane vesicles is directly correlated to toxicity. *Journal of Biology Chemical*, Vol. (270): 24719-24724.

[72] Fiuza, L.M. (2009). Mecanismo de ção de *Bacillus thuringiensis*. *Biotecnologia Ciência & Desenvolvimento*, Vol. (38): 32-35.

Chapter 11

Neuronal and Mixed Neuronal-Glial Tumors of the Central Nervous System

Mohammed M.A. Al Barbarawi,
Mohammed Z. Allouh and Suhair M.A. Qudsieh

Additional information is available at the end of the chapter

http://dx.doi.org/10.5772/50733

1. Introduction

Objective: Neuronal and Mixed Neuronal-glial Tumors of the Central Nervous System are frequently encountered in the neurosurgical practice. *Differentiation of neuronal tumors from the more common glial tumors is crucial because neuronal tumors have favorable clinical outcomes and are generally curable with total surgical resection alone, whereas gliomas typically require further chemo-radiotherapy depending on their histologic grade and have poor prognosis. At histopathologic analysis, neuronal tumors are usually classified as pure neuronal cell tumors (gangliocytoma, Lhermitte-Duclos disease (dysplastic cerebellar gangliocytoma], central neurocytoma) and mixed neuronal-glial tumors (ganglioglioma, desmoplastic infantile ganglioglioma, dysembryoplastic neuroepithelial tumor, ganglioneuroma) In this chapter, we review the WHO classification of each type of neuroepithelial cell tumours and the incidence and distribution. The clinical presentation and neuroimaging will also be briefed, then we describe the specific histopathologic characteristics, immunohistochemestry and genetic suscipitability of the various neuronal tumors of the central nervous system and finally demonstrate the outcome of these lesions.*

2. Contents

2.1. Ganglioglioma and gangliocytoma

Ganglioglioma and gangliocytoma are well-differentiated, slowly growing benign neuroepithelial tumors. with World Health Organization (WHO) grade I. higher grade is based on the degree of malignancy in the glial-cell component. They represent around 1% of all central nervous system (CNS) tumors, However it is frequently oencountered in children and young adults between age 8 and 25 years. Gangliogliomas contain mature neoplastic neuronal cells, neoplastic glial cells, astrocytic cells, and ganglion cells, and may display mitotic activity. These lesions are curable by total removal.

2.2. Central neurocytoma and extraventricular neurocytoma

Central neurocytoma and extraventricular neurocytoma are WHO grade II tumors composed of regular rounded cells that have undergone neuronal differentiation. Central neurocytomas are typicaly located within the lateral ventricles just next to the foramen of Monro, whereas extraventricular neurocytomas are located within the brain parenchyma. Both characteristically occur in young adults. The outcome is favorable after complete resectioning.

2.3. Dysembryoplastic neuroepithelial tumor

Dysembryoplastic neuroepithelial tumor (DNT) is frequently a benign, supratentorial glial-neuronal WHO grade I tumor. DNT occur mainly in children or young adults, who usually present with intractable partial complex seizure. Characterized by a predominantly cortical location, DNT histopathologically exhibits a complex columnar and multinodular architecture, and is often associated with cortical dysplasia.

2.4. Desmoplastic infantile astrocytoma and desmoplastic infantile ganglioglioma

Desmoplastic infantile astrocytomas (DIAs) and desmoplastic infantile gangliogliomas (DIGs) are almost WHO grade I tumors that are often cystic and commonly occur in infants. Composed of a prominent desmoplastic stroma with neuroepithelial components, mainly neoplastic astrocytes in DIAs or astrocytes together with variable neuronal components in DIGs, they involve the cerebral cortex and leptomeninges, and are often adherent to the dura. The natural course is benign.

2.5. Rosette-forming glioneuronal tumor of the fourth ventricle

Rosette-forming glioneuronal tumor of the fourth ventricle (RGNT) is a usually rare and slowly growing WHO grade I tumor. It is commonly affecting young adults, RGNT is composed of two distinct histological cells types; uniform neurocytes which form rosettes and/or perivascular pseudorosettes and astrocytic cells similar to pilocytic astrocytomas. The prognosis is good upon surgical removal.

2.6. Cerebellar liponeurocytoma

This rare type of cerebellar tumors is WHO grade II tumor that typically occurs in adults. It is Composed of neuronal, astrocytic, and some lipomatous cells, they tend to recur after initial treatment.

2.7. Papillary glio-neuronal tumor

Papillary glio-neuronal tumors is a well defined and benign with WHO grade I. the natural course is insidius. It is composed of flat to cuboidal, GFAP-positive astrocytes lining hyalinized vascular pseudo-papillae and synaptophysin-positive interpapillary sheets of neuronal cells. Upon microscopy, it exhibits different sizes of large and intermediate neuron "ganglioid" cells.

2.8. Spinal paraganglioma

Spinal paraganglioma is encapsulated, benign, neuro-endocrine WHO grade I tumor. Arising from neural crest cells and composed of segmental or collateral autonomic ganglia (paraganglia), It is primarily involving the cauda equine and filum terminale region. The uniform main cells exhibit neuronal differentiation and forming compact nests (Zellballen) surrounded by cells and a delicate capillary network within the CNS.

3. Gangliogliomas and gangliocytomas

3.1. Definition

Gangliogliomas and gangliocytomas are well-differentiated, slowly growing benign neuroepithelial neoplasms that consist of neoplastic, mature ganglion cells. Both gangliogliomas and gangliocytomas are a type of neuroepithelial tumor that is the most frequent pathology observed in patients with long-term epilepsy. A gangliocytoma in the absence of neoplastic glial-cell development and a ganglioglioma in the presence of neoplastic glial-cell development. (1)

3.2. WHO grading

Gangliocytomas and most gangliogliomas are categorized as WHO grade I tumors (1).

Some gangliogliomas with anaplastic features of the glial component are categorized as WHO grade III tumors (anaplastic gangliogliomas). Criteria for grade II types has also been suggested (2, 3).

3.3. Incidence and gender distribution

These uncommon neoplastic lesions represent only 0.4% of all CNS tumors and 1.3% of all brain tumors (3,4). The age of patients is variable, ranging from 2 months to 70 years. Data from 5 large series of a total of 626 patients indicate an average age at diagnosis ranging from 8.5 to 25 years and a male: female ratio ranging from 1.1:1 to 1.9:1 (5,6,7,8). In one study, the mean age in children at diagnosis is 9.5 years, with a slight female prevalence (9).

3.4. Localization

The vast majority of gangliogliomas (>70%) occur in the temporal lobe. However, Gangliocytomas and most gangliogliomas may occur throughout the CNS, including in the cerebrum, brain stem, cerebellum, spinal cord, optic nerves, and pituitary and pineal glands. (2, 6, 7, 8, 10).

3.5. Clinical features

Variable clinical symptoms of gangliocytomas and most gangliogliomas are encountered and related to tumor size and site. Seizure is usually the initial presenting symptoms. Gangliocytomas and gangliogliomas are the most common tumors associated with chronic and intractable temporal lobe epilepsy and observed in 15% to 25% of patients undergoing epilepsy surgery (11,12).duration of symptoms ranging from 1 month to 50 years before diagnosis, with a median interval of 6 to 25 years (6,7,8). Tumors affecting the brain stem or spinal cord frequently present with crossed paresis or long-tract lesion and sphincteric disorder of a mean duration of 1.25 and 1.4 years, respectively (6).

3.6. Neuroimaging

Computed tomography (CT) of a ganglioglioma or gangliocytoma may indicate a well-circumscribed solid mass or cyst with a mural nodule and some calcification, and slight or absent contrast enhancement. Skull scalloping may be noted adjacent to superficial cerebral tumors. These lesions appear hypointense on T1-weighted and hyperintense on T2-weighted magnetic resonance imaging (MRI), with well-defined masses showing enhancement absorption that can range from none to vivid and may be solid or only on the rim or nodular (13,14) . **Figure 1**

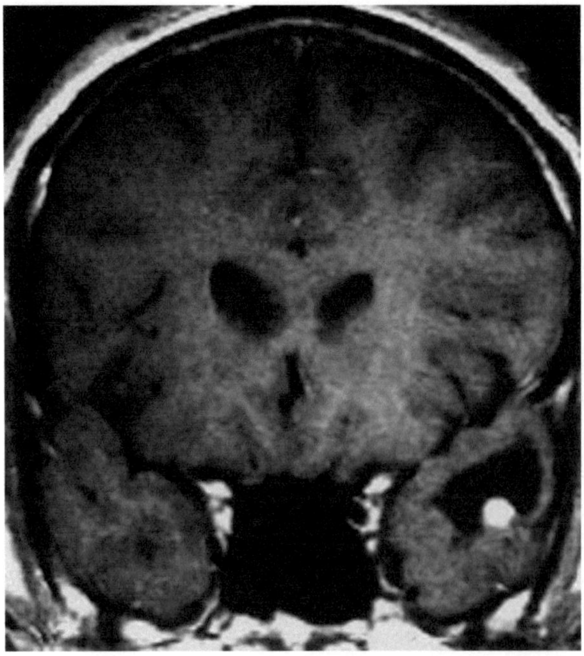

Figure 1. MRI

3.7. Macroscopical features

Gangliogliomas are solid or cystic lesions, characteristically with little mass effect. Calcification may be observed, whilst hemorrhage and necrosis are rare (8)

3.8. Histopathology

A primary characteristic of gangliogliomas is a mixture of neuronal and glial-cell elements that may display a striking heterogeneity. Gangliocytomas consist of clusters of large, multipolar neurons with immature features. The matrix contains non-neoplastic glial components and a network of reticulin fibers. Immature neurons are characterized by the loss of cyto-architectural arrangement of subcortical localization, a grouped appearance, enlargement of cells, and aggregation of Nissl bodies. Multinucleated neurons may present in 50% of cases. On the other hand, the glial element in gangliogliomas, which comprises the proliferation part of the tumor, shows considerable inconsistency, and may include any glial-cell type with Rosenthal fibers and eosinophilic granular bodies. Thestroma is typically fibrillary and may contain a microcystic component with mucous material. Occasional mitotic activity may be noted, and is typically compatible with the diagnosis of ganglioglioma, whereas necrosis is absent unless the glial component is undergoing malignant transformation. Other histopathological features that may be seen in gangliogliomas are calcifications, extensive lymphatic infiltrates with perivascular spaces or within the tumor substance or brain tissue, and a capillary network that forms an angiomatous constituent. In high-grade (anaplastic) gangliogliomas, malignant changes almost always involve the glial component and may be seen at the site of a previously removed ganglioglioma (2, 3, 5, 7, 8). **Figure 2A**

3.9. Immunohistochemistry

No specific marker is available to differentiate dysplastic and neoplastic neurons from normal and mature neurons. Neuronal protein markers, such as synaptophysin, neurofilaments, MAP2, and Neu N, are used to reveal the neuronal component in gangliogliomas.. However, use of the onco-fetal CD34 antigen can be positive, as CD34 is absent in neural cells of the adult brain but consistently expressed in 70% to 80% of gangliogliomas, especially those arising from the temporal lobe (15). Staining for GFAP reveals the astrocytic component the neoplastic glial element of gangliogliomas. Contrary to that seen in diffuse gliomas, MAP2 immunoreactivity is usually weak or absent in the astrocytic component of gangliogliomas (16). **Figure 2B**

3.10. Electron microscopy

The presence of neurons with dense core granules is a characteristic feature of gangliogliomas and gangliocytomas. Neuronal synaptic junctions may be few or completely absent (5,17). Observation of round protein bodies in gangliogliomas has also been mentioned (18).

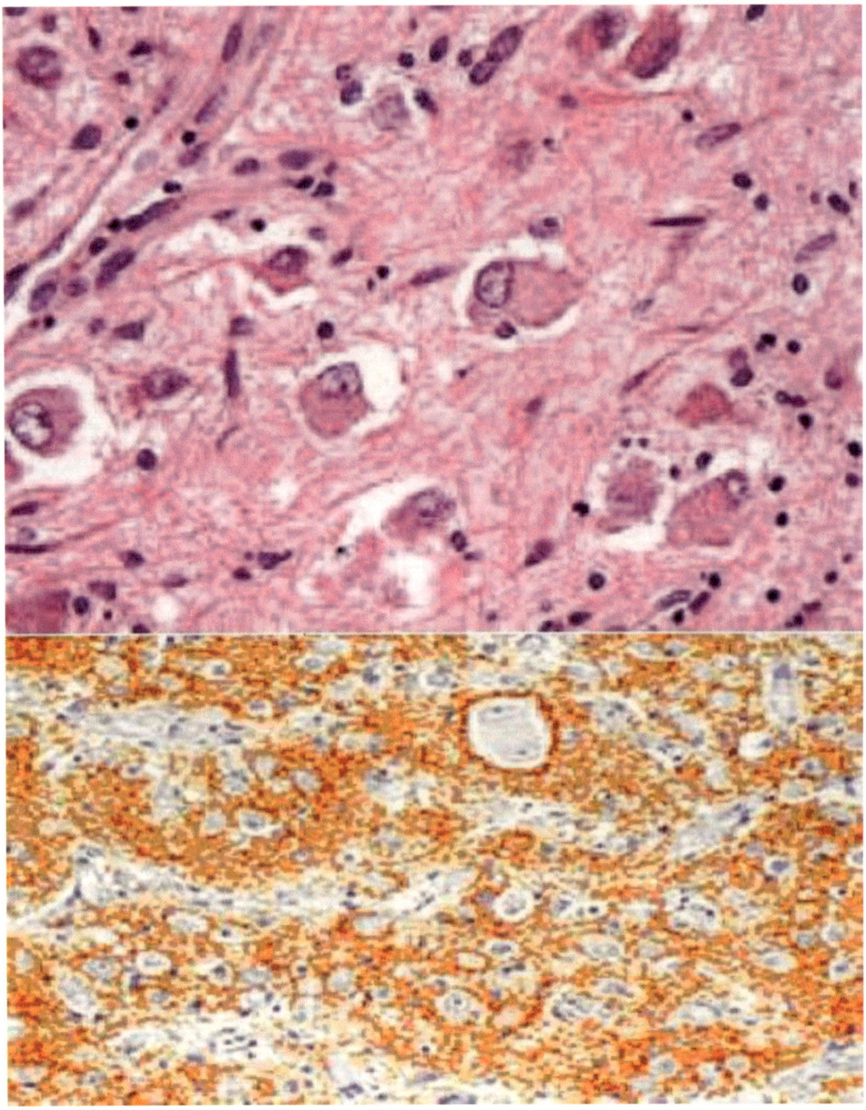

Figure 2. A and B

3.11. Proliferation index

Ki-67/MIB-1 labeling the glial component has shown values ranging from 1.1 to 2.7%. Mitotic activity is low (5,7).

3.12. Genetic susceptibility

Genetic vulnerability to the development of gangliogliomas and gangliocytomas has not been well established. Previous studies reported a ganglioglioma of the optic nerve in a patient with neurofibromatosis type 1 (19) and a ganglioglioma in a Peutz-Jeghers patient

(20).. Mutational analysis of the tuberous sclerosis 1 (TSC1) and TSC2 genes revealed significant sequence alterations in the TSC2 gene, including polymorphisms in intron 4 and exon 41, in patients with gangliogliomas. In a further study of ezrin and radixin genes, coding for the interaction partners of TSC1 and TSC2 was not observed (30,31,32).

Chromosomal abnormalities have been recorded in one-third of cases, in the approximately 30 cases of gangliogliomas that have been studied cytogenetically, a change in chromosome 7 was the most one observed. The karyotype was found to be abnormal in 3 cases with unfavorable outcomes. (21,22,23,24,25,26). Chromosomal imbalances have been detected in 5/5 gangliogliomas by comparative genomic hybridization. Although partial loss of chromosome 9p and gain of chromosome 7 has been observed in several patients, abnormal epidermal growth factor receptor (EGFR) expression was not observed in these cases (27). A study of 14 cases (11 WHO grade I and 3 WHO grade III) failed to show TP53 mutation, PTEN mutation, or CDK4 and EGFR amplification, whereas CDKN2A deletion was observed in two-thirds of cases of anaplastic ganglioglioma (28). However, TP53 mutation was only noted in the recurrence of a WHO grade I ganglioglioma (29).

3.13. Histogenesis

The histogenesis of gangliogliomas and gangliocytomas still not understood. However, evolution from a dysplastic, abnormal glio-neuronal precursor with subsequent neoplastic transformation of the glial element has been proposed (33).

3.14. Prognosic factors

Favorable prognosis is observed in patients with long-standing epilepsy with temporal localization and complete surgical resectioning. These lesions are typically benign tumors with a 7.5-year recurrence-free survival rate of 94%.. Anaplastic changes, such as mitotic activity and microvascular proliferation and necrosis, in the glial component similar to those observed in high-grade gliomas.

4. Central neurocytomas and extraventricular neurocytomas

4.1. Definition

Central neurocytomas and extraventricular neurocytomas are neoplasms composed of uniform round cells with neuronal differentiation. Central neurocytomas are typically located in the lateral ventricles in the region of the foramen of Monro and extraventricular neurocytomas in the brain parenchyma. These tumors are usually seen in young adults and have a favorable prognosis.

4.2. WHO grading

Central neurocytomas correspond histologically to WHO grade II tumors (1).

4.3. Historical background

"Central neurocytoma" expression was used by Hassoun et al. (34) to describe a neuronal tumor with pathological features to differentiate it from cerebral neuroblastomas that occurs in young adults, it is commonly located in the third ventricle, and histologically may resemble oligodendrogliomas. They were also reported in other locations. The term central neurocytoma should be restricted to neoplasms located within the intracerebral ventricles. Tumors similar to central neurocytomas but occurring within the cerebral hemispheres ("cerebral neurocytomas") or the spinal cord (35, 36,37) have subsequently been mentioned and described as "extraventricular neurocytoma" these tumours are now given to neoplasms that arise within the CNS parenchyma and have histological features with the more common central neurocytomas but exhibit a wider morphological spectrum. Neurocytic differentiation has been reported in an increasing number of tumors with specific morphological characteristics, some of these have been categorized as new entities, such as cerebellar liponeurocytomas, papillary glioneuronal tumors, or their variants (38, 39, 40).

4.4. Incidence and sex distribution

The incidence ranged from 0.25% to 0.5% of all intracranial tumors. In an analysis of 243 cases, age at clinical manifestation is almost variable ranging from 8 days to 67 years (mean age, 29 years), with 69% between the ages of 20 and 40 year. Both sexes are equally affected (40, 34).

4.5. Localization

Central neurocytomas are usually located supratentorially in the lateral or the third ventricle. With most common site is the anterior part of the lateral ventricles (50%), more frequently on the left, followed by combined extension into the lateral and third ventricles and a bilateral intraventricular location. Attachment to the septum pellucidum is common, but isolated third-ventricular occurrence is rare. (40, 41)

4.6. Clinical features

The majority of patients present with symptoms of increased intracranial pressure rather than with other neurological deficit. The clinical history is short (mean 3.2 months). Central neurocytomas may present as acute hemorrhage or as an incidental finding on imaging (41).

4.7. Neuroimaging

On CT scans, mass is typically isodense or slightly hyperdense. Enhancement is common . Calcifications and cystic changes may be observed. MRI scan shows heterogeneous hypointensity on T1-weighted images and fluid- attenuated inversion recovery (FLAIR) and hyperintensity on T2-weighted images and FLAIR, with a well-defined margin mild to strong enhancement after gadolinum injection (42). **Figure 3**

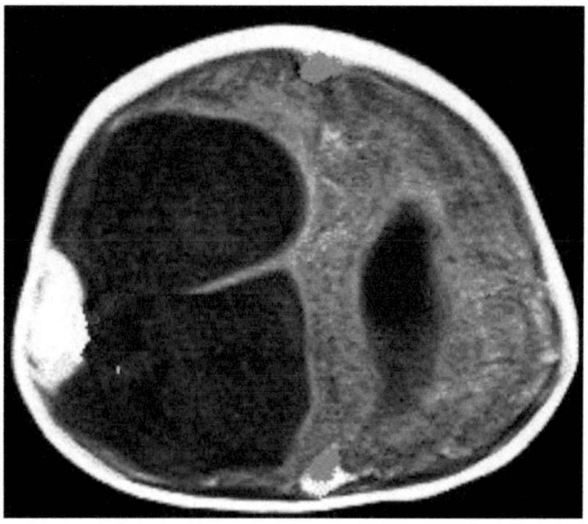

Figure 3.

4.8. Macroscopical appearance

Intraventricular tumors are typically grey in color and friable with varying calcifications, these tumours are vascular and with occasional hemorrhage. (43,44)

4.9. Histopathology

Central neurocytomas have a benign histological appearance and may display various architectural patterns, even within the same specimen, including an oligodendroglioma-like honeycomb appearance, large fibrillary areas mimicking the irregular "rosettes" in pineocytomas. These lesions are neuroepithelial tumors composed of uniform round cells that show immunohistochemical and ultrastructural features of neuronal differentiation, fibrillary areas mimicking neuropils, and a low proliferation rate. Cells are isomorphous, having a round or oval nucleus with a finely speckled chromatin and an occasional nucleolus, cells arranged in straight lines, or perivascular pseudorosettes similar to those noted in ependymoma tumours. Calcifications are usually seen in around 50% of cases, normally distributed throughout the tumor. Blood vessels, classically arranged in a linear architecture pattern, giving an endocrine appearance. Rarer findings may include Homer Wright rosettes and ganglioid cells (43,44).

These tumour may mimic, and must be distinguished from, oligodendroglioma, ependymoma, pineocytoma, and dysembryoplastic neuroepithelial . In rare cases, anaplastic histological features, including high mitotic activity and microvascular proliferation, have been observed. In some conditions, necrosis was associated with anaplastic features. Necrosis may also be observed in rare cases that are otherwise without malignant features, may be s as a vascular effect (41, 44, 46, 47, 48,49). **Figure 4A**

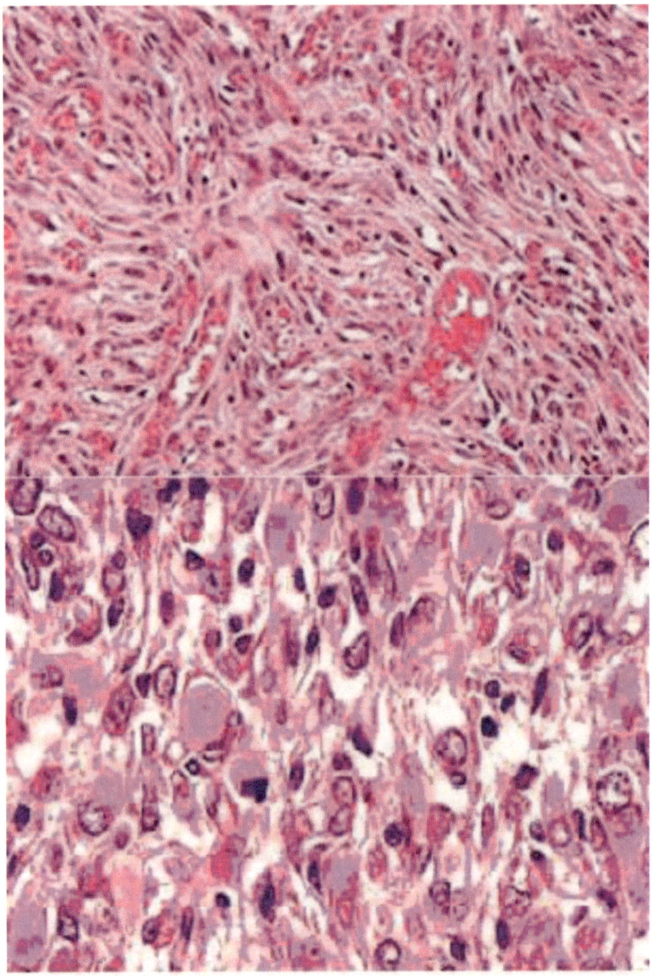

Figure 4. A and B

4.10. Immunohistochemistry

Synaptophysin is the most suitable and reliable diagnostic marker, with immunoreactivity diffusely present in neuropils, especially in fibrillary zones and perivascular nuclei-free cuffs (48). A significant number of nuclei are immunopositive for NeuN in almost all cases (50). The mean labeling index was 74% in one series of 11 cases, with a significantly lower Ki-67 staining rate for cells expressing NeuN (51). In extraventricular lesions, intracytoplasmic and para-nuclear immunolabeling must be cautiously inferred whenever other histological, immunohistochemical, or ultrastructural data of neuronal differentiation is lacking. Of particular interest is the anti-Hu antibody because it labels the nuclei of neurocytes (52). Chromogranin A and neurofilament staining are typically absent except when ganglion cells are present Although most studies found that GFAP was expressed only in trapped reactive astrocytes, the antigen has been detected by some studies in tumor cells (44, 45, 53 ,54). **Figure 4B**

4.11. Electron microscopy

Electron microscopy may be required when expression of specific neuronal markers (synaptophysin, NeuN) is questionable and in other extraventricular neoplasms mimicking central neurocytomas. The central neurocytoma cells show uniform round nuclei with a finely discreted chromatin and a small nucleolus in a few cells. The cytoplasm contains mitochondria, a prominent Golgi apparatus, and several rough endoplasmic reticulum cisternae, often arranged in concentric lamellae. copious thin and combined cell processes containing microtubules and dense core and clear vesicles are always observed (41,55).

4.12. Proliferation index

MIB-1 labeling indices are classically low, usually less than 2%. However, Tumors with indices greater than 2%, as in one series in which they were found to be 3% , are referred to as "atypical neurocytomas" and associated with a significantly shorter recurrence-free interval (53, 56, 57).

4.13. Genetic susceptibility

Unclear, but central neurocytoma was observedin patients with von Hippel-Lindau disease (58). The molecular pathogenesis of central neurocytomas remains unknown, the observation of several genetic alterations, mainly chromosomal gains, has been reported. In one study, gain on chromosome 7 was observed in 3 of 9 neurocytomas (59). However, another study found no EGFR amplification in central neurocytomas (60). In related studies, gains on chromosomes 2p, 10q, 18q, and 13q were found in over 20% of tumors in one study ; an isochromosome 17 and complex karyotype were observed in 2 studies (61, 62, 63); and TP53 mutations and MYCN amplification were reported to be rare or absent in several studies (45, 60, 63, 64, 65).there are two studies that reported loss of 1p and 19q, 1 study reported allelic loss on 1p as well as an inability to detect 19q (64), whereas the other study reported 6 of 9 tumors showed loss at 1 or more loci on 1p and that 5 tumors showed 19q loss. These data suggest that central neurocytomas are genetically distinct from oligodendrogliomas. Although the expression profiles of cerebellar liponeurocytomas appear to have a closer relationship to those of central neurocytomas, the lack of TP53 mutations in central neurocytomas suggests the involvement of different genetic pathways (60, 66,67).

4.14. Histogenesis

Central neurocytomas were previously thought to be derived from precurssor cells of the septum pellucidum (34). Still, the indication of both astrocytic and neuronal differentiation in some tumor cells by various approaches in vivo and in vitro has suggested that they are derived from neuroglial precursor cells with a potential to undergo dual differentiation. These precursor cells might arise from the subependymal layer of the lateral ventricle or from the ventricular region. (45,54, 68).

4.15. Prognostic factors

The natural course of central neurocytoma is classically benign. Total surgical resection is the most important prognostic factor. recurrence is frequent with incomplete removal, but the residual tumor growth can be treated with radiotherapy. CNS dissemination is rare. (57, 66, 69, 70). central neurocytomas is rarely aggressive (44,47). Patients with central neurocytomas and a MIB-1 labeling index (LI) >2% or >3% have significantly shorter recurrence-free intervals. Involvement of the periventricular parenchyma involvement may be associated with poor outcome (71, 72).

4.16. Extraventricular neurocytomas

Extraventricular neurocytomas are usually well-defined and contrast-enhancing lesions that often have a cyst–mural nodule complex which is usually useful in distinguishing them from histologically similar neoplasms, such as oligodendrogliomas. Histologically, extraventricular neurocytomas may be identical to central lesions, but are often more complex, less cellular, and more likely to contain ganglion cells or ganglioid cells with nuclei that are larger than those of neurocytes. Lower cellularity, in combination with the presence of perinuclear haloes, may give these lesions the appearance of oligodendrogliomas. Although GFAP-positive glial cells have been observed, it has been difficult to identify them as clearly neoplastic. Hyalinized vessels and dense calcification are common (73).

5. Dysembryoplastic neuroepithelial tumors

5.1. Definition

Dysembryoplastic neuroepithelial tumors (DNTs) are usually benign. They are supratentorial glio- neuronal neoplasms that seen in children or young adults. Characterized by a cortical location and intractable partial complex seizures, they ideally demonstrate a complex columnar and multinodular structural design and are often associated with cortical dysplasia (74).

5.2. WHO grading

DNTs correspond histologically to WHO grade I tumors. (1)

5.3. Historical background

DNTs were first recognized as lesions in patients who had undergone epilepsy surgery for the treatment of longstanding, drug-resistant partial seizure sand showed unusual morphological features, including cortical topography, multinodular architecture, a "specific glioneuronal component" with a columnar structure. No recurrence with long term follow up even in patients with incomplete partia resection. Several factors strongly suggested a dysembryoplastic origin, the term "dysembryoplastic neuroepithelial tumor" was proposed for these lesions (74).

In the 1993 WHO Classification of Tumors Affecting the Central Nervous System (36), DNTs were included in the category of "neuronal and mixed neuronal-glial tumors." With

"complex form," and "simple type" (75). Later , "non-specific histological forms" were addedd. Furthermore, it has been indicated that DNTs may be seen in the infratentorial location (76, 77, 78,79).

5.4. Incidence

Incidence is variable. In a study of patients who were treated surgically for epilepsy, the incidence of "typical" DNTs was reported to be 12% in adults and 13.5% in children (80), whereas it was reported to be 19% to 22% in all patients in a series that included "non-specific" histological variants (78,81,82). Among all neuroepithelial tumors diagnosed in a single institution, DNTs were identified in about 0.2% among patients aged more than 20 years and in 1.2% of the patients under the age of 20 years (83).

5.5. Age and sex distribution

In about 90% of cases, the first seizure attack occurs before 20 years of age, but it may present from 3 weeks to 38 years (84,85). though patients are often diagnosed in the 2ed or 3rd decade of life, detection of DNTs by imaging in children or young adults with recent onset seizures has become more common, leading to more surgical intervention for treatment of DNTs in pediatric neurosurgery. It was observe that males are more slightly affected. (86, 87, 88, 89,90).

5.6. Localization

There is a predilection for the temporal lobe and for involvement with mesial structures although DNTs may be located in any part of the supratentorial cortex, (80, 81,82,83,84). In one series of patients treated in a general practice, temporal lobe involvement was found in 50% or fewer of cases (85,86). DNTs have also been found in the area of the caudate nucleus (76,77) or lateral ventricle, the septum pellucidum, the trigonoseptal region (88), the midbrain and tectum , and the cerebellum or cerebellum and brain stem (89,90,91,92). In total, 25 extracortical cases have been reported. In addition, 4 cases of multifocal DNTs have been reported, indicating that these tumors may arise in the region of the third ventricle, the basal ganglia, and the pons (93, 94,95).

5.7. Clinical presentation

Drug -resistant partial complex seizure is the typical presentation with or without secondary generalization, and no focal neurological deficit. The duration of seizures prior to surgical resection can vary from weeks to many years, leading to variability in patient age at pathologic diagnosis(79, 73,74, 97,98).

5.8. Neuroimaging

The cortical location of the lesion in the absence of both mass effect and peritumoral edema are important criteria in differentiating between DNTs and gliomas. DNTs typically encompass the thickness of the normal cortex and, in a minority of the cases, have an area of signal abnormality that extends into the subcortical white matter. The cortical location of the lesion is easily identified on MRI than on CT. DNTs appear hyperintense on T2-weighted images and hypointense or iso-intense on T1-weighted images. They often have a pseudo-cystic or multi-cystic appearance although true cyst formations are rare and small (91). In tumors located at the convexity, scalloping of the overlying bone is often observed on scans , a finding supports the diagnosis of DNT(, 77, 99,100, 101,102). Calcifications are rare. Contrast enhancement on CT or MRI is not common, it is often appearing as rings rather than homogeneous enhancement. Such ring-shaped contrast enhancement may be observed on a previously non-enhancing tumor on scans (96, 102). Increased tumour size, without peritumoral edema, may also be observed on imaging follow-up. However, these changes are naturally not signs of malignant transformation but rather as a result of ischemic or hemorrhagic changes (103,104).

5.9. Macroscopy

DNTs vary in size from several millimeters to several centimeters. In their typical location, they are often easily identified superficially at the cortical, and may show exophytic development, but indicate no involvement of leptomeninges. The most typical feature is viscous consistency of the glioneuronal component, which may be associated with multiple or single firmer nodules, and spreading out of the affected cortex (68).

5.10. Histopathology

The histological hallmark of a classical DNT is the presence of a "specific glio-neuronal constituent." This element is characterized by columns formed by bundles of axons lined by small oligodendroglia-like cells that are oriented perpendicularly to the cortical surface between which neurons with normal cytology appear to float in a pale, eosinophilic medium. There are also elements of scattered GFAP-positive stellate astrocytes. Depending on the amount of fluid extravasation, subtle variation from a columnar to o a more packed in structure may be observed . Several histological forms of DNTs have been mentioned, but their subclassification has no clinical or therapeutic implications (76,77). **Figure 5A.B**

5.11. Complex and non specific forms

In the complex form of a DNT, glial nodules, which give the tumor a feature of multinodular pattern, are seen in association with a specific glio-neuronal element. The variable appearance of these tumors is due to the presence of multiple cells of astrocytic, oligodendrocytic, and neuronal components. The glial components seen in the complex forms of DNTs have a highly variable form due to many causes : 1- they may form typical nodules with diffuse pattern; 2- they may mimic usual categories of gliomas and may illustrate unusual features; 3- they usually resemble low-grade gliomas, but may demonstrate nuclear atypia, some mitotic activity, or microvascular-like proliferation and ischemic necrosis; 4- they display a microvascular network. Within the glial components, typically calcified vessels are frequent that may behave as vascular malformations and be responsible for bleeding (65,66,86, 99,101,103, 104,105).

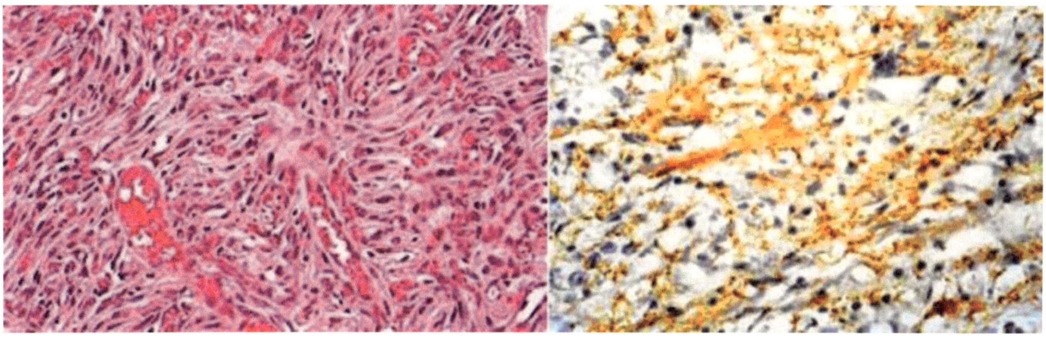

Figure 5. A and B

"Non-specific" histological variants of DNTs, identified according to clinical presentation as well as their cortical location, neuroimaging features, and steadiness on long-term preoperative imaging follow-up, have been described (77). Due to lackness the specific glioneuronal element and multinodular architecture, these variants are often histologically indistinguishable from low-grade gliomas. The diagnosis of these tumors thus requires that the clinical presentation and neuro-imaging appearance of the lesion be taken into consideration. Non-specific histological types account for 20% to 50% of DNTs in many studies (79,106,). Although gliomas identified in patients with long-term epilepsy during epilepsy surgery are typically associated with a distinctly benign course the diagnosis of "non-specific" histological variants of DNTs still debatable (107,108,110).

5.12. Simple form

Morphologically, the simple form of a DNT consists of a unique glioneuronal component it shows a patchy pattern owing to the proximity of foci of tumor and a well-defined cortex (76),.

5.13. Cortical dysplasia and Neuronal distribution of DNTs

Dysplastic disorganization of the cortex has been observed in up to 80% of DNT cases in studies with adequate sampling (111,112). Supratentorial cortical DNTs contain mature neurons that, both in the tumor itself and in the area of cortical dysplasia, may show different degrees of cytological anomaly. Thoug, DNTs do not have atypical or immature neurons that look like dysplastic ganglion cells as observed in gangliogliomas. Some tumor cells with an oligodendrocytic appearance have been found to occasionally express neuronal markers and display axo-somatic synapses suggesting that what is called "oligodendroglial-like cells" of DNTs and it may undergo early neuronal differentiation. However, using in-situ hybridization indicates that oligodendro-glial-like cells copy myelin genes and express myelin oligodendrocyte glycoprotein protein, indicating oligodendro-glial demarcation (113, 114,115, 116).

5.14. Cortical topography

The borders of the tumor often match with those of the cortex to a very large degree. it also appears to involve the adjoining white matter. However, as neurons are typically found in even the deeper parts of the tumor and in the neighboring white matter, such association is high likely indicates disordered neuronal migration (117).

5.15. Diagnostic criteria

The diagnosis of DNT should be taken into consideration in every case in which all of the following criteria (76, 77, 80. 81) are present:

1. the presence of partial complex seizures with/ without secondary generalization beginning before age 20
2. the absence of progressive neurological deficit.
3. the presence of a supratentorial lesion with a predominantly cortical topography, best indicated on MRI
4. the absence of mass effect on CT or MRI, except if related to a cyst
5. the absence of peritumoral edema on the scans

5.16. Comparison between DNTs and gangliogliomas

Differential diagnosis of DNTs and gangliogliomas may be tricky on account of several factors: 1- the clinical presentation of gangliogliomas is often similar to that of DNTs. 2- the immature ganglion cells of gangliogliomas may not be present in a small or inadequate sample. 3- Gangliogliomas may show a multinodular arrangement, 4- small gangliogliomas may show a predominant cortical topography.

A ganglioglioma is suspected when a tumor shows perivascular lymphocytic infiltration, a network of reticulin fibers, and a large cystic component. as gangliogliomas may undergo malignant transformation, their distinction from DNTs is important from a prognostic point of view. (118, 119, 120,121).

5.17. Comparison between DNTs and low-grade gliomas

The above clinical and radiological criteria help in distinguishing benign DNTs from diffuse gliomas. In diagnosis, it is important to consider that 1- in diffuse gliomas, so-called "floating" neurons may be present, 2- in low-grade diffuse gliomas, infiltrative microcystic activity may cause to the formation of a construction that mimics a "specific glio-neuronal element"; 3- some oligodendrogliomas, a nodular pattern may be seen, 4- in diffuse gliomas, secondary architectural changes in the cortex caused by the expansion of gliomas into the cortex may be not easy to differentiate from the presence of dysplastic cortical disorganization (76,77,80.81)..

5.18. Genetic susceptibility

DNTs have reported in patients with neurofibromatosis type 1 (NF1) and with XYY syndrome (122,123,124).

5.19. Proliferation index

Variable MIB-1 labeling indices of DNTs have been reported from 0% to 8% focally (79, 81, 84).

5.20. Histogenesis

Many factors have suggested that DNTs are a malformative origin, including the presence of focal cortical dysplasia and migrated neurons in the adjacent white matter, young age of symptom onset, and bone deformity adjacent to the tumor. Some observations indicate that they may be derived from secondary germinal layers. the histogenesis of DNTs remains unknown (74,77,81, 125)

5.21. Prognostic factors

DNTs are benign lesions. Their stability was indicated in a study of 53 patients for whom successive pre-operative CT or MRI was available with a mean duration of follow-up of 4.5 years (102). Long-term clinical follow-up typically shows no evidence of recurrence, even in patients with incomplete surgical resection (76, 97,99, 102, 107, 126). Risk factors for post operative recurrent seizures at long-term follow-up include longer pre-operative history of seizures, cortical dysplasia next to DNT and residual tumour (85, 100, 127, 128). Malignant transformation is extremely rare, only 2 cases reported from 700 cases of DNTs (129).

6. Desmoplastic infantile astrocytomas and desmoplastic infantile gangliogliomas

Desmoplastic infantile astrocytomas (DIAs) and desmoplastic infantile gangliogliomas (DIGs) are usually large cystic tumors occurring in infantile period that typically affect the cerebral cortex and leptomeninges and are often attached to the dura. DIGs contain neoplastic astrocytes and neuronal components while DIAs contain only neoplastic astrocytes.

6.1. WHO grading

Histologically, DIAs and DIGs correspond to WHO grade I tumors.

6.2. Historical annotation

DIAs were originally described by Taratuto et al in 1982. (130) as meningocerebral astrocytomas attached to the dura displaying a desmoplastic reaction. Their subsequent description as superficial cerebral astrocytomas attached to the dura (131) led to the delineation of a previously unknown entity. In 1993, this entity was included in the WHO Classification of Tumors Affecting the Central Nervous System (132) under the term "desmoplastic cerebral astrocytoma of infancy." In 1987, VandenBerg et al reported observation of desmoplastic supratentorial neuroepithelial tumors of infancy with diverse differentiation ("desmoplastic infantile gangliogliomas") in the same clinical setting. They described the histopathology of DIGs as differing from that of DIAs due to the presence of a neuronal component with variable differentiation in the former. (133). Since both types of lesions have similar clinical and neuroimaging features they have been currently categorized together as DIAs or DIGs in the WHO Classification.

6.3. Incidence

DIAs and DIGs are rare tumours and only observed in childhood whose rate can only be estimated from their reported frequency in institutional series. One series of 6500 CNS tumors in patients of all ages reported only 22 cases of DIG at a rate of 0.3% (134). In a series of CNS intracranial tumors limited only to the pediatric age group reported 6 cases of DIA, accounting for 1.25% of all childhood brain neoplasm. While, reports limited to brain tumors of infancy have found that DIAs and DIGs account for 16% of intracranial tumors (131,135).

6.4. Age and sex allocation

In a study, the age range for 84 reported cases of DIA and DIG was found to be 1 to 24 months. Males ae more commonly affected, with Male:female ratio is 1.5:1. The large majority of infantile cases present within the first year of life. However, several non-infantile DIA, DIG between 5 to 25 years have been reported (136, 137).

6.5. Localization

DIAs and DIGs invariably arise in the supratentorial region and commonly involve more than one lobe, most frequently the frontal and parietal lobes, followed by the temporal and less commom the occipital lobe (137).

6.6. Clinical presentation

The clinical features of DIAs and DIGs are of short duration and include increasing head circumference, tense and bulging fontanelles, lethargy, and sun set sign. Patients may also present with seizuresor focal motor signs, calvarial bulging over the tumor may also be observed (136).

6.7. Neuroimaging

On CT, these lesions are seen as large, hypodense cystic masses with a solid isodense or slightly hyperdense superficial portion that extends into the overlying meninges and shows contrast enhancement. The cystic portion is typically located deep within the tumor, where the solid portion is peripheral. The MRI T1-weighted images are characterized by a hypointense cystic component with an isointense peripheral solid component that takes contrast. On T2-weighted images, the cystic component is hyperintense and the solid portion is heterogeneous. Edema is usually absent or light (138). **Figure 6**

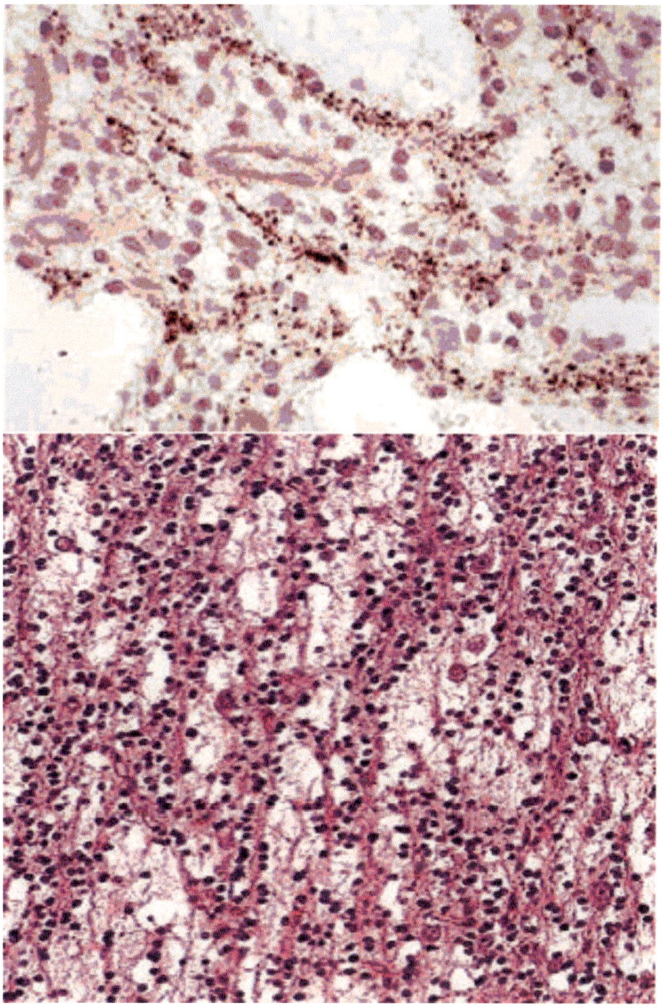

Figure 6. A and B

6.8. Macroscopy

DIAs and DIGs are typically large tumors, measuring up to 13 cm in diameter, with deep multiloculated cysts filled with clear or xanthochromic fluid. The solid superficial portion is primarily extracerebral, attached to leptomeninges and the superficial cortex, it is firm or rubbery in consistency, and grey or white in color.

6.9. Histopathology

The DIA or DIG composed of neuroepithelial tumor with 3 characteristic components: a main desmoplastic leptomeningeal component, a poorly differentiated neuroepithelial component, and a cortical component. The desmoplastic leptomeningeal component consists of a mixture of fibroblast-like spindle-shaped cells and pleomorphic, neoplastic, and neuroepithelial cells with eosinophilic cytoplasm, both of which are arranged in fascicles or in a whorled pattern. Reticulin impregnations show a prominent reticulin-positive network surrounding almost every cell and mimicking that of a mesenchymal tumor. Astrocytes are the main tumor-cell feature in DIAs or the predominant neoplastic population associated with immature neurons in DIGs. The type of neoplastic neuron may range from atypical ganglionic cell to a small polygonal cell (133,139).

In addition to this desmoplastic leptomeningeal component, both DIAs and DIGs contain a group of poorly differentiated neuroepithelial cells with small, round, deeply basophilic nuclei and minimal surrounding perikarya. Such an immature component lacking desmoplasia may predominate in some areas. A cortical component devoid of desmoplasia may also be seen that is often multinodular, with some nodules being microcystic (139).There is a sharp delineation between the cortical surface and the desmoplastic neoplasm, Virchow-Robin spaces in the underlying cortex are often occupied with tumor cells. Calcifications are frequent. Mitotic activity and necrosis are rare. Some tumors may be slightly vascular (137, 140, 141, 142). **Figure 7A.B**

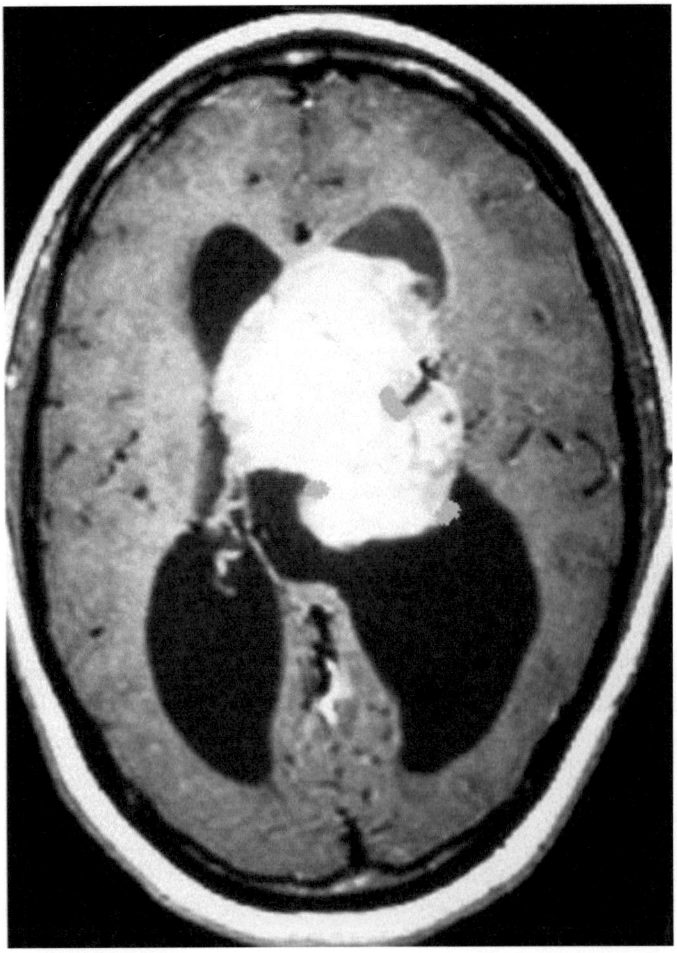

Figure 7.

6.10. Immunohistochemistry

In the desmoplastic leptomeningeal component, fibroblast-like cells express vimentin. As most other neuroepithelial tumor cells react with GFAP, astrocytes predominate in this component. Antibodies to collagen typr VI react in a reticulin-like pattern around tumor cells (143,144). Expression of neuronal markers (synaptophysin, NF-H, and class III ß-tubulin) has been observed in both the neoplastic neuronal cells as well as cells lacking apparent neuronal differentiation (145). In the poorly differentiated neuroepithelial component, cells react with not only GFAP and vimentin but also with neuronal markers and MAP2 Desmin expression may be present (134,145, 146, 148); but epithelial markers (CAM 5.2, AE1/AE3, and EMA) are usually absent (145). **Figure 8A.B**

6.11. Electron microscopy

Astrocytic tumor cells are characterized by intermediate filaments typically arranged in bundles as well as scattered cisternae of rough endoplasmic reticulum and mitochondria with extensive basal lamina. Fibroblasts containing granular endoplasmic reticulum and well-developed Golgi complexes (141, 142). The neuronal cells of DIGs contain dense core secretory granules and neurofilaments. Immunoelectron microscopy has shown filamentous reactivity to NF-H in these neuronal cell bodies as well as processes lacking involvement of the basal lamina. (149).

6.12. Proliferation index

Mitotic activity is rare and, when present, is mostly restricted to the undifferentiated, small-cells in DIGs (134,139). Ki-67 labeling indices reported in the literature range from less than 0.5% to 5%, with the majority of studies reporting them as less than 2% (150). Proliferation does not appear to be related to clinical behavior in completely resected tumors but may expect more aggressive nature in subtotally resected cases. In 3 cases analyzed by flow cytometry, the S-phase fraction ranged from 3.7% to 12%, with a mean of 6.6% (151, 152, 153).

6.13. Histogenesis

The cellular origins of DIAs and DIGs is yet to be known. The presence of primitive small-cell populations that express both glial and neuronal proteins suggest that these cells are progenitor cells to the more differentiated neuroepithelial components and supports the contention that DIAs and DIGs are embryonal neoplasms programmed to progressive maturation (42,155). Origination from the specialized subpial astrocytes that form a continuous, limiting basal lamina providing their terminal processes could account for a comparable phenomenon occurring in desmoplastic infantile tumors and for their superficial localization. The lack of genetic alterationsas observed in most diffuse astrocytomas suggests they are not related to these neoplasms (142,143).

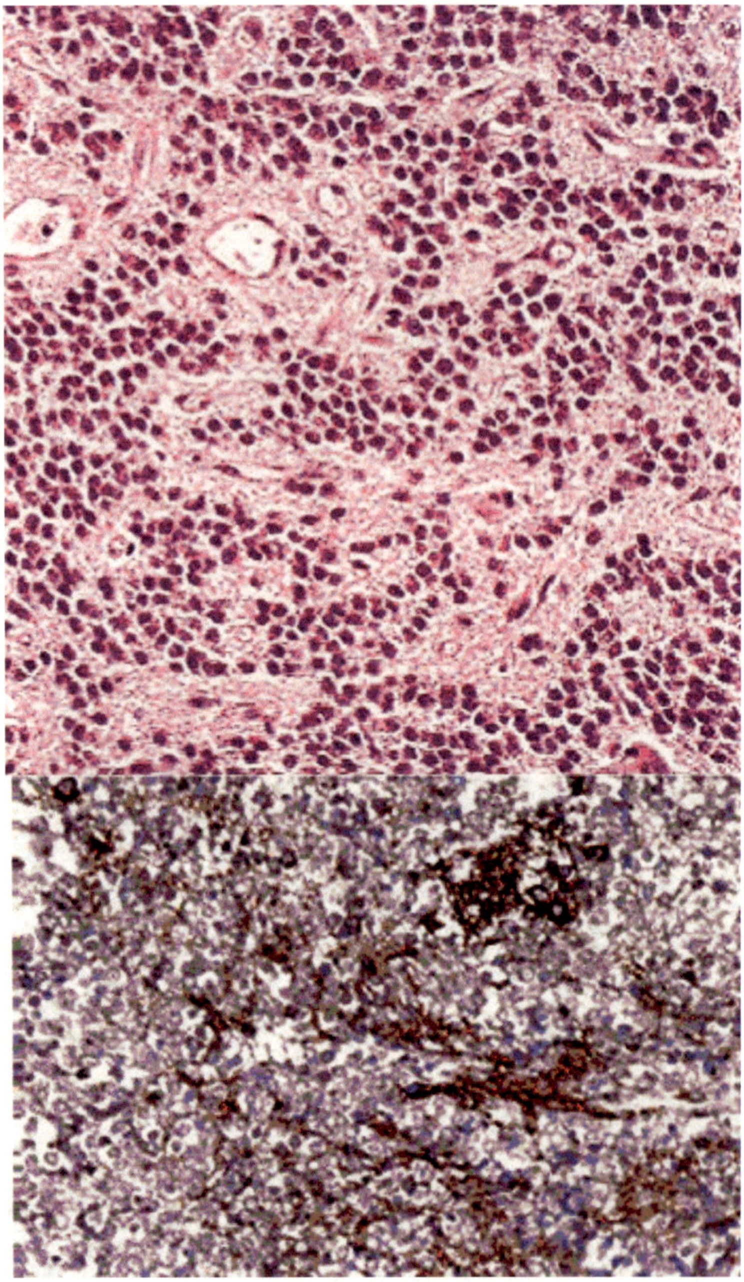

Figure 8. A and B

6.14. Genetics susceptibility

A comparative genomic hybridization study of 3 cases of DIA and DIG revealed no consistent chromosomal gains or losses (150). Molecular studies of DIAs revealed no loss of heterozygosity on chromosomes 10 and 17 and the absence of TP53 mutations (142,152). One case of DIG showed a loss on 8p22-pter, whereas one case of DIA showed a gain on 13q21. (154).

6.15. Prognostic factors and outcome

Follow-up studies indicate that gross total removal is the treatment of choice. In a study 14 of patients with DIGs (median follow-up, 8.7 years), no mortality or evidence of tumor recurrence was observed (134).. In cases of subtotal resectioning or biopsy, most tumors are stable or recurre slowly. In 1 study, 2 tumors showed radiologic evidence of tumor regression following incomplete resectioning . Dissemination of these tumors through the CSF has been reported but rare,(151,156) Long-term tumor control in cases of DIA and DIG can be achieved by total surgical resectioning despite the presence of primitive-appearing cellular aggregates with mitotic activity or foci of necrosis.. However, tumor evolution has been reported in cases of DIG that underwent subtotal removal , including those with high proliferative indices and anaplastic features (149,157,158)

7. Rosette-forming glioneuronal tumor of the fourth ventricle

7.1. Definition

This type of posterior fossa tumours is a rare and slowly growing neoplasm in the fourth ventricular region, predominantly affecting young adults, and composed of uniform neurocytes forming rosettes or perivascular pseudorosettes and astrocytes mimic pilocytic astrocytoma.

7.2. Grading

The rosette-forming glioneuronal tumor (RGNT) corresponds to WHO grade I (1).

7.3. Synonyms

A neoplasm displaying features of RGNT was early reported as a "dysembryoplastic neuroepithelial tumor (DNT) of the cerebellum" . However, Komori et al. described RGNT as a distinct entity as a variant of mixed glio-neuronal tumor (159,160). Wheares, Preusser et al. confirmed RGNT as a tumor entity (161).

7.4. Age and sex distribution

The age range at disease presentation is 12–59 years (mean, 33 years). With a slight female preference.

7.5. Incidence and localization

RGNT is a rare brain tumor. In five different studies, only 17 cases were reported. These lesions arise in the midline and occupy the fourth ventricle and may be the aqueduct, it may extend to involve the adjacent brain stem, cerebellar vermis, pineal gland, or thalamus(160,161, 163, 164,165).

7.6. Neuroimaging

MR imaging reveals a relatively circumscribed, solid tumor in the fourth ventricular region, showing low intensity on T1-weighted images and high intensity on T2-weighted images, , and focal or heterogenous gadolinium enhancement. Secondary hydrocephalus is common (164,165) .

7.7. Clinical features

The clinical presentation of RGNT is most often with headache due to of obstructive hydrocephalus, and unsteadiness. Cervical pain is occasionally experienced. Rarely discovered incidentally. **Figure 9**.

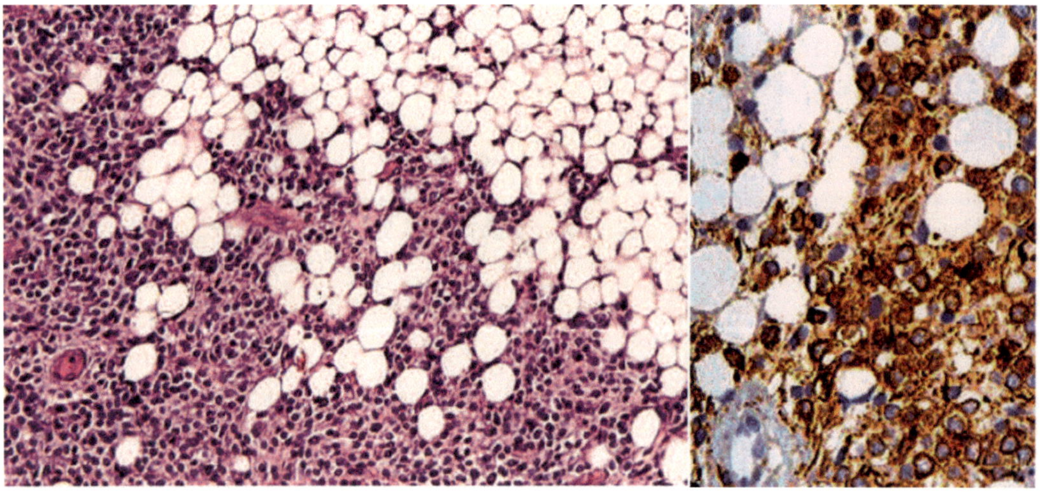

Figure 9.

7.8. Histopathology

RGNTs are well demarcated, but some infiltration into the brain stem and cerebellar parenchyma may be observed. They are characterized by a biphasic neurocytic and glial architecture. The neurocytic component consists of a uniform group of neurocytes. these cells have spherical nuclei with finely granular chromatin, inconspicuous nucleoli, scant cytoplasm, and delicate cytoplasmic processes forming neurocytic rosettes and/or perivascular pseudorosettes. Neurocytic rosettes feature ring-like arrays of neurocytic nuclei surrounding delicate eosinophilic neuropil cores. While the perivascular pseudorosettes feature delicate cell processes radiating toward vessels. The neurocytic rosettes and perivascular pseudorosettes when viewed longitudinally, may show a columnar arrangement.. These neurocytic structures may lie in a partly microcystic, mucinous matrix.

The glial component of RGNT typically dominates, and in some areas may resemble pilocytic astrocytoma. Astrocytic tumor cells are spindle to stellate in shape, with elongated to oval nuclei and moderately dense chromatin. Cytoplasmic processes often form a compact to loosely textured fibrillary background. Rosenthal fibers, eosinophilic granular bodies, microcalcifications, and hemosiderin deposits may be observed. In some areas, the glial component may be microcystic, containing round, oligodendroglia-like cells with some perinuclear halos. Vessels may be thin-walled and dilated or hyalinized. Thrombosed vessels and glomeruloid vasculature may also be noted. The adjacent cerebellar cortex has no features of dysplasia (160,162, 164, 165). **Figure 10A**

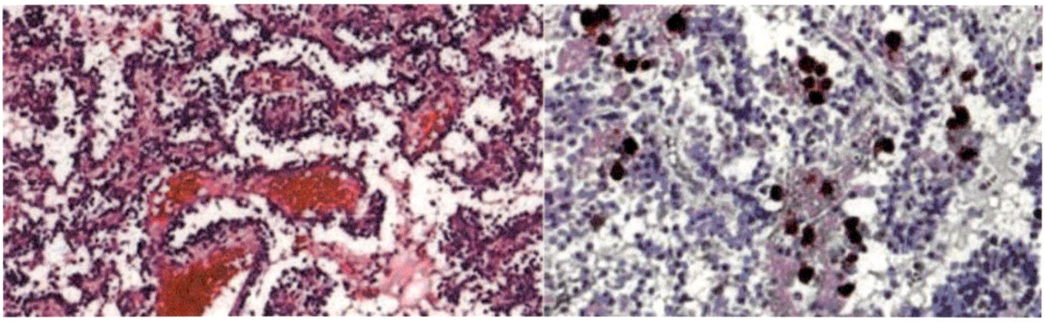

Figure 10. A and B

7.9. Immunohistochemistry

Immunoreactivity for synaptophysin is present at the centers of neurocytic rosettes and in the neuropil of perivascular pseudorosettes.furthermore, the cytoplasm and processes of neurocytic tumor cells may express MAP-2 and neuron-specific enolase. GFAP and S-100 immunoreactivity is shown in the glial part, but absent in the rosettes and pseudorosettes. (160, 162, 164). **Figure 10 B.**

7.10. Proliferation index

Ki-67 labeling indices are low, being less than 3% in reported cases, Mitosis is absent (165).

7.11. Genetic susceptibility

One reported patient with RGNT had a Chiari type I malformation (160). No other evidence of an underlying neurological disorder or association with a familial tumor syndrome has been reported.

7.12. Histogenesis

The histological investigations indicate that RGNTs arise from the brain tissue surrounding the infratentorial ventricular system. An origin of RGNT from the subependymal plate; the remnants of the periventricular germinal matrix has been suggested (160).

7.13. Outcome

The clinical outcome of these primary benign neoplasm is favorable in terms of survival, but disabling cerebellar features postoperatively have been reported in approximately half the cases (160).

8. Papillary glio-neuronal tumor

8.1. Definition

A well circumscribed, clinically insidius and histologically biphasic cerebral neoplasm composed of flat to cuboidal, GFAP-positive astrocytes lining hyalinized vascular pseudopapillae and synaptophysin-positive interpapillary collections of sheets of neurocytes, large neurons, and ganglioid cells.

8.2. Grading

Papillary glioneuronal tumors is corresponding to WHO grade I. late aggressive behavior has been reported (1,165).

8.3. Historical annotation

The papillary glioneuronal tumor, was first established as a distinct clinicopathological entity by Komori et al. in 1998 and listed in the 2000 WHO classification as a variant of ganglioglioma, (166). Some tumors were previously described under a variety of names, including pseudopapillary gangliogliONeurocytoma and pseudopapillary neurocytoma with glial differentiation (167,168).

8.4. Incidence, age and sex distribution

They are very rare neoplasms; and only a few cases have been reported (169.170). These tumors may occur at any age. There is no gender preference. The mean age at presentation is 27 years; the oldest and youngest patient reported was 75 and 4 years, respectively (171,172)..

8.5. Localization

These tumors are generally seen in the cerebral hemispheres, with a predilection for the temporal lobe.

8.6. Neuroimaging

On MRI and CT imaging, the tumors appear as well defined, solid and/ or cystic, with some contrast-enhancement there is usually little mass effect. A cyst-mural nodule architecture may be observed (166, 169.173).

8.7. Clinical features

Mainly headache and seizures. Focal deficits, cognition, and emotional disorder may also be encountered. (174).

8.8. Histopathology and immunohistochemistry

Papillary glioneuronal neoplasms is characterized by a prominent pseudopapillary manner in which a single or pseudostratified layer of small, cuboidal glial cells with rounded nuclei and scant cytoplasm covers hyalinized blood vessels, as well as interpapillary sheets or focal collections of neurocytes, and occasionally ganglion cells or medium-sized ganglioid cells with accompanying neuropil.

At the immunohistochemical level, vessels with mural hyalinization are ensheathed by a layer of small, uniform, GFAP-positive cells with rounded nuclei and scant cytoplasm. In some cases, OLIG2-positive, GFAP-negative glial cells surround this layer. These glial elements lack both nuclear atypia and mitotic activity. Interpapillary neuronal elements show considerable variation in size and shape. all get stained with antisera to synaptophysin, NSE, and class III-tubulin. The majority of neuronal cells are positive for NeuN, but NFP expression is mostly confined to larger ganglioid and ganglion cells. Membranous immunoreactivity for NCAM is also found (166, 172, 175), but chromogranin-A expression is lacking. Minigemistocytes which show intense GFAP immunoreactivity, are occasionally noted in the interpapillary spaces. Microvascular proliferation or necrosis is rare. Even in cases with increased proliferative activity. At the periphery of the lesion, scattered tumor cells are mixed with gliotic brain tissue containing Rosenthal fibers, eosinophilic granular bodies, hemosiderin, and microcalcifications are encountered; this results in a a blurred tumor edge (165, 175). **Figure 11 A.B**

8.9. Electron microscopy

The ultrastructure of few papillary glioneuronal tumors has been studied. Three cell types have been reported: astrocytic; neuronal; and poorly differentiated neurons. Neurons vary in size: large forms with abundant organelles lie between the papillae; their neuronal processes filled with parallel microtubules showed terminations containing clear vesicles and occasional synapses. The poorly differentiated cells contain mitochondria, ribosomes, occasional dense bodies, intermediate filaments and microtubules, but no well-formed dense core granules. Astrocytes contain bundles of intermediate filaments, and are separated from vessels by a basal lamina. Minigemistocytes and OLIG-2-expressing oligodendrocyte-like cells may also be present (165, 166, 171).

8.10. Proliferation index

MIB-1 labeling indices are usually low, in the range of 1–2%. Only 1 tumor featuring minigemistocytes showed an increased (10%) labeling index in that unusual element (165).

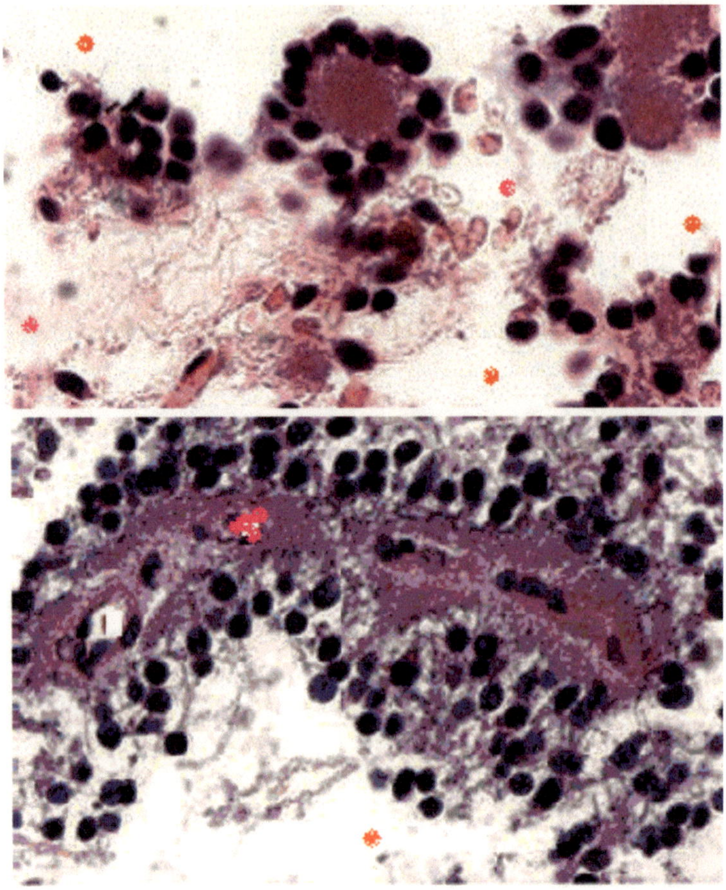

Figure 11. A and B

8.11. Genetic susceptibility

Papillary glioneuronal tumors reported to date have been sporadic in occurrence. (175).

8.12. Histogenesis

The histogenesis of papillary glioneuronal tumors is uncertain, but an origin from multipotent precursors capable of divergent glioneuronal differentiation is supposed. (166).

8.13. Prognosis

The cystic formation, indolent course and low proliferative activity are given a favorable clinical outcome. In most cases, gross total resection without adjuvant therapy is curable with long-term survival. (165).

9. Cerebellar liponeurocytoma

9.1. Definition

A very rare cerebellar neoplasm with variable neuronal, astrocytic, and focal lipomatous differentiation, and low proliferative potential; the tumor usually has a favorable clinical course.

9.2. Grading

Data available advocate that this tumor typically corresponded to WHO grade I (1). However, recurrences have been reported in almost 50% cases, typically without the histological features of malignant transformation. (176).

9.3. Synonyms and historical annotation

Bechtel et al. Reported a case of lipomatous medulloblastoma in a 44-year-old man. in 1978 (177). Subsequently 28 more cases were reported. The terms neurolipocytoma (178), medullocytoma (179), lipomatous glioneurocytoma (180), and lipidized mature neuroectodermal tumor of the cerebellum (181). The WHO Classification in 2000 (1) included the term "cerebellar liponeurocytoma". However, This term is now widely accepted, and is supported by genetic analyses indicating that this lesion is not a variant of medulloblastoma (170). Clinical, histopathological, immunohistochemical, and genetic data strongly suggest that the cerebellar liponeurocytoma comprise a rare but distinct clinico-pathological entity. Some tumors with features of liponeurocytoma have also been observed in supratentorial locations. (182, 183, 184)..

9.4. Age and sex distribution

In the 29 patients with cerebellar liponeurocytoma reported (182, 185, 186, 187,188,189), the mean age was around 50 years (range, 24–77 years), with a peak in the third to sixth decade of life. This is in contrast with the age distribution of cerebellar medulloblastomas, more than 70% of which occur in children (178). There is no significant gender predilection (13 men and 16 women) in patients with cerebellar Liponeurocytoma (186, 187,188,189).

9.5. Clinical features

Non specific symptoms such as Headache and signs of raised intracranial pressure may be the initial presentation, resulting from either the lesion itself or obstructive hydrocephalus. Cerebellar signs are also frequent (188).

9.6. Neuroimaging

MRI appearance is variable, and may be related to the distribution and proportion of lipidized tissue. On T1-weighted MRI, the mass is generally hyperintense but heterogeneous. Hyperintense streaks on T2-weighted images have been associated with the macroscopic appearance of adipose tissue at surgery. Enhancement with gadolinium is usually irregular. Peritumoral edema is usually absent (,190, 191).

9.7. Localization

These neoplasms are predominantly located in the cerebellar hemispheres, followed by in the vermis. And rarely in the cerebellopontine angle. Raely, liponeurocytomas have been diagnosed in the supratentorial ventricular system at a rate to approximately 3% of central neurocytomas. There are 2 cases of cerebellar neurocytomas without adipose tissue have been reported (182, 185, 192, 193). In 1 case, it was shown that the lipid vacuoles progressively accumulate and coalesce within cells, maintaining neurocytic features, and indicating tumoral lipidization rather than true adipose metaplasia. These observations justify the description of central liponeurocytoma as a separate entity, and these lesions contribute to histogenetic and biological characteristics with cerebellar liponeurocytoma (194, 195,196).

9.8. Histopathology

Biphasic in appearance, the tumor consists of small neuronal cells with the cytology of neurocytes and focal lipomatous differentiation, characterized by lipidized cells resembling mature adipose tissue. Tumor cells have round or oval nuclei, and often show a clear cytoplasm resembling neoplastic oligodendrocytes, but also have many morphological similarities to medulloblastoma and clear cell ependymoma. Despite the cellularity of the lesion, tumor cells have a uniform cytological appearance, with absent or very few mitotic figures and aggressive features. No malignant transformation noted (194, 195,196). **Figure 12A**

9.9. Immunohistochemistry

Neuronal differentiation is observed by a reliable, diffuse expression of NSE, synaptophysin, and MAP-2. Accordingly, several reported cases were diagnosed as neurocytoma or neuroblastoma, rather than medulloblastoma. Focal GFAP expression by tumor is also seen, indicating astrocytic differentiation (184). Immunoreactivity for neuronal markers and GFAP is also seen in the adipose cells, indicating an abnormal differentiation of tumor cells rather than an entrapped adipocytes. It is crucial to note that xanthomatous histiocytes, as are occasionally observed in ordinary medulloblastomas, are not considered evidence of lipomatous differentiation. Two reports mention additional immunoreactivity to desmin, and morphological features of incipient myogenic differentiation (177,181). **Figure 12 B**

9.10. Differential diagnosis

The most important differential diagnosis is medulloblastoma with lipidized cells. The distinction between these 2 lesions is crucial, since medulloblastomas with lipidized cells

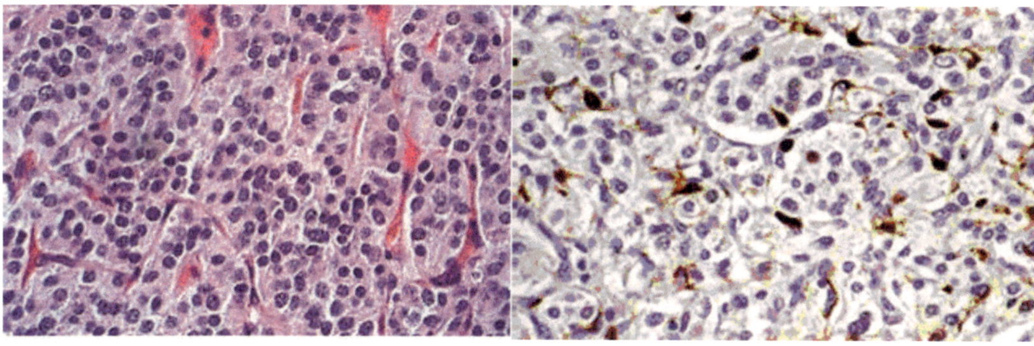

Figure 12.

require adjuvant radio/chemotherapy. Most importantly, the growth fraction is in the range of 15–40%, which is incompatible with a diagnosis of liponeurocytoma. Cerebellar liponeurocytoma is a neoplasm of adults, while lipidized medulloblastomas also occur in children (186, 188, 197, 198, 199). The liponeurocytomas may also mimic neoplastic oligodendrocytes and clear cell ependymoma (199).

9.11. Proliferation index

The Ki-67/ MIB-1 labeling index, is usually in the range of 1–3%, but may be as high as 6%, with a mean value of 2.5% . In the adipose component, the MIB-1 labeling index is even lower (184, 200).

9.12. Histogenesis

An origin from the external granular layer of the cerebellum cannot be ruled out, Immunoreactivity to neuronal antigens and GFAP includes cell bodies embracing fat globules. This suggests that the fat-containing cells result from lipomatous differentiation of tumor cells. The cell of origin is most likely a precursor cell with a preferential commitment to neuronal differentiation. (184,185,200).

9.13. Genetics susceptibility

Genetic analysis of 20 cerebellar liponeurocytomas revealed TP53 missense mutations in 4 cases (20%), a frequency significantly higher than that in medulloblastomas (6%). There was no case with a PTCH, APC, or ß-catenin mutation, each of which can be present in subsets of medulloblastomas. FISH analysis showed that isochromosome 17q, a genetic hallmark present in 40% of cerebellar medulloblastomas, was not enountered in any of the cases investigated. This finding supports the view that the cerebellar liponeurocytoma is a distinct entity and not a variant of medulloblastoma. cDNA expression profiles showed a relationship to central neurocytoma, but the presence of TP53 mutations, which are absent in central neurocytomas, suggests that they develop through different genetic pathways (182).

9.14. Prognostis

A review of published cases indicates that this lesion generally carries a favorable prognosis. Because of the rarity of this tumor and the lack of systematic follow-up data, survival and recurrence rates must be interpreted with some caution (182, 185).

Of 21 patients with follow-up data, 6 (29%) died within 6 months to 2 years, 5 (24%) died after 2–4 years and 10 (48%) survived 5–16 years after surgical intervention. The 5-year survival rate was 48% and the mean overall survival was 5.8 years. However, 62% of patients developed a recurrence from 1 to 12 years, and in 3 patients there was a second relapse 1 to 5 years later. Despite its aggressive course there is no malignant transformation observed. (176).

10. Filum terminale and spinal paraganglioma

10.1. Definition

A distinctive neuroendocrine neoplasm, usually encapsulated, slowgrowing, and benign, arising from specialized neural crest cells associated with segmental autonomic ganglia (paraganglia); it is composed of uniform chief cells displaying neuronal differentiation and forming compact nests (Zellballen), surrounded by sustentacular cells and a delicate capillary network. This type of neoplasm is mostly affecting the cauda equine and filum terminale

10.2. Grading

Paragangliomas of the cauda equine/filum terminale correspond histologically to WHO grade I (1).

10.3. Synonyms and historical annotation

The early terminology of paragangliomas is not well known. Early authors divided them into chromaffin and nonchromaffin on the basis of their reaction with chromic acid. However, since this reaction does not reliably reflect their functional activity, current terminology is based upon anatomical location as seen in carotid body paraganglioma (chemodectoma), jugulotympanic paraganglioma (glomus jugulare tumor).

10.4. Incidence and location

Paragangliomas of the CNS are infrequent, the vast majority present as lumber spinal intradural tumors in the cauda equina region. Since the first description of cauda equina region paraganglioma in 1970 (201), more than 210 cases have been reported. And 174 cases reported prior to 2003 (202). Paragangliomas of the cauda equine region comprise 3.4% to 3.8% of all tumors affecting this region (203, 204). Other spinal levels are involved far less often; 14 paragangliomas were reported in the thoracic region, most being extradural with an intravertebral and paraspinal component (205, 206), and 2 tumors involved the cervical region (207, 208).

Intracranial paragangliomas are usually located in the posterior fossa; jugulotympanic paragangliomas (209). However, intracranial tumors have also been described. These locations include sellar region, the cerebellopontine angle, cerebellar parenchyma, and the fronto-temporal lobes (210, 211, 212, 213).

10.5. Age and sex distribution

Cauda equina paragangliomas generally affect adults. Patient age ranges from 9 to 74 years (mean, 46 years), with a slight predominance in males with Male:Female ratio at 1.4:1. Jugulotympanic paragangliomas are more common in Caucasians, with a strong female preference, and occur mainly in the fifth and sixth decades (209).

10.6. Clinical features

The most common presenting symptoms include a long standing history of low-back pain and sciatica. Sensory deficit, paraparesis, and sphincter disturbances are common in the later stage, while complete cauda equina syndrome is rare. An intracranial hypertension symptoms and signs was reported in 8 cases. Only 3 endocrinologically functional paragangliomas of the cauda equine region have been reported (214, 215, 216). The few reported paragangliomas of the thoracic spine presented with short term of signs of spinal cord compression (217). About 36% of glomus jugulare paragangliomas extend into the cranial cavity and produce headache, pulsatile tinnitus and lower cranial nerve involvement; rarely, signs of catecholamine secretion may be seen (209).

10.7. Neuroimaging

Cauda equina paragangliomas has no specific features. Most appear as isodense, homogeneously enhancing masses on CT. However, since CT without contrast may miss the lesion, MRI is the investigation of choice. MRI images typically show a well marked, may be with cystic component mass that is hypo- or isointense to spinal cord on T1-weighted images, with a vivd contrast enhancemnet. It appears as hyperintense on T2-weighted images. The presence of ecstatic and dilated vessels and a low signal intensity rim ("cap sign") on T2-weighted images are considered diagnostically important feature. Plain radiographs are usually helpful, and show some scalloping of the vertebral bod y due to chronic bone compression (204, 218). **Figure 13**

10.8. Histopathology

Tumors are well differentiated, mimicking normal paraganglia, nearly half of cauda equina paragangliomas contain mature ganglion cells, as well as cells transitional between chief and ganglion cells. These lesions are composed of chief (type I) cells disposed in nests or lobules

(Zellballen pattern), and surrounded by a single layer of sustentacular (type II) cells. The Zellballen are surrounded by a delicate capillary network that may undergo sclerosis. The uniform round or polygonal chief cells possess central, round-to-oval nuclei, with finely stippled chromatin and inconspicuous nucleoli. Cytoplasm varies somewhat in quantity and is usually eosinophilic and finely granular. In some conditions, it is amphophilic or clear. Sustentacular cells are spindle-shaped. Encompassing the lobules, their long processes are often so attenuated that they are undetectable by routine light microscopy, and visible only on immunostains for S-100 protein. (219). Such "gangliocytic paragangliomas" are also found in other sites such as the duodenum and are analogous to phaeochromocytoma with neuronal differentiation. Some paragangliomas of the cauda equina region show architectural features similar to carcinoid tumors, including angiomatous, adenomatous, and pseudorosette patterns. Tumors composed predominantly of spindle and melanin-containing cells (melanotic paragangliomas) have also been described at this site, as has oncocytic paraganglioma (220, 221, 222). hemorrhagic necrosis may also occur, and scattered mitotic figures can be seen. these features are not of prognostic implication (223). **Figure 14A**

10.9. Immunohistochemistry

Chief and sustentacular cells can be identified by biomarkers. Chief cells are marked with Neuron-specific enolase (NSE), synaptophysin and chromogranin (228, 229). Chromogranin A reactivity parallels the Grimelius (argyrophil) reaction (219, 223,224). Neurofilament proteins are also useful markers of chief cells. Expression of serotonin (5H-T) and of various neuropeptides (somatostatin, leu, and metenkephalin) has been demonstrated in paraganglioma of the cauda equina region. Paranuclear cytkeokeratin immunoreactivity is particularly prominent in cauda equina examples. Sustentacular cells are uniformly reactive for S-100 protein, and usually show staining for glial fibrillary acidic protein (GFAP). Chief cells may also show variable S-100 immunoreactivity (220, 223, 225). **Figure 14B**

10.10. Electron microscopy

The characteristic ultrastructural features of chief cells is the presence of dense core (neurosecretory) granules measuring 100 to 400 nm (mean, 140 nm). Depending on their cytoplasmic electron density, "light" and "dark" chief cells are recognized. A layer of basal lamina is present at the interface of Zellballen and surrounding stroma. In addition to well-developed Golgi, extensive smooth endoplasmic reticulum, and lysosomes, chief cells may contain numerous atypical mitochondria, as well as paranuclear whorls of intermediate filaments (223, 226). Sustentacular cells are characterized by an elongated nucleus with marginal chromatin, increased cytoplasmic electron density, relative profusion of intermediate filaments, and low core granules (225, 226, 227).

10.11. Genetics susceptibility

It is not clear, there is no reported association of spinal paragangliomas with genetic abnormalit. However, Systemic paragangliomas may be multifocal, The association of spinal paraganglioma with brain tumors, spinal epidural haemangioma, syringomyelia, and intramedullary cysts are encountered (228, 229, 230, 231), but these associations may be coincidental. Several autosomal dominant inherited syndromes predispose to paraganglioma or phaeochromocytomaas noted in von Hippel- Lindau disease (VHL); multiple endocrine neoplasia type 2 (RET mutations); neurofibromatosis type 1 (NF1). Multiple, benign, head and neck paragangliomas are often caused by SDHD mutations, while SDHB mutations are associated with phaeochromocytoma. There are only 4 families with the SDHC mutation have been identified. Spinal paragangliomas are considered non-familial, but a study of 22 spinal paragangliomas showed an SDHD germline mutation in 1 patient with recurrent spinal paraganglioma and a cerebellar metastasis (232).

10.12. Histogenesis

The histogenesis is unknow. Some authors favor an origin from paraganglion cells associated with regional autonomic nerves and blood vessels (233). Others have suggested that peripheral neuroblasts usually present in the adult filum terminale may undergo paraganglionic differentiation (229). Jugulotympanic paragangliomas presumably arise from microscopic paraganglia within the temporal bone. Some interesting cases have reported the coexistence of a paraganglioma and myxopapillary ependymoma in the cauda equina region (234, 235).

10.13. Prognostic factors

Tumor location is the most important predictive prognostic factor rather than histology of paragangliomas. For instance, the metastasis rate of para-aortic paraganglioma is high (28 to 42%), whereas that of carotid body tumors is only 2 to 9% (236). About 50% of the glomus jugulare tumors recur locally, but only 5% with distant metastastases (234, 237). The tumor vascularity has no significant value. The vast majority of cauda equina paragangliomas are slowly growing and curable by total excision. Based on long-term follow-up, it is estimated that 4% will recur following gross total removal (238, 239). Metastasis outside the CNS is rare (220). CSF seeding of spinal paragangliomas has been reported (240).

11. Conclusion

CNS neuroepithelial and neuronal tumours are usually benign and slow growing neoplasms with WHO grade I-II. They comprise a low percentage of the whole CNS neoplasms and may affect any part of the CNS. These lesions present with non specific symptoms and signs; but tend to cause intractable epilepsy when affecting the cerebral cortex. Along with clinical presentation and neuroimaging; the histopathology and immunochemistry confirm the diagnosis. Surgical resctioning is the treatment of choice with favorable prognosis and long term cure; adjuvant treatment is preserved to recurrent tumours or to high grade lesions

12. Table of summary

	Location	WHO	Type of cells	Specific features	prognosis
Ganglioglioma and Gangliocytoma	Throughout the CNS more common in Supratentorial. Temporal lobe predilection	Grade I Garde III	Immature ganglion cells and/ or astrocyte	Large neoplastic ganglion cells with/without glial components	Low grade favorable Higher grade : variable
Central Neurocytoma and extraventricular Neurocytoma	Supratentorial. Paraventricular	Grade I-II	Uniform ferentiated neurocyte	Oligodendroglioma-like honeycomb appearance, irregular "rosettes" perivascular pseudorosettes	Favorable
Dysembryoplastic Neuroepithelial tumour	Temporal lobe and mesial region	Grade I	glio-neuronal constituent	columns formed by bundles of axons lined by small oligodendroglia-like cells	Favorable
DIA , DIG	Supratentorial with frontal and parietal lobes predilection	Grade I	desmoplastic leptomeningeal, poorly differentiated neuroepithelial cells	Astrocytes are the main tumor-cell in DIAs. immature neurons in DIGs	Favorable
RGNT	4th ventricle and aqueduct cerebellar and brain stem	Grade I	a biphasic neurocytic and glial architecture.	The neurocytic rosettes ,perivascular pseudorosettes.	Favorable
Papillary Glio-neuronal tumour	Temporal lobe	Grade I	small, cuboidal glial cells,collections of neurocytes,and occasionally ganglion cells	pseudopapillary manner and pseudostratified layer of small, cuboidal glial cells, interpapillary sheets collections of neurocytes, ganglion cells.	Favorable
Cerebellar Liponeurocytoma	Cerebellar hemisphere , vermis CP angle, rarely supratentorial	Grade I	small neuronal cells with focal lipomatous differentiation,	small neuronal cells with the cytology of neurocytes and focal lipomatous cella, resembling mature adipose tissue	Favorable
Filum terminale and spinal paraganglioma	Cauda equine region. Jugulotympaniirial arely supratento	Grade I	mature ganglion cells, transitional cells between chief and ganglion cells	mature ganglion cells, cells transitional cells. Chief (type I) cells disposed in nests or lobules (Zellballen pattern) surrounded a delicate capillary network, and sustentacular (type II) cells.	Favorable

Table 1. Summary

Author details

Mohammed M.A. Al Barbarawi
Section of Neurosurgery, Department of Neuroscience, Faculty of Medicine, Jordan University of Science & Technology, Jordan

Mohammed Z. Allouh
Department of Anatomy, Faculty of Medicine, Jordan University of Science & Technology, Jordan

Suhair M.A. Qudsieh
Clinical department, Faculty of medicine, Hashemite University, Jordan

13. References

[1] Louis DN, Ohgaki H, Wiestler OD, Cavenee WK (*eds.*) (2007). World Health Organization Classification of Tumours of the Nervous System. International Agency for Research on Cancer IARC Press: Lyon-France.
[2] Blumcke I, Wiestler OD (2002). Gangliogliomas: an intriguing tumor entity associated with focal epilepsies. J Neuropathol Exp Neurol 61: 575-584.
[3] Luyken C, Blumcke I, Fimmers R, Urbach H, Wiestler OD, Schramm J (2004). Supratentorial gangliogliomas: histopathologic grading and tumor recurrence in 184 patients with a median follow-up of 8 years. Cancer 101: 146-155.
[4] Kalyan R, Olivero WC (1987). Ganglioglioma: a correlative clinicopathological and radiological study of ten surgically treated cases with follow-up. Neurosurgery 20: 428-433.
[5] Hirose T, Scheithauer BW, Lopes MBS, Gerber HA, Altermatt HJ, VandenBerg SR(1997). Ganglioglioma: An ultrastructural and immunohistochemical study. Cancer 79: 989- 1003.
[6] Lang FF, Epstein FJ, Ransohoff J, Allen JC, Wisoff J, Abbott IR, Miller DC (1993). Central nervous system gangliogliomas. Part 2: Clinical outcome. J Neurosurg 79: 867-873.
[7] Prayson RA, Khajavi K, Comair YG (1995). Cortical architectural abnormalities and MIB1 immunoreactivity in gangliogliomas: a study of 60 patients with intracranial tumors. J Neuropathol Exp Neurol 54: 513-520.
[8] Wolf HK, Muller MB, Spanle M, Zentner J, Schramm J, Wiestler OD (1988). Ganglioglioma: a detailed histopathological and immunohistochemical analysis of 61 cases. Acta Neuropathol 166-173.
[9] Johnson JHJ, Hariharan S, Berman J, Sutton LN, Rorke LB, Molloy P, Phillips PC (1997). Clinical outcome of pediatric gangliogliomas: ninety-nine cases over 20 years. Pediatr Neurosurg 27: 203-207
[10] Barbarawi, M., Qudsieh S., Saa'd, S. Conus medullaris ganglioglioma (2008). Pan Arab Journal of Neurosurgery. 12, (2): 114-117. 10 .
[11] Wolf HK, Wiestler OD (1995). Surgical pathology of chronic epileptic seizure disorders. Brain Pathol 3: 371-
[12] Luyken C, Blumcke I, Fimmers R, Urbach H, Elger CE, Wiestler OD, Schramm J(2003). The spectrum of long-term epilepsyassociated tumors: long-term seizure andtumor outcome and neurosurgical aspects. Epilepsia 44: 822-830.

[13] Grossman RI, Yousem DM (1994). Neuroradiology. The Requisites. Mosby-Yearbook: St Louis.
[14] Osborne AG (1994). Diagnostic Neuroradiology. Mosby, St Louis.
[15] Blumcke I, Giencke K, Wardelmann E, Beyenburg S, Kral T, Sarioglu N, Pietsch T, Wolf HK, Schramm J, Elger CE, Wiestler OD (1999). The CD34 epitope is expressed in neoplastic and malformative lesions associated with chronic, focal epilepsia. Acta Neuropathol 97: 481-490.
[16] Blumcke I, Muller S, Buslei R, Riederer BM, Wiestler OD (2004). Microtubule-associated protein-2 immunoreactivity: a useful tool in the differential diagnosis of low-grade neuroepithelial tumors. Acta Neuropathol 108: 89-96.
[17] Miller DC, Lang FF, Epstein FJ (1993). Central nervous system gangliogliomas. Part 1: Pathology. J Neurosurg 79: 859-866.
[18] Issidorides MR, Havaki S, Chrysanthou-Piterou M, Arvanitis DL (2000). Ultrastructural identification of protein bodies, cellular markers of human catecholamine neurons, in a temporal lobe ganglioglioma. Ultrastruct Pathol 24: 399-405.
[19] Meyer P, Eberle MM, Probst A, Tolnay M (2000). [Ganglioglioma of optic nerve in neurofibromatosis type 1. Case report and review of the literature]. Klin Monatsbl Augenheilkd 217: 55-58.
[20] Resta N, Lauriola L, Puca A, Susca FC, Albanese A, Sabatino G, Di Giacomo MC, Gessi M, Guanti G (2006). Ganglioglioma arising in a Peutz-Jeghers patient: a case report with molecular implications. Acta Neuropathol 112: 106-111.
[21] Bhattacharjee MB, Armstrong DD, Vogel H, Cooley LD (1997). Cytogenetic analysis of 120 primary pediatric brain tumors and literature review. Cancer Genet Cytogenet 97: 39-53.
[22] Squire JA, Arab S, Marrano P, Bayani J, Karaskova J, Taylor M, Becker L, Rutka J, Zielenska M (2001). Molecular cytogenetic analysis of glial tumors using spectral karyotyping and comparative genomic hybridization. Mol Diagn 6: 93-108.
[23] Wacker MR, Cogen PH, Etzell JE, Daneshvar L, Davis RL, Prados MD (1992). Diffuse leptomeningeal involvement by a ganglioglioma in a child. Case report. J Neurosurg 77: 302-306.
[24] Yin XL, Hui AB, Pang JC, Poon WS, Ng HK (2002). Genome-wide survey for chromosomal imbalances in ganglioglioma using comparative genomic hybridization. Cancer Genet Cytogenet 134: 71-76.
[25] Jay V, Squire J, Becker LE, Humphreys R (1994). Malignant transformation in a ganglioglioma with anaplastic neuronal and astrocytic components. Report of a case with flow cytometric and cytogenetic analysis. Cancer 73: 2862-2868.
[26] Jay V, Squire J, Blaser S, Hoffman HJ, Hwang P (1997). Intracranial and spinal metastases from a ganglioglioma with unusual cytogenetic abnormalities in a patient with complex partial seizures. Childs Nerv Syst 13: 550-555.
[27] Yin XL, Hui AB, Pang JC, Poon WS, Ng HK (2002). Genome-wide survey for chromosomal imbalances in ganglioglioma using comparative genomic hybridization. Cancer Genet Cytogenet 134: 71-76.

[28] von Deimling A, Fimmers R, Schmidt MC, Bender B, Fassbender F, Nagel J, Jahnke R, Kaskel P, Duerr EM, Koopmann J, Maintz D, Steinbeck S, Wick W, Platten M, Muller DJ, Przkora R, Waha A, Blumcke B, Wellenreuther R, Meyer-Puttlitz B, Schmidt O, Mollenhauer J, Poustka A, Stangl AP, Lenartz D, von Ammon K (2000). Comprehensive allelotype and genetic analysis of 466 human nervous system tumors. J Neuropathol Exp Neurol 59: 544-558.
[29] Hayashi Y, Iwato M, Hasegawa M, Tachibana O, von Deimling A, Yamashita J (2001). Malignant transformation of a gangliocytoma/ ganglioglioma into a glioblastoma multiforme: a molecular genetic analysis. Case report. J Neurosurg 95: 138-142.
[30] Becker AJ, Lobach M, Klein H, Normann S, Nothen MM, von Deimling A, Mizuguchi M, Elger CE, Schramm J, Wiestler OD, Blumcke I (2001). Mutational analysis of TSC1 and TSC2 genes in gangliogliomas. Neuropathol Appl Neurobiol 27: 105-114.
[31] Parry L, Maynard JH, Patel A, Hodges AK, von Deimling A, Sampson JR, Cheadle JP (2000). Molecular analysis of the TSC1 and TSC2 tumour suppressor genes in sporadic glial and glioneuronal tumours. Hum Genet 107: 350-356.
[32] Majores M, Schick V, Engels G, Fassunke J, Elger CE, Schramm J, Blumcke I, Becker AJ (2005). Mutational and immunohistochemical analysis of ezrin-, radixin-, moesin (ERM) molecules in epilepsy-associated glioneuronal lesions. Acta Neuropathol 110: 537-546.
[33] Zhu JJ, Leon SP, Folkerth RD, Guo SZ, Wu JK, Black PM (1997). Evidence for clonal origin of neoplastic neuronal and glial cells in gangliogliomas. Am J Pathol 151: 565-571
[34] Hassoun J, Gambarelli D, Grisoli F, Pellet W, Salamon G, Pellisier JF, Toga M(1982). Central neurocytoma. An electronmicroscopic study of two cases. Acta Neuropathol 56: 151-156.
[35] Nishio S, Takeshita I, Kaneko Y, Fukui M (1992). Cerebral neurocytoma. A new subset of benign neuronal tumors of the cerebrum. Cancer 70: 529-537.
[36] Coca S, Moreno M, Martos JA, Rodriguez J, Barcena A, Vaquero J (1994). Neurocytoma of spinal cord. Acta Neuropathol 87: 537-540.
[37] Tatter SB, Borges LF, Louis DN (1994). Central neurocytomas of the cervical spinal cord. Report of two cases. J Neurosurg 81: 288-293.
[38] Giangaspero F, Cenacchi G, Losi L, Cerasoli S, Bisceglia M, Burger PC (1997).Extraventricular neoplasms with Neurocytoma features: A clinicopathological study of11 cases. Am J Surg Pathol 21: 206-212.
[39] Komori T, Scheithauer BW, Anthony DC, Rosenblum MK, McLendon RE, Scott RM, Okazaki H, Kobayashi M (1998). Papillary glioneuronal tumor: a new variant of mixed neuronal- glial neoplasm. Am J Surg Pathol 22: 1171-1183.
[40] Cenacchi G, Giangaspero F (2004). Emerging tumor entities and variants of CNS neoplasms. J Neuropathol Exp Neurol 63: 185-192.
[41] Hassoun J, Soylemezoglu F, Gambarelli D, Figarella B, von Ammon K, Kleihues P (1993). Central neurocytoma: a synopsis of clinical and histological features. Brain Pathol 3: 297-306.
[42] Zhang D, Wen L, Henning TD, Feng XY, Zhang YL, Zou LG, Zhang ZG (2006). Central neurocytoma: clinical, pathological and neuroradiological findings. Clin Radiol 61: 348-357.

[43] Roberts RO, Lynch CF, Jones MP, Hart MN (1991). Medulloblastoma: a populationbased study of 532 cases. J Neuropathol Exp Neurol 50: 134-144.
[44] von Deimling A, Janzer R, Kleihues P, Wiestler OD (1990). Patterns of differentiation in central neurocytoma. An immunohistochemical study of eleven biopsies. Acta Neuropathol 79: 473-479.
[45] von Deimling A, Kleihues P, Saremaslani P, Yasargil MG, Spoerri O, Sudhof TC, Wiestler OD (1991). Histogenesis and differentiation potential of central neurocytomas. Lab Invest 64: 585-591.
[46] Kubota T, Hayashi M, Kawano H, Kabuto M, Sato K, Ishise J, Kawamoto K, Shirataki K, Iizuka H, Tsunoda S (1991). Central neurocytoma: immunohistochemical and ultrastructural study. Acta Neuropathol 81: 418-427.
[47] Yasargil MG, von Ammon K, von Deimling A, Valavanis A, Wichmann W, Wiestler OD (1992). Central neurocytoma: histopathological variants and therapeutic approaches. J Neurosurg 76: 32-37.
[48] Figarella B, Pellissier JF, Daumas D, Delisle MB, Pasquier B, Parent M, Gambarelli D, Rougon G, Hassoun J (1992). Central neurocytomas. Critical evaluation of a small-cell neuronal tumor. Am J Surg Pathol 16: 97-109.
[49] Hessler RB, Lopes MB, Frankfurter A, Reidy J, VandenBerg SR (1992). Cytoskeletal immunohistochemistry of central neurocytomas. Am J Surg Pathol 16: 1031-1038.
[50] Soylemezoglu F, Onder S, Tezel GG, Berker M (2003). Neuronal nuclear antigen (NeuN): a new tool in the diagnosis of central neurocytoma. Pathol Res Pract 199: 463-468.
[51] Englund C, Alvord EC, Jr., Folkerth RD, Silbergeld D, Born DE, Small R, Hevner RF (2005). NeuN expression correlates with reduced mitotic index of neoplastic cells in central neurocytomas. Neuropathol Appl Neurobiol 31: 429-438.
[52] Gultekin SH, Dalmau J, Graus Y, Posner JB, Rosenblum MK (1998). Anti-Hu immunolabeling as an index of neuronal differentiation in human brain tumors: a study of 112 central neuroepithelial neoplasms. Am J Surg Pathol 22: 195-200.
[53] oylemezoglu F, Kleihues P, Esteve J, Scheithauer BW (1997). Atypical central neurocytoma. J Neuropath Exp Neurol 56: 551-556.
[54] Tsuchida T, Matsumoto M, Shirayama Y, Imahori T, Kasai H, Kawamoto K (1996). Neuronal and glial characteristics of central neurocytoma: electron microscopical analysis of two cases. Acta Neuropathol 91: 573-577.
[55] Cenacchi G, Giangaspero A, Cerasoli S, Manetto V, Martinelli GN (1996). Ultrastructural characterization of oligodendroglial- like cells in central nervous system tumors. Ultrastruct Pathol 20: 537-547.
[56] Mackenzie IR (1999). Central neurocytoma: histologic atypia, proliferation potential, and clinical outcome. Cancer 85: 1606-1610.
[57] Kim DG, Kim JS, Chi JG, Park SH, Jung HW, Choi KS, Han DH (1996). Central neurocytoma: proliferative potential and biological behavior. J Neurosurg 84: 742-747.
[58] Pearl GS, Takei Y, Bakay RA, Davis P (1985). Intraventricular primary cerebral neuroblastoma in adults: report of three cases. Neurosurgery 16: 847-849.
[59] Taruscio D, Danesi R, Montaldi A, Cerasoli S, Cenacchi G, Giangaspero F (1997).Nonrandom gain of chromosome 7 in central neurocytoma: a chromosomal analysis and fluorescence in situ hybridization study. Virchows Arch 430: 47-51.

[60] Tong CY, Ng HK, Pang JC, Hu J, Hui AB, Poon WS (2000). Central neurocytomas are genetically distinct from oligodendrogliomas and neuroblastomas. Histopathology 37: 160-165

[61] Yin XL, Pang JC, Hui AB, Ng HK (2000). Detection of chromosomal imbalances in central neurocytomas by using comparative genomic hybridization. J Neurosurg 93: 77-81.

[62] Cerda-Nicolas M, Lopez-Gines C, Peydro O, Llombart-Bosch A (1993). Central neurocytoma: a cytogenetic case study. Cancer Genet Cytogenet 65: 173-174.

[63] Jay V, Edwards V, Hoving E, Rutka J, Becker L, Zielenska M, Teshima I (1999). Central neurocytoma: morphological, flow cytometric, polymerase chain reaction, fluorescence in situ hybridization, and karyotypic analyses. Case report. J Neurosurg 90: 348-354.

[64] Fujisawa H, Marukawa K, Hasegawa M, Tohma Y, Hayashi Y, Uchiyama N, Tachibana O, Yamashita J (2002). Genetic differences between neurocytoma and dysembryoplastic neuroepithelial tumor and oligodendroglial tumors. J Neurosurg 97: 1350-1355.

[65] Ohgaki H, Eibl RH, Schwab M, Reichel MB, Mariani L, Gehring M, Petersen I, Holl T, Wiestler OD, Kleihues P (1993). Mutations of the p53 tumor suppressor gene in neoplasms of the human nervous system. Mol Carcinog 8: 74-80.

[66] Rades D, Fehlauer F, Lamszus K, Schild SE, Hagel C, Westphal M, Alberti W (2005). Well-differentiated neurocytoma: what is the best available treatment? Neuro-oncol 7: 77-83.

[67] Horstmann S, Perry A, Reifenberger G, Giangaspero F, Huang H, Hara A, Masuoka J, Rainov NG, Bergmann M, Heppner FL, Brandner S, Chimelli L, Montagna N, Jackson T, Davis DG, Markesbery WR, Ellison DW, Weller RO, Taddei GL, Conti R, Del Bigio MR, Gonzalez-Campora R, Radhakrishnan VV, Soylemezoglu F, Uro-Coste E, Qian J, Kleihues P, Ohgaki H (2004). Genetic and expression profiles of cerebellar liponeurocytomas. Brain Pathol 14: 281-289.

[68] Jouvet A, Lellouch-Tubiana A, Boddaert N, Zerah M, Champier J, Fevre-Montange M (2005). Fourth ventricle Neurocytoma with lipomatous and ependymal differentiation. Acta Neuropathol 109: 346-351.

[69] Eng DY, DeMonte F, Ginsberg L, Fuller GN, Jaeckle K (1997). Craniospinal dissemination of central neurocytoma - report of two cases. J Neurosurg 86: 547-552

[70] Tomura N, Hirano H, Watanabe O, Watarai J, Itoh Y, Mineura K, Kowada M (1997). Central neurocytoma with clinically malignant behavior. AJNR Am J Neuroradiol 18: 1175- 1178.

[71] Rades D, Schild SE, Fehlauer F (2004). Prognostic value of the MIB-1 labeling index for central neurocytomas. Neurology 62: 987-989.

[72] Robbins P, Segal A, Narula S, Stokes B, Lee M, Thomas W, Caterina P, Sinclair I, Spagnolo D (1995). Central neurocytoma. A clinicopathological, immunohistochemical and ultrastructural study of 7 cases. Pathol Res Pract 191: 100-111.

[73] Brat DJ, Scheithauer BW, Eberhart CG, Burger PC (2001). Extraventricular neurocytomas: pathologic features and clinical outcome. Am J Surg Pathol 25: 1252-1260.

[74] Daumas-Duport C, Scheithauer BW, Chodkiewicz JP, Laws ER, Jr., Vedrenne C (1988). Dysembryoplastic neuroepithelial tumor: a surgically curable tumor of young patients with intractable partial seizures. Report of thirty-nine cases. Neurosurgery 23: 545-556.

[75] Russell DS, Rubinstein LJ (1989). Pathology of Tumours of the Nervous System.Edward Arnold: London.
[76] Daumas-Duport C (1993). Dysembryoplastic neuroepithelial tumours. Brain Pathol 3: 283-295.
[77] Daumas-Duport C, Varlet P, Bacha S, Beuvon F, Cervera-Pierot P, Chodkiewicz JP (1999). Dysembryoplastic neuroepithelial tumors: nonspecific histological forms — a study of 40 cases. J Neurooncol 41: 267-280.
[78] Honavar M, Janota I (1994). 73 cases of dysembryoplastic neuroepithelial tumour: the range of histological appearances. Brain Pathol 4: 428
[79] Pasquier B, Peoc'h M, Fabre- Bocquentin B, Bensaadi L, Pasquier D, Hoffmann D, Kahane P, Tassi L, Le Bas JF, Benabid AL (2002). Surgical pathology of drugresistantpartial epilepsy. A 10-year-experience with a series of 327 consecutive resections. Epileptic Disord 4: 99-119.
[80] Daumas-Duport C (1995). Dysembryoplastic neuroepithelial tumours in epilepsy surgery. In: Dysplasia of Cerebral Cortex and Epilepsy. Guerrini R, ed. Raven Press: New York, pp. 125-147.
[81] Daumas Duport C (1995). Patterns of tumor growth and problems associated with histological typing of low-grade gliomas. In: Benign Cerebral Gliomas. Apuzzo LJ, ed. AANS: Park Ridge, pp. 125-147.
[82] Rosemberg S, Vieira GS (1998). [Dysembryoplastic neuroepithelial tumor. An epidemiological study from a single institution]. Arq Neuropsiquiatr 56: 232-236.
[83] Degen R, Ebner A, Lahl R, Leonhardt S, Pannek HW, Tuxhorn I (2002). Various findings in surgically treated epilepsy patients with dysembryoplastic neuroepithelial tumors in comparison with those of patients with other low-grade brain tumors and other neuronal migration disorders. Epilepsia 43: 1379-1384.
[84] Prayson RA, Estes ML (1992). Dysembryoplastic neuroepithelial tumor. Am J Clin Pathol 97: 398-401.
[85] Taratuto AL, Pomata H, Sevlever G, Gallo G, Monges J (1995). Dysembryoplastic neuroepithelial tumor: morphological, immunocytochemical, and deoxyribonucleic acid analyses in a pediatric series. Neurosurgery 36: 474- 481.
[86] Tatke M, Suri VS, Malhotra V, Sharma A, Sinha S, Kumar S (2001). Dysembryoplastic neuroepithelial tumors: report of 10 cases from a center where epilepsy surgery is not done. Pathol Res Pract 197: 769-774.
[87] Cervera-Pierot P, Varlet P, Chodkiewicz JP, Daumas D (1997). Dysembryoplastic neuroepithelial tumors located in the caudate nucleus area: report of four cases. Neurosurg 40: 1065-1069.
[88] Guesmi H, Houtteville JP, Courtheoux P, Derlon JM, Chapon F (1999). [Dysembryoplastic neuroepithelial tumors. Report of 8 cases including two with unusual localization]. Neurochirurgie 45: 190-200.
[89] Kurtkaya-Yapicier O, Elmaci I, Boran B, Kilic T, Sav A, Pamir MN (2002). Dysembryoplastic neuroepithelial tumor of the midbrain tectum: a case report. Brain Tumor Pathol 19: 97-100.

[90] Kuchelmeister K, Demirel T, Schlorer E, Bergmann M, Gullotta F (1995). Dysembryoplastic neuroepithelial tumour of the cerebellum. Acta Neuropathol 89: 385-390.

[91] Yasha TC, Mohanty A, Radhesh S, Santosh V, Das S, Shankar SK (1998). Infratentorial dysembryoplastic neuroepithelial tumor (DNT) associated with Arnold-Chiari malformation. Clin Neuropathol 17: 305-310.

[92] Fujimoto K, Ohnishi H, Tsujimoto M, Hoshida T, Nakazato Y (2000). Dysembryoplastic neuroepithelial tumor of the cerebellum and brainstem. Case report. J Neurosurg 93: 487-489.

[93] Lellouch-Tubiana A, Bourgeois M, Vekemans M, Robain O (1995). Dysembryoplastic neuroepithelial tumors in two children with neurofibromatosis type 1. Acta Neuropathol 90: 319-322.

[94] Leung SY, Gwi E, Ng HK, Fung CF, Yam KY (1994). Dysembryoplastic neuroepithelial tumor. A tumor with small neuronal cells resembling oligodendroglioma. Am J Surg Pathol 18: 604-614.

[95] Whittle IR, Dow GR, Lammie GA, Wardlaw J (1999). Dsyembryoplastic neuroepithelial tumour with discrete bilateral multifocality: further evidence for a germinal origin. Br J Neurosurg 13: 508-511.

[96] Nolan MA, Sakuta R, Chuang N, Otsubo H, Rutka JT, Snead OC, III, Hawkins CE, Weiss SK (2004). Dysembryoplastic neuroepithelial tumors in childhood: long-term outcome and prognostic features. Neurology 62: 2270-2276.

[97] Raymond AA, Halpin SF, Alsanjari N, Cook MJ, Kitchen ND, Fish DR, Stevens JM, Harding BN, Scaravilli F, Kendall B (1994). Dysembryoplastic neuroepithelial tumor. Features in 16 patients. Brain 117: 461-475.

[98] Rosenberg DS, Demarquay G, Jouvet A, Le Bars D, Streichenberger N, Sindou M, Kopp N, Mauguiere F, Ryvlin P (2005). [11C]- Methionine PET: dysembryoplastic neuroepithelial tumours compared with other epileptogenic brain neoplasms. J Neurol Neurosurg Psychiatry 76: 1686-1692.

[99] Fernandez C, Girard N, Paz PA, Bouvier-Labit C, Lena G, Figarella-Branger D (2003). The usefulness of MR imaging in the diagnosis of dysembryoplastic neuroepithelial tumor in children: a study of 14 cases. AJNR Am J Neuroradiol 24: 829-834.

[100] Kuroiwa T, Bergey GK, Rothman MI, Zoarski GH, Wolf A, Zagardo MT, Kristt DA, Hudson LP, Krumholz A, Barry E (1995). Radiologic appearance of the dysembryoplastic neuroepithelial tumor. Radiology 197: 233-238.

[101] Ostertun B, Wolf HK, Campos MG, Matus C, Solymosi L, Elger CE, Schramm J, Schild HH (1996). Dysembryoplastic neuroepithelial tumors: MR and CT evaluation. AJNR Am J Neuroradiol 17: 419-430.

[102] Stanescu CR, Varlet P, Beuvon F, Daumas DC, Devaux B, Chassoux F, Fredy D, Meder JF (2001). Dysembryoplastic neuroepithelial tumors: CT, MR findings and imaging follow-up: a study of 53 cases. J Neuroradiol 28: 230-240.

[103] Daumas-Duport C, Varlet P (2003). [Dysembryoplastic neuroepithelial tumors]. Rev Neurol (Paris) 159: 622-636.

[104] Jensen RL, Caamano E, Jensen EM, Couldwell WT (2006). Development of contrast enhancement after long-term observation of a dysembryoplastic neuroepithelial tumor. J Neurooncol 78: 59-62.

[105] Thom M, Gomez-Anson B, Revesz T, Harkness W, O'Brien CJ, Kett-White R, Jones EW, Stevens J, Scaravilli F (1999). Spontaneous intralesional haemorrhage in dysembryoplastic neuroepithelial tumours: a series of five cases. J Neurol Neurosurg Psychiatry 67: 97-101.

[106] Valenti MP, Froelich S, Armspach JP, Chenard MP, Dietemann JL, Kerhli P, Marescaux C, Hirsch E, Namer IJ (2002). Contribution of SISCOM imaging in the presurgical evaluation of temporal lobe epilepsy related to dysembryoplastic neuroepithelial tumors. Epilepsia 43: 270-276.

[107] uyken C, Blumcke I, Fimmers R, Urbach H, Elger CE, Wiestler OD, Schramm J(2003). The spectrum of long-term epilepsyassociated tumors: long-term seizure and tumor outcome and neurosurgical aspects. Epilepsia 44: 822-830.

[108] Bartolomei JC, Christopher S, Vives K, Spencer DD, Piepmeier JM (1997). Low-grade gliomas of chronic epilepsy: a distinct clinical and pathological entity. J Neurooncol 34: 79-84.

[109] Blumcke I, Luyken C, Urbach H, Schramm J, Wiestler OD (2004). An iso morphic subtype of long-term epilepsy-associated astrocytomas associated with benign prognosis. Acta Neuropathol 107: 381-388.

[110] Clusmann H, Kral T, Fackeldey E, Blumcke I, Helmstaedter C, von Oertzen J, Urbach H, Schramm J (2004). Lesional mesial temporal lobe epilepsy and limited resections: prognostic factors and outcome. J Neurol Neurosurg Psychiatry 75: 1589-1596.

[111] Sakuta R, Otsubo H, Nolan MA, Weiss SK, Hawkins C, Rutka JT, Chuang NA, Chuang SH, Snead OC, III (2005). Recurrent intractable seizures in children with cortical dysplasia adjacent to dysembryoplastic neuroepithelial tumor. J Child Neurol 20: 377-384.

[112] Takahashi A, Hong SC, Seo DW, Hong SB, Lee M, Suh YL (2005). Frequent association of cortical dysplasia in dysembryoplastic neuroepithelial tumor treated by epilepsy surgery.Surg Neurol 64: 419-427.

[113] Hirose T, Scheithauer BW, Lopes MB, VandenBerg SR (1994). Dysembryoplastic neuroeptihelial tumor (DNT): an immunohistochemical and ultrastructural study. J Neuropathol Exp Neurol 53: 184-195.

[114] Honavar M, Janota I, Polkey CE (1999). Histological heterogeneity of dysembryoplastic neuroepithelial tumour: identification and differential diagnosis in a series of 74 cases. Histopathology 34: 342-356.

[115] Wolf HK, Buslei R, Blumcke I, Wiestler OD, Pietsch T (1997). Neural antigens in oligodendrogliomas and dysembryoplastic neuroepithelial tumors. Acta Neuropathol 94: 436-443.

[116] Wong K, Gyure KA, Prayson RA, Morrison AL, Le TQ, Armstrong RC (1999).Dysembryoplastic neuroepithelial tumor: in situ hybridization of proteolipid protein (PLP) messenger ribonucleic acid (mRNA). J Neuropath Exp Neurol 58: 542-542.

[117] Wolf HK, Wellmer J, Muller MB, Wiestler OD, Hufnagel A, Pietsch T (1995).Glioneuronal malformative lesions and dysembryoplastic neuroepithelial tumors in patients with chronic pharmacoresistant epilepsies. J Neuropathol Exp Neurol 54: 245-254.

[118] Chan CH, Bittar RG, Davis GA, Kalnins RM, Fabinyi GC (2006). Long-term seizure outcome following surgery for dysembryoplastic neuroepithelial tumor. J Neurosurg 104: 62-69.

[119] Hirose T, Scheithauer BW (1998). Mixed dysembryoplastic neuroepithelial tumorand ganglioglioma. Acta Neuropathol 95: 649- 654.

[120] Prayson RA (1999). Composite ganglioglioma and dysembryoplastic neuroepithelial tumor. Arch Pathol Lab Med 123: 247-250.

[121] Shimbo Y, Takahashi H, Hayano M, Kumagai T, Kameyama S (1997). Temporallobe lesion demonstrating features of dysembryoplastic neuroepithelial tumor and ganglioglioma: a transitional form? Clin Neuropathol 16: 65-68.

[122] Kannuki S, Bando K, Soga T, Matsumoto K, Hirose T (1996). [A case report of dysembryoplastic neuroepithelial tumor associated with neurofibromatosis type 1]. No Shinkei Geka 24: 183-188.

[123] Krossnes BK, Wester K, Moen G, Mork SJ (2005). Multifocal dysembryoplastic neuroepithelial tumour in a male with the XYY syndrome. Neuropathol Appl Neurobiol 31: 556-560.

[124] Lellouch-Tubiana A, Bourgeois M, Vekemans M, Robain O (1995). Dysembryoplastic neuroepithelial tumors in two children with neurofibromatosis type 1. Acta Neuropathol 90: 319-322.

[125] Fujisawa H, Marukawa K, Hasegawa M, Tohma Y, Hayashi Y, Uchiyama N, Tachibana O, Yamashita J (2002). Genetic differences between neurocytoma and dysembryoplastic neuroepithelial tumor and oligodendroglial tumors. J Neurosurg 97: 1350-1355.

[126] Kirkpatrick PJ, Honavar M, Janota I, Polkey CE (1993). Control of temporal lobe epilepsy following en bloc resection of lowgrade tumors. J Neurosurg 78: 19-25.

[127] Hennessy MJ, Elwes RD, Rabe- Hesketh S, Binnie CD, Polkey CE (2001). Prognostic factors in the surgical treatment of medically intractable epilepsy associated with mesial temporal sclerosis. Acta Neurol Scand 103: 344-350.

[128] Giulioni M, Galassi E, Zucchelli M, Volpi L (2005). Seizure outcome of lesionectomy in glioneuronal tumors associated with epilepsy in children. J Neurosurg 102: 288-293.

[129] Rushing EJ, Thompson LD, Mena H (2003). Malignant transformation of a dysembryoplastic neuroepithelial tumor after radiation and chemotherapy. Ann Diagn Pathol 7: 240-244.

[130] Taratuto AL, Monges J, Lylyk P, Leiguarda R (1982). Meningocerebral astrocytoma attached to dura with "desmoplastic" reaction. Proceedings of the IX International Congress of Neuropathology (Viena) 5-10.

[131] Taratuto AL, Monges J, Lylyk P, Leiguarda R (1984). Superficial cerebral astrocytoma attached to dura. Report of six cases in infants. Cancer 54: 2505-2512.

[132] Kleihues P, Burger PC, Scheithauer BW eds. (1993). Histological Typing of Tumours of the Central Nervous System. World Health Organization International Histological Classification of Tumours. Springer Verlag: Berlin Heidelberg.

[133] VandenBerg SR, May EE, Rubinstein LJ, Herman MM, Perentes E, Vinores SA,Collins VP, Park TS (1987). Desmoplastic supratentorial neuroepithelial tumors of infancy with divergent differentiation potential ("desmoplastic infantile gangliogliomas"). Report on 11 cases of a distinctive embryonal tumor with favorable prognosis. J Neurosurg 66: 58-71.

[134] VandenBerg SR (1993). Desmoplastic infantile ganglioglioma and desmoplastic cerebral astrocytoma of infancy. Brain Pathol 3: 275-281.

[135] Zuccaro G, Taratuto AL, Monges J (1986). Intracranial neoplasms during the first year of life. Surg Neurol 26: 29-36.

[136] Ganesan K, Desai S, Udwadia-Hegde A (2006). Non-infantile variant of desmoplastic ganglioglioma: a report of 2 cases. Pediatr Radiol 36: 541-545.

[137] Zulch KJ (1957). Brain Tumours. Their Biology and Pathology. Springer-Verlag: New York.

[138] Trehan G, Bruge H, Vinchon M, Khalil C, Ruchoux MM, Dhellemmes P, Ares GS (2004). MR imaging in the diagnosis of desmoplastic infantile tumor: retrospective study of six cases. AJNR Am J Neuroradiol 25: 1028-1033.

[139] VandenBerg SR (1991). Desmoplastic infantile ganglioglioma: a clinicopathologic review of sixteen cases. Brain Tumor Pathol 8: 25-31.

[140] Pommepuy I, Delage-Corre M, Moreau JJ, Labrousse F (2006). A report of a desmoplastic ganglioglioma in a 12-year-old girl with review of the literature. J Neurooncol 76: 271-275.

[141] de Chadarevian JP, Pattisapu JV, Faerber EN (1990). Desmoplastic cerebral astrocytoma of infancy. Light microscopy, immunocytochemistry, and ultrastructure. Cancer 66: 173-179.

[142] Louis DN, von Deimling A, Dickersin GR, Dooling EC, Seizinger BR (1992). Desmoplastic cerebral astrocytomas of infancy: a histopathologic, immunohistochemical, ultrastructural, and molecular genetic study. Hum Pathol 23: 1402-1409

[143] Aydin F, Ghatak NR, Salvant J, Muizelaar P (1993). Desmoplastic cerebral astrocytoma of infancy. A case report with immunohistochemical, ultrastructural and proliferation studies. Acta Neuropathol 86: 666-670.

[144] Cushing H (1931). Experiences with the cerebellar astrocytomas. A critical review of seventy-six cases. Surg Gynecol Obstet 52: 1129-1204.

[145] Paulus W, Schlote W, Perentes E, Jacobi G, Warmuth Metz M, Roggendorf W (1992). Desmoplastic supratentorial neuroepithelial tumours of infancy. Histopathology 21: 43-49.

[146] Ng TH, Fung CF, Ma LT (1990). The pathological spectrum of desmoplastic infantile gangliogliomas. Histopathology 16: 235-241.

[147] aratuto AL, Sevlever G, Schultz M (1987). Monoclonal antibodies in superficial desmoplastic cerebral astrocytoma attached to dura in infants. J Neuropathol Exp Neurol 46: 395-395.

[148] Rushing EJ, Rorke LB, Sutton L (1993). Problems in the nosology of desmoplastic tumors of childhood. Pediatr Neurosurg 19: 57-62.

[149] Komori T, Scheithauer BW, Parisi JE, Watterson J, Priest JR (2001). Mixed conventional and desmoplastic infantile ganglioglioma: an autopsied case with 6-year follow-up. Mod Pathol 14: 720-726.

[150] Kros JM, Delwel EJ, de Jong TH, Tanghe HL, van Run PR, Vissers K, Alers JC(2002). Desmoplastic infantile astrocytoma and ganglioglioma: a search for genomic characteristics. Acta Neuropathol 104: 144-148.

[151] De Munnynck K, Van Gool S, Van Calenbergh F, Demaerel P, Uyttebroeck A, Buyse G, Sciot R (2002). Desmoplastic infantile ganglioglioma: a potentially malignant tumor? Am J Surg Pathol 26: 1515-1522.

[152] Taratuto AL, Sevlever G, Schultz M, Gutierrez M, Monges J, Sanchez M (1994).Desmoplastic cerebral astrocytoma of infancy (DCAI). Survival data of the original series and report of two additional cases, DNA, kinetic and molecular genetic studies. Brain Pathol 4: 423.

[153] Tenreiro P, Kamath SV, Knorr JR, Ragland RL, Smith TW, Lau KY (1995). Desmoplastic infantile ganglioglioma: CT and MRI features. Pediatr Radiol 25: 540-543.

[154] Cerda-Nicolas M, Lopez-Gines C, Gil- Benso R, Donat J, Fernandez-Delgado R, Pellin A, Lopez-Guerrero JA, Roldan P, Barbera J (2006). Desmoplastic infantile ganglioglioma. Morphological, immunohistochemical and genetic features. Histopathology 48: 617-621.

[155] Rutka JT, Giblin JR, Apodaca G, DeArmond SJ, Stern R, Rosenblum ML (1987). Inhibition of growth and induction of differentiation in a malignant human glioma cell line by normal leptomeningeal extracellular matrix proteins. Cancer Res 47: 3515-3522.

[156] Takeshima H, Kawahara Y, Hirano H, Obara S, Niiro M, Kuratsu J (2003). Postoperative regression of desmoplastic infantile gangliogliomas: report of two cases. Neurosurgery 53: 979-983.

[157] Kuchelmeister K, Schonmeyr R, Albani M, Schachenmayr W (1998). Anaplastic desmoplastic infantile ganglioglioma. Clin Neuropathol 17: 269-269.

[158] Kuchelmeister K, Steinhauser A, Korf B, Wagner D, Prey N, Schachenmayr W (1996). Anaplastic desmoplastic infantile ganglioglioma: a case report. Clin Neuropathol 15: 280-280.

[159] Kuchelmeister K, Demirel T, Schlorer E, Bergmann M, Gullotta F (1995). Dysembryoplastic neuroepithelial tumour of the cerebellum. Acta Neuropathol 89: 385-390.

[160] Komori T, Scheithauer BW, Hirose T (2002). A rosette-forming glioneuronal tumor of the fourth ventricle: infratentorial form of dysembryoplastic neuroepithelial tumor? Am J Surg Pathol 26: 582-591.

[161] Preusser M, Dietrich W, Czech T, Prayer D, Budka H, Hainfellner JA (2003). Rosette-forming glioneuronal tumor of the fourth ventricle. Acta Neuropathol 106: 506-508.

[162] Albanese A, Mangiola A, Pompucci A, Sabatino G, Gessi M, Lauriola L, Anile C (2005). Rosette-forming glioneuronal tumour of the fourth ventricle: report of a case with clinical and surgical implications. J Neurooncol 71: 195-197.

[163] acques TS, Eldridge C, Patel A, Saleem NM, Powell M, Kitchen ND, Thom M, Revesz T (2006). Mixed glioneuronal tumour of the fourth ventricle with prominent rosette formation. Neuropathol Appl Neurobiol 32: 217-220.

[164] Johnson M, Pace J, Burroughs JF (2006). Fourth ventricle rosette-forming glioneuronal tumor. Case report. J Neurosurg 105: 129-131.

[165] Ishizawa T, Komori T, Shibahara J, Ishizawa K, Adachi J, Nishikawa R, Matsutani M, Hirose T (2006). Papillary glioneuronal tumor with minigemistocytic components and increased proliferative activity. Hum Pathol 37: 627-630.

[166] Komori T, Scheithauer BW, Anthony DC, Rosenblum MK, McLendon RE, Scott RM, Okazaki H, Kobayashi M (1998). Papillary glioneuronal tumor: a new variant of mixed neuronal- glial neoplasm. Am J Surg Pathol 22: 1171-1183.

[167] Komori T, Scheithauer BW, Anthony DC, Scott RM, Okazaki H, Kobayashi M (1996). Pseudopapillary ganglioneurocytoma. J Neuropathol Exp Neurol 55: 654-654.

[168] Kim DH, Suh YL (1997). Pseudopapillary neurocytoma of temporal lobe with glial differentiation. Acta Neuropathol 94: 187- 191.

[169] Broholm H, Madsen FF, Wagner AA, Laursen H (2002). Papillary glioneuronal tumor—a new tumor entity. Clin Neuropathol 21: 1-4.

[170] Dim DC, Lingamfelter DC, Taboada EM, Fiorella RM (2006). Papillary glioneuronal tumor: a case report and review of the literature. Hum Pathol 37: 914-918.

[171] Bouvier-Labit C, Daniel L, Dufour H, Grisoli F, Figarella-Branger D (2000). Papillary glioneuronal tumour: clinicopathological and biochemical study of one case with 7-year follow up. Acta Neuropathol 99: 321-326.

[172] Vajtai I, Kappeler A, Lukes A, Arnold M, Luthy AR, Leibundgut K (2006). Papillary glioneuronal tumor. Pathol Res Pract 202: 107-112.

[173] Prayson RA (2000). Papillary glioneuronal tumor. Arch Pathol Lab Med 124: 1820-1823.

[174] Buccoliero AM, Giordano F, Mussa F, Taddei A, Genitori L, Taddei GL (2006). Papillary glioneuronal tumor radiologically mimicking a cavernous hemangioma with hemorrhagic onset. Neuropathology 26: 206-211.

[175] Tanaka Y, Yokoo H, Komori T, Makita Y, Ishizawa T, Hirose T, Ebato M, Shibahara J, Tsukayama C, Shibuya M, Nakazato Y (2005). A distinct pattern of Olig2-positive cellular distribution in papillary glioneuronal tumors: a manifestation of the oligodendroglial phenotype? Acta Neuropathol 110: 39-47.

[176] Jenkinson MD, Bosma JJ, Du PD, Ohgaki H, Kleihues P, Warnke P, Rainov N(2003). Cerebellar liponeurocytoma with an unusually aggressive clinical course: case report. Neurosurgery 53: 1425-1427

[177] Bechtel JT, Patton JM, Takei Y (1978). Mixed mesenchymal and neuroectodermal tumor of the cerebellum. Acta Neuropathol 41: 261-263.

[178] Ellison DW, Zygmunt SC, Weller RO (1993). Neurocytoma/lipoma (neurolipocytoma) of the cerebellum. Neuropathol Appl Neurobiol 19: 95-98.

[179] Giangaspero F, Cenacchi G, Roncaroli F, Rigobello L, Manetto V, Gambacorta M,Allegranza A (1996). Medullocytoma (lipidized medulloblastoma): a cerebellar neoplasm of adults with favorable prognosis. Am J Surg Pathol 20: 656-664.

[180] Alleyne CH, Jr., Hunter S, Olson JJ, Barrow DL (1998). Lipomatous glioneurocytoma of the posterior fossa with divergent differentiation: case report. Neurosurgery 42: 639-643.

[181] Gonzalez-Campora R, Weller RO (1998). Lipidized mature neuroectodermal tumour of the cerebellum with myoid differentiation. Neuropathol Appl Neurobiol 24: 397-402.

[182] Horstmann S, Perry A, Reifenberger G, Giangaspero F, Huang H, Hara A, Masuoka J, Rainov NG, Bergmann M, Heppner FL, Brandner S, Chimelli L, Montagna N, Jackson T, Davis DG, Markesbery WR, Ellison DW, Weller RO, Taddei GL, Conti R, Del Bigio MR, Gonzalez-Campora R, Radhakrishnan VV, Soylemezoglu F, Uro-Coste E, Qian J, Kleihues P, Ohgaki H (2004). Genetic and expression profiles of cerebellar liponeurocytomas. Brain Pathol 14: 281-289.

[183] Budka H, Chimelli L (1994). Lipomatous medulloblastoma in adults: a new tumor type with possible favorable prognosis [letter]. Hum Pathol 25: 730-731.

[184] Soylemezoglu F, Soffer D, Onol B, Schwechheimer K, Kleihues P (1996). Lipomatous medulloblastoma in adults: a distinct clinicopathological entity. Am J Surg Pathol 20: 413-418.

[185] Aker FV, Ozkara S, Eren P, Peker O, Armagan S, Hakan T (2005). Cerebellar liponeurocytoma/lipidized medulloblastoma. J Neurooncol 71: 53-59.

[186] Buccoliero AM, Caldarella A, Bacci S, Gallina P, Taddei A, Di Lorenzo N, Romagnoli P, Taddei GL (2005). Cerebellar liponeurocytoma: morphological, immunohistochemical, and ultrastructural study of a relapsed case. Neuropathology 25: 77-83.

[187] Megdiche BH, Nagi S, Zouauoi W, Belghith L, Sebai R, Touibi S (2005). [Cerebellar liponeurocytoma. Case report]. Tunis Med 83: 120-122.

[188] Owler BK, Makeham JM, Shingde M, Besser M (2005). Cerebellar liponeurocytoma. J Clin Neurosci 12: 326-329.

[189] Valery CA, Sakka LJ, Poirier J (2004). Problematic differential diagnosis between cerebellar liponeurocytoma and anaplastic oligodendroglioma. Br J Neurosurg 18: 300-303.

[190] Hubbard JL, Scheithauer BW, Kispert DB, Carpenter SM, Wick MR, Laws ER, Jr. (1989). Adult cerebellar medulloblastomas: the pathological, radiographic, and clinical disease spectrum. J Neurosurg 70: 536-544.

[191] Akhaddar A, Zrara I, Gazzaz M, El Moustarchid B, Benomar S, Boucetta M (2003). Cerebellar liponeurocytoma (lipomatous medulloblastoma). J Neuroradiol 30: 121-126.

[192] Kuchelmeister K, Nestler U, Siekmann R, Schachenmayr W (2006). Liponeurocytoma of the left lateral ventricle—case report and review of the literature. Clin Neuropathol 25: 86-94.

[193] Mena H, Morrison AL, Jones RV, Gyure KA (2001). Central neurocytomas express photoreceptor differentiation. Cancer 91: 136-143.

[194] Brandis A, Heyer R, Hori A, Walter GF (1997). Cerebellar neurocytoma in an infant: an important differential diagnosis from cerebellar neuroblastoma and medulloblastoma? Neuropediatrics 28: 235-238.
[195] Enam SA, Rosenblum ML, Ho KL (1997). Neurocytoma in the cerebellum. Case report. J Neurosurg 87: 100-102.
[196] George DH, Scheithauer BW (2001). Central liponeurocytoma. Am J Surg Pathol 25: 1551-1555.
[197] Giordana MT, Schiffer P, Boghi A, Buoncristiani P, Benech F (2000). Medulloblastoma with lipidized cells versus lipomatous medulloblastoma. Clin Neuropathol 19: 273-277.
[198] Sharma MC, Agarwal M, Suri A, Gaikwad S, Mukhopadhyay P, Sarkar C (2002).Lipomedulloblastoma in a child: a controversial entity. Hum Pathol 33: 564-569.
[199] Jackson TR, Regine WF, Wilson D, Davis DG (2001). Cerebellar liponeurocytoma. Case report and review of the literature. J Neurosurg 95: 700-703.
[200] Kachhara R, Bhattacharya RN, Nair S, Radhakrishnan VV (2003). Liponeurocytoma of the cerebellum—a case report. Neurol India 51: 274-276.
[201] Miller CA, Torack RM (1970). Secretory ependymoma of the filum terminale. Acta Neuropathol 15: 240-250.
[202] Gelabert-Gonzalez M (2005). Paragangliomas of the lumbar region. Report of two cases and review of the literature. J Neurosurg Spine 2: 354-365.
[203] Wippold FJ, Smirniotopoulos JG, Pilgram TK (1997). Lesions of the cauda equina: a clinical and pathology review from the Armed Forces Institute of Pathology. Clin Neurol Neurosurg 99: 229-234.
[204] Yang SY, Jin YJ, Park SH, Jahng TA, Kim HJ, Chung CK (2005). Paragangliomas in the cauda equina region: clinicopathoradiologic findings in four cases. J Neurooncol 72: 49-55.
[205] Conti P, Mouchaty H, Spacca B, Buccoliero AM, Conti R (2006). Thoracic extradural paragangliomas: a case report and review of the literature. Spinal Cord 44: 120- 125.
[206] Telera S, Carosi M, Cerasoli V, Facciolo F, Occhipinti E, Vidiri A, Pompili A (2006). Hemothorax presenting as a primitive thoracic paraganglioma. Case illustration. J Neurosurg Spine 4: 515.
[207] Sundgren P, Annertz M, Englund E, Stromblad LG, Holtas S (1999). Paragangliomas of the spinal canal. Neuroradiology 41: 788-794.
[208] Blades DA, Hardy RW, Cohen M (1991). Cervical paraganglioma with subsequentintracranial and intraspinal metastases. Case report. J Neurosurg 75: 320-323.
[209] Jackson CG (2001). Glomus tympanicum and glomus jugulare tumors. Otolaryngol Clin North Am 34: 941-970..
[210] Naggara O, Varlet P, Page P, Oppenheim C, Meder JF (2005). Suprasellar paraganglioma: a case report and review of the literature. Neuroradiology 47: 753-757.
[211] Deb P, Sharma MC, Gaikwad S, Gupta A, Mehta VS, Sarkar C (2005). Cerebellopontine angle paraganglioma - report of a case and review of literature. J Neurooncol 74: 65-69
[212] Prayson RA, Chahlavi A, Luciano M (2004). Cerebellar paraganglioma. Ann Diagn Pathol 8: 219-223.

[213] Reithmeier T, Gumprecht H, Stolzle A, Lumenta CB (2000). Intracerebral paraganglioma. Acta Neurochir 142: 1063-1066.
[214] Bannykh S, Strugar J, Baehring J (2005). Paraganglioma of the lumbar spinal
[215] Gelabert-Gonzalez M (2005). Paragangliomas of the lumbar region. Report of two cases and review of the literature. J Neurosurg Spine 2: 354-365.
[216] Sankhla S, Khan GM (2004). Cauda equina paraganglioma presenting with intracranial hypertension: case report and review of the literature. Neurol India 52: 243-244.
[217] Jeffs GJ, Lee GY, Wong GT (2003). Functioning paraganglioma of the thoracic spine: case report. Neurosurgery 53: 992-994.
[218] Levy RA (1993). Paraganglioma of the filum terminale: MR findings. AJR Am J Roentgenol 160: 851-852.
[219] Burger PC, Scheithauer BW (1994). Tumors of paraganglionic tissue. In: Tumors of the Central Nervous System. Atlas of Tumor Pathology. Tumors of the Central Nervous System. Atlas of Tumor Pathology. Armed Forces Institute of Pathology: Washington D.C., pp. 317-320.
[220] Moran CA, Rush W, Mena H (1997). Primary spinal paragangliomas: a clinicopathological and immunohistochemical study of 30 cases. Histopathology 31: 167-173.
[221] Gaffney EF, Doorly T, Dinn JJ (1986). Aggressive oncocytic neuroendocrine tumour ('oncocytic paraganglioma') of the cauda equina. Histopathology 10: 311-319.
[222] Sonneland PR, Scheithauer BW, LeChago J, Crawford BG, Onofrio BM (1986). Paraganglioma of the cauda equina region. Clinicopathologic study of 31 cases with special reference to immunocytology and ultrastructure. Cancer 58: 1720-1735.
[223] Kliewer KE, Cochran AJ (1989). A review of the histology, ultrastructure, immunohistology, and molecular biology of extra-adrenal paragangliomas. Arch Pathol Lab Med 113: 1209-1218.
[224] Chetty R (1999). Cytokeratin expression in cauda equina paragangliomas [letter]. Am J Surg Pathol 23: 491.
[225] Erlandson RA (1994). Paragangliomas. In: Diagnostic Transmission Electron Microscopy of Tumors. Diagnostic Transmission Electron Microscopy of Tumors. Raven Press: New York, pp. 615-622.
[226] Yokoo H, Tanaka G, Isoda K, Hirato J, Nakazato Y, Fujimaki H, Watanabe K, Saito N, Sasaki T (2003). Novel crystalloid structures in suprasellar paraganglioma. Clin Neuropathol 22: 222-228.
[227] Wester DJ, Falcone S, Green BA, Camp A, Quencer RM (1993). Paraganglioma of the filum: MR appearance. J Comput Assist Tomogr 17: 967-969.
[228] Caccamo DV, Ho KL, Garcia JH (1992). Cauda equina tumor with ependymal and paraganglionic differentiation. Hum Pathol 23: 835- 838.
[229] Constantini S, Soffer D, Siegel T, Shalit MN (1989). Paraganglioma of the thoracic spinal cord with cerebrospinal fluid metastasis. Spine 14: 643-645.
[230] Steel TR, Botterill P, Sheehy JP (1994). Paraganglioma of the cauda equina with associated syringomyelia: case report. Surg Neurol 42: 489-493.

[231] Faro SH, Turtz AR, Koenigsberg RA, Mohamed FB, Chen CY, Stein H (1997). Paraganglioma of the cauda equina with associated intramedullary cyst: MR findings. AJNR Am J Neuroradiol 18: 1588-1590.

[232] Masuoka J, Brandner S, Paulus W, Soffer D, Vital A, Chimelli L, Jouvet A, Yonekawa Y, Kleihues P, Ohgaki H (2001). Germline SDHD mutation in paraganglioma of the spinal cord. Oncogene 20: 5084-5086.

[233] Lipper S, Decker RE (1984). Paraganglioma of the cauda equina. A histologic, immunohistochemical, and ultrastructural study and review of the literature. Surg Neurol 22: 415-420.

[234] Lack EE (1994). Paragangliomas. In: Diagnostic Surgical Pathology. Sternberg SS, ed. Raven Press: New York, pp. 559-621.

[235] Keith J, Lownie S, Ang LC (2006). Coexistence of paraganglioma and myxopapillary ependymoma of the cauda equina. Acta Neuropathol 111: 617-618.

[236] Kliewer KE, Wen DR, Cancilla PA, Cochran AJ (1989). Paragangliomas: assessment of prognosis by histologic, immunohistochemical, and ultrastructural techniques. Hum Pathol 20: 29-39.

[237] Masuoka J, Brandner S, Paulus W, Soffer D, Vital A, Chimelli L, Jouvet A, Yonekawa Y, Kleihues P, Ohgaki H (2001). Germline SDHD mutation in paraganglioma of the spinal cord. Oncogene 20: 5084-5086.

[238] Lack EE, Cubilla AL, Woodruff JM (1979). Paragangliomas of the head and neck region. A pathologic study of tumors from 71 patients. Hum Pathol 10: 191-218.

[239] Brown HM, Komorowski RA, Wilson SD, Demeure MJ, Zhu YR (1999). Predicting metastasis of pheochromocytomas using DNA flow cytometry and immunohistochemical markers of cell proliferation: A positive correlation between MIB-1 staining and malignant tumor behavior. Cancer 86: 1583-1589.

[240] Clarke MR, Weyant RJ, Watson CG, Carty SE (1998). Prognostic markers in pheochromocytoma. Hum Pathol 29: 522-526.

[241] Ohji H, Sasagawa I, Iciyanagi O, Suzuki Y, Nakada T (2001). Tumour angiogenesis and Ki-67 expression in phaeochromocytoma. BJU Int 87: 381-385

[242] Strommer KN, Brandner S, Sarioglu AC, Sure U, Yonekawa Y (1995). Symptomatic cerebellar metastasis and late local recurrence of a cauda equina paraganglioma. Case report. J Neurosurg 83: 166-169.

[243] Constantini S, Soffer D, Siegel T, Shalit MN (1989). Paraganglioma of the thoracic spinal cord with cerebrospinal fluid metastasis. Spine 14: 643-645.

[244] Roche PH, Figarella B, Regis J, Peragut JC (1996). Cauda equina paraganglioma with subsequent intracranial and intraspinal metastases. Acta Neurochir 138: 475-479.

[245] Thines L, Lejeune JP, Ruchoux MM, Assaker R (2006). Management of delayed intracranial and intraspinal metastases of intradural spinal paragangliomas. Acta Neurochir 148: 63-66.

Chapter 12

Calcitonin Expression in the Metastatic Tissue of Medullary Thyroid Carcinoma

Wei-Wen Hung, Kun-Bow Tsai and Pi-Jung Hsiao

Additional information is available at the end of the chapter

http://dx.doi.org/10.5772/51959

1. Introduction

Medullary thyroid carcinoma (MTC) is an uncommon primary thyroid carcinoma accounting for as much as 10% of all thyroid malignancies and as much as 14% of thyroid cancer-related deaths.[1] It is a neuroendocrine malignancy arising from the C cell or parafollicular cell of the thyroid.[2] The sporadic and hereditary forms of MTC account for 80% and 20% of all cases, respectively.[3] The hereditary form is part of the multiple endocrine neoplasia (MEN) syndromes including MEN 2A (MTC, pheochromocytoma, and hyperparathyroidism), MEN 2B (MTC, pheochromocytoma, mucosal neuroma, and marfanoid habitus), and familial MTC (FMTC).[4] About 40% to 50% of sporadic MTC cases present with distant metastasis involving cervical lymph nodes, lungs, liver, and/or bones at initial diagnosis.[5] The literature reports other rare metastatic sites including pituitary metastasis, [6] choroidal and optic disc metastasis, [7,8] breast metastasis, [9] and skin metastasis. [10]

Certain diagnostic tools such as calcitonin and REarranged during Transfection (RET) proto-oncogene tests enable the discovery of hereditary MTC cases in the preclinical stage, allowing for early surgical interventions and resulting in high cure rates. [5] In contrast to hereditary MTC, early detection of sporadic MTC is difficult, making prognosis more unfavorable. [11] The initial presentation of a metastatic tumor may be difficult to diagnose if the clinician is unaware of the occult primary thyroid cancer. Immunohistochemical staining with calcitonin for the metastatic tumor has been used as a diagnostic marker for MTC. [12] However, no consensus exists regarding calcitonin expression by metastatic MTC tissues. Still calcitonin staining is routinely used to make a differential diagnosis of MTC. This poses particular challenges when metastatic MTC occurs without the expression of calcitonin.

We had encountered a case of sporadic MTC in a 73-year-old man who initially presented with two ill-defined pulmonary opacities on chest radiography (CXR). Computed tomography (CT) of the chest inadvertently found a thyroid nodule, which led to the ultimate diagnosis of primary MTC with pulmonary metastasis. This atypical histopathologic presentation of pulmonary metastasis from MTC made diagnosis particularly challenging.

2. Body

The patient was a 73-year-old man with an unremarkable medical history. He had the initial presentation of intermittent anterior chest pain for more than 20 days. The CXR showed two ill-defined opacities in the upper lobe and the hilum of the right lung (Figure 1B). Chest CT findings highly suggested bronchogenic carcinoma localized in the upper and middle lobes of the right lung with extension and encasement to the adjacent hilum and the segmental bronchus of right upper lobe (Figure 1A). We discovered lymph node metastases to the right anterior mediastinum and subcarinal region and an accidental thyroid nodule over the right lobe. Initial pathological examination of a transbronchoscopic lung biopsy favored poorly-differentiated carcinoma with desmoplastic stroma infiltrated by sheets of cancer cells that had hyperchromatic nuclei with no distinct nucleoli (Figure 2A, x40).

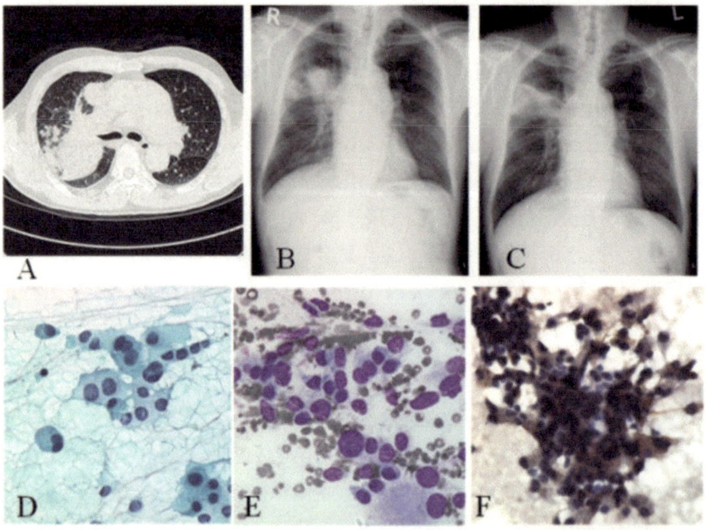

Figure 1. (A) chest CT at diagnosis: higly suggested bronchogenic carcinoma (B) chest PA at diagnosis: two ill-defined opacities over the right upper lobe and the right hilum of the lung (C) chest PA after chemotherapy: partial shrinkage of the tumor opacity. Thyroid aspiration (x100 objective lens) with (D) Papanicolau's stain: dispersed cell pattern with nuclear eccentricity and "salt-and-pepper" chromatin (E) Riu's stain: plasmacytoid cells with binucleation and basophilic stippling in the cytoplasm (F) positive calcitonin stain using liquid-based cytology (LBC) method

Sonography revealed a calcified heterogenous right thyroid tumor greatest diameter 2.9cm. Fine-needle aspiration cytology with Papanicolaou's stain showed cells arranged in dispersed pattern with nuclear eccentricity and "salt-and-pepper" chromatin (Figure 1D, x100). Characteristic plasmacytoid cells with binucleation and basophilic stippling in the cytoplasm were also noted in the aspiration cytology with Riu's stain (Figure 1E, x100). MTC was highly suspected because there was a positive immunocytochemical staining for calcitonin as detected by liquid-based cytology (LBC) with Ligui-Prep™ (LGM International, Fort Lauderdale) (Figure 1F, x100), and because serum calcitonin level was above 950 pg/ml (normal range: 0-42 pg/ml) and carcinoembryonic antigen (CEA) level at 259 ng/ml (normal range: 0-3 ng/ml).

After total thyroidectomy, the diagnosis of MTC was confirmed by positive immunohistochemical staining for chromogranin-A (Figure 2F, x40), synaptophysin (Figure 2G, x40), calcitonin (Figure 2H, x40), and Congo-red stain for amyloid. Because of the similarity between the histopathologic patterns of focal vascular invasions in the thyroid (Figure 2E, x40) and the lung carcinoma (Figure 2A, x40), MTC metastasis to the lung was further diagnosed based on a positive finding of chromogranin-A (Figure 2B, x40) and synaptophysin (Figure 2C, x40), though there was no staining of calcitonin (Figure 2D, x40).

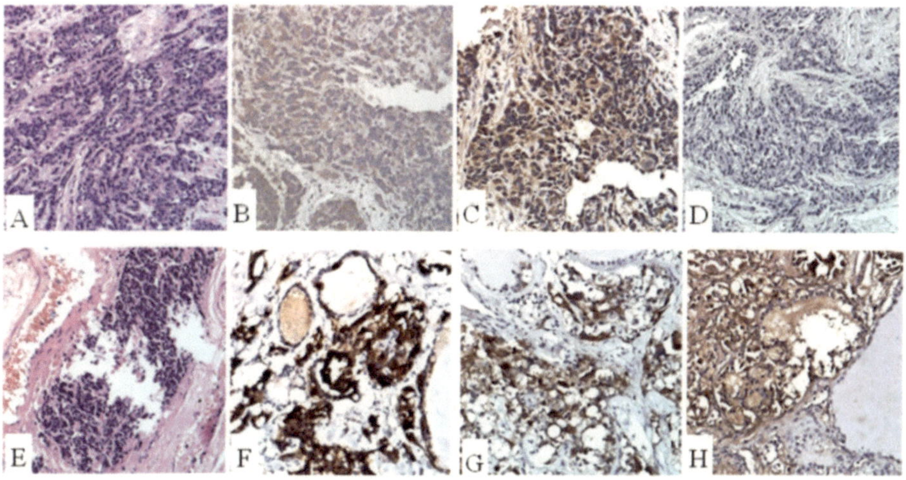

Figure 2. (x40 objective lens) Lung sections staining with H.E. (A) showing poorly-differentiated cancer cells infiltrating in desmoplastic stroma, with strong expressions for chromogranin-A (B) and synaptophysin (C), but negative calcitonin (D). Thyroid sections staining with H.E. (E) showing focal vascular invasions in the thyroid with poorly-differentiated cancer cell morphology resembling that in the lung section, with positive expressions for chromogranin – A (F), synaptophysin (G), and calcitonin (H).

Because the patient had no family history of MTC and no evidence of pheochromocytoma and hyperparathyroidism, he was diagnosed with sporadic MTC. As for the treatment, post-operation chemotherapy with Gemcitabine was administered to treat pulmonary metastasis of the MTC. After total thyroidectomy and one course of gemcitabine, serum CEA and calcitonin levels decreased to 135 ng/ml and 766.7 pg/ml, respectively. CXR showed partial shrinkage of the tumor opacity (Figure 1C).

To our knowledge, this is the first reported case of accidental MTC initially presenting as pulmonary metastasis without calcitonin expression in the metastatic lesions. A correct diagnosis might have been missed if the thyroid nodule had not been discovered. The atypical histopathologic patterns in this MTC case could have led to a misdiagnosis of double cancer.

We presented this case with several issues worth discussing. First, the absence of calcitonin expression in the pulmonary metastases in our case did not exclude the possibility of primary MTC. Calcitonin has been recognized as a specific and sensitive tumor marker for MTC. Although the disparity between tissue and serum calcitonin in patient with medullary thyroid carcinoma were reported, [13] the follow-up of patients with MTC before and after total thyroidectomy by the measurement of calcitonin is still widely used in clinical condition. Calcitonin is a small polypeptide hormone of 32 amino acids that is produced almost exclusively by neuroendocrine C cells in the thyroid. [14] However, little was known about the calcitonin expression in the metastatic tissue of MTC. Only four of 142 MTC cases in a retrospective study were described as "atypical", characterized by cytomorphologic features and positive neuroendocrine markers of chromogranins and synaptophysin. Among the four cases, three had very little expression of calcitonin and one had no expression of this tumor marker. [15] Previous reports have also postulated that the metastatic lesion may lose the ability to express calcitonin, [12] which is consistent with the patient in this report who exhibited poorly differentiated cancer cell morphology (Figure 2A, x40) similar to that seen in the focal vascular invasion of thyroid (Figure 2E, x40). The pathological mechanisms of the poorly-differentiated MTC cells without calcitonin expression are not well understood. Oncocytic variant of MTC seen in the recurrent tumor has been documented in the literature to represent a further step in tumor progression and may be indicative of a poor prognosis. [16] But regarding the absence of calcitonin expression in the metastatic tissue of MTC, no references have been found. Thus we postulated two possible mechanisms for the absence of calcitonin expression in the metastatic tissue of medullary thyroid carcinoma: the first one is that the potential for metastasis increases as cancer cells lose their ability to secrete calcitonin during dedifferentiation, and the second explanation is that the secondary environment (metastatic site) may have disabled the cancer cells' ability to secret calcitonin. Further research will be needed to elucidate the exact mechanism.

Second, the radiographic patterns of pulmonary metastasis from MTC in this patient were hard to differentiate from primary lung carcinoma. The patient presented with elevated serum CEA level and two ill-defined pulmonary opacities in the right upper lobe and the right hilum, which clinically resembled primary lung carcinoma. Pulmonary metastases from MTC generally exhibit a macronodular, or "cannonball" appearance with clear-cut margins.[17] Reticulonodular perihilar lesions,[17] calcified pulmonary metastases,[18] and micronodular patterns[17] have also been reported in the literature. The diverse radiographic manifestations of pulmonary MTC metastases pose as a diagnostic challenge for clinicians. Because 40% to 50% of sporadic MTC cases are initially discovered through distant metastasis,[5] the clinician may need to test the patient's serum calcitonin level to rule out MTC if a thyroid nodule and a pulmonary lesion coexist. We believe that immunohistochemical staining with neuroendocrine markers (chromogranin and synaptophysin) are more useful than calcitonin expression for testing transbronchoscopic lung biopsy specimens, even if elevated serum CEA may favor the possibility of lung (adeno)carcinoma. In addition to calcitonin, CEA can be secreted and released by the malignant transformed C cells. Although CEA is not specific for the diagnosis of MTC, as its levels can be elevated in several types of tumors, the serum levels of CEA is an excellent test for monitoring disease progression once the diagnosis of MTC has been confirmed. [14]

In our case, liquid-based cytology (LBC) was particularly helpful in facilitating immunocytochemical staining. Although most MTC can be easily diagnosed based on cytomorphologic findings in aspirates with Pap-staining[12,19] or Riu's stain,[20,21] calcitonin staining has been regarded as the gold standard for the definitive diagnosis of MTC.[12] LBC allows ancillary tests, including immunocytochemical staining, to be conducted on residual cell samples.[22] To our knowledge, this is the first reported case of a primary thyroid carcinoma confirmed by LBC. Although cervical smear using LBC preparation has been described,[23] the role of LBC in thyroid aspiration cytology has yet to be explored. We expect the clinical application of LBC in thyroid fine needle aspiration cytology to help in establishing correct preoperative diagnoses.

The five-year and ten-year survival rates of MTC with distant metastasis have been estimated at 60% and 40%, respectively.[24] Cancer staging of MTC at initial diagnosis is highly predictive of future mortality in long-term follow-up.[25] Radioactive iodine, external beam radiation therapy, and conventional chemotherapy have not resulted in satisfactory response in metastatic MTC.[26] Combination chemotherapy regimens used to treat metastatic MTC, including doxorubicin, cisplatin, fluorouracil, dacarbazine, streptozocin, cyclophosphamide, and vincristine have yielded limited outcomes with tumor response rates less than 20%.[27] Gemcitabine, a pyrimidine antimetabolite, has not been described in the literature as a treatment for MTC.[27] Based on an in vitro study in which gemcitabine inhibited proliferation and neuroendocrine activity of human TT cells derived from MTC,[28] we used gemcitabine to treat the pulmonary metastasis of MTC in this patient. This is the first case report demonstrating partial response to gemcitabine in a patient with pulmonary metastasis of MTC.

3. Conclusion

In conclusion, metastatic medullary thyroid carcinoma with atypical chest radiography and calcitonin-free histopathlogic lung lesions can be difficult to diagnose. This unique case report demonstrates that MTC metastatic lesions may not express its routine biomarker, calcitonin.

Author details

Wei-Wen Hung and Pi-Jung Hsiao
Division of Endocrinology and Metabolism, Department of Internal Medicine,
Kaohsiung Medical University Hospital, Kaohsiung Medical University, Kaohsiung, Taiwan

Kun-Bow Tsai
Department of Pathology, Kaohsiung Municipal Hsiao-Kang Hospital,
Kaohsiung Medical University, Kaohsiung, Taiwan

Acknowledgement

The authors thank Min-Jan Tsai, Wan-Chen Hsieh, Ya-Chun Tseng in Kaohsiung Municipal Hsiao-Kang Hospital for their assistances with the immunocytochemical and immunohistochemical studies

4. References

[1] Roman S, Lin R, Sosa JA (2006) Prognosis of medullary thyroid carcinoma: demographic, clinical, and pathologic predictors of survival in 1252 cases. Cancer. 107 (9): 2134-42.

[2] Kebebew E, Ituarte PH, Siperstein AE, Duh QY, Clark OH (2000) Medullary thyroid carcinoma: clinical characteristics, treatment, prognostic factors, and a comparison of staging systems. Cancer. 88 (5): 1139-48.

[3] Lewis CE, Yeh MW (2008) Inherited endocrinopathies: an update. Mol Genet Metab. 94 (3): 271-82.

[4] Fialkowski EA, Moley JF (2006) Current approaches to medullary thyroid carcinoma, sporadic and familial. J Surg Oncol. 94 (8): 737-47.

[5] Martins RG, Rajendran JG, Capell P, Byrd DR, Mankoff DA (2006) Medullary thyroid cancer: options for systemic therapy of metastatic disease? J Clin Oncol. 24 (11): 1653-5.

[6] Bhatoe HS, Badwal S, Dutta V, Kannan N (2008) Pituitary metastasis from medullary carcinoma of thyroid: case report and review of literature. J Neurooncol. 89 (1): 63-7.

[7] Bianciotto CG, Demirci HY, Shields CL, Shields JA (2008) Simultaneous eyelid and choroidal metastases 36 years after diagnosis of medullary thyroid carcinoma. Ophthal Plast Reconstr Surg. 24 (1): 62-3.

[8] Yildiz I, Sen F, Tuncer S, Kilic L, Basaran M, Bavbek S (2011) Optic disc and choroidal metastasis from sporadic medullary thyroid carcinoma: case report and review of the literature. Onkologie. 34 (11): 630-3.

[9] Nofech-Mozes S, Mackenzie R, Kahn HJ, Ehrlich L, Raphael SJ (2008) Breast metastasis by medullary thyroid carcinoma detected by FDG positron emission tomography. Ann Diagn Pathol. 12 (1): 67-71.

[10] Sanii S, Tavangar SM (2011) Cutaneous metastasis of medullary thyroid carcinoma as the initial manifestation of an otherwise limited malignancy: a case report. Am J Dermatopathol. 33 (7): 716-8.

[11] Bergholm U, Bergstrom R, Ekbom A (1997) Long-term follow-up of patients with medullary carcinoma of the thyroid. Cancer. 79 (1): 132-8.
[12] Bhanot P, Yang J, Schnadig VJ, Logrono R (2007) Role of FNA cytology and immunochemistry in the diagnosis and management of medullary thyroid carcinoma: report of six cases and review of the literature. Diagn Cytopathol. 35 (5): 285-92.
[13] Alapat DV, Ain KB, Sloan DA, Monaghan KG, Karabakhtsian RG (2011) Disparity between tissue and serum calcitonin and carcinoembryonic antigen in a patient with medullary thyroid carcinoma. Endocrine. 39 (2): 148-52.
[14] Elisei R, Pinchera A (2012) Advances in the follow-up of differentiated or medullary thyroid cancer. Nat Rev Endocrinol. 8(8): 466-75.
[15] Schmid KW, Ensinger C (1998) Atypical" medullary thyroid carcinoma with little or no calcitonin expression. Virchows Arch. 433 (3): 209-15.
[16] Tranchida P, Estigarribia J, Sethi S, Giorgadze T (2011) Cytologic diagnosis of recurrent medullary thyroid carcinoma with oncocytic change twenty-one years post-thyroidectomy: case report and review of the literature. Diagn Cytopathol. 39 (9): 641-6.
[17] Afshar K, Alalawi R, Boylen CT (2007) Micronodular radiographic pulmonary pattern in metastatic medullary thyroid carcinoma. J Natl Med Assoc. 99 (5): 575-7.
[18] Jimenez JM, Casey SO, Citron M, Khan A (1995) Calcified pulmonary metastases from medullary carcinoma of the thyroid. Comput Med Imaging Graph. 19 (4): 325-8.
[19] Green I, Ali SZ, Allen EA, Zakowski MF (1997) A spectrum of cytomorphologic variations in medullary thyroid carcinoma. Fine-needle aspiration findings in 19 cases. Cancer. 81 (1): 40-4.
[20] Tsou MH, Lin HH, Ko JS (1997) Riu's stain and the cytologic diagnosis of thyroid fine-needle aspiration: a single cancer center experience. Diagn Cytopathol. 16 (6): 543-7.
[21] Hsieh MH, Hsiao YL, Chang TC (2007) Fine needle aspiration cytology stained with Rius method in quicker diagnosis of medullary thyroid carcinoma. J Formos Med Assoc. 106 (9): 728-35.
[22] Pinto AP, Maia HF, di Loretto C, Krunn P, Tulio S, Collaco LM (2007) Repeating cytological preparations on liquid-based cytology samples: A methodological advantage? Diagn Cytopathol. 35 (10): 663-9.
[23] Herbert A, Johnson J . Personal view (2001) Is it reality or an illusion that liquid-based cytology is better than conventional cervical smears? Cytopathology. 12 (6): 383-9.
[24] Cupisti K, Wolf A, Raffel A, Schott M, Miersch D, Yang Q, Eisenberger CF, Roher HD, Knoefel WT (2007) Long-term clinical and biochemical follow-up in medullary thyroid carcinoma: a single institution's experience over 20 years. Ann Surg. 246 (5): 815-21.
[25] Ball DW (2007) Medullary thyroid cancer: monitoring and therapy. Endocrinol Metab Clin North Am. 36 (3): 823-37.
[26] Moley JF, Fialkowski EA (2007) Evidence-based approach to the management of sporadic medullary thyroid carcinoma. World J Surg. 31 (5): 946-56.
[27] Schlumberger M, Carlomagno F, Baudin E, Bidart JM, Santoro M (2008) New therapeutic approaches to treat medullary thyroid carcinoma. Nat Clin Pract Endocrinol Metab. 4 (1): 22-32.

[28] Dadan J, Wolczynski S, Sawicki B, Chyczewski L, Azzadin A, Dzieciol J, Puchalski Z (2001) Preliminary evaluation of influence of gemcitabine (Gemzar) on proliferation and neuroendocrine activity of human TT cell line: immunocytochemical investigations. Folia Histochem Cytobiol. 39 (2):187-8.

Chapter 13

Molecular Histopathology

Hussein A. Kaoud

Additional information is available at the end of the chapter

http://dx.doi.org/10.5772/52919

1. Introduction

Traditional pathology concentrates on the morphological manifestations of disease. Molecular pathology, in addition, integrates tools of molecular biology to: isolate and identify the causative agents in infectious disease, understand the role of differential gene expression in disease etiology, provide more accurate means of disease diagnosis and provide more individualized approaches to therapy.

Molecular pathology is a branch of the biomedical sciences which focuses on the progress, development, and evolution of diseases on the molecular level. It can be applied practically to patients in addition to being utilized in biomedical research to learn more about specific diseases, ranging from cancer to genetic conditions. Usually, molecular pathology is treated as a subset of the field of pathology, but it also involves genetics, immunology, and many other aspects of the medical field, and people can approach it from a number of perspectives.

A molecular pathologist can conduct a variety of tests to learn about the fundamental components of a cell, including the array of amino acids which makes up cellular DNA. In addition to performing amino acid sequencing, people in this field also look at samples of cellular tissue, and they perform a variety of tests to learn more about the progress of disease in specific patients and in general.

To understand the causes and molecular basis of the development of disease, with particular reference to cancer, and to apply this knowledge to improving disease prevention, detection, diagnosis and treatment. Improving the outlook for cancer patients can only come from an understanding of molecular and cell biology. There has been a dramatic increase in knowledge of the molecular genetics of cancers over the last few years and already we have reached the point where this can be translated into clinical application.

Many diseases are caused by inherited gene mutations, for example, cystic fibrosis, muscular dystrophy and lysosomal storage diseases. Other gene alterations confer a greater susceptibility to disease – for example, cancer or heart disease.

One common use for a molecular pathologist is in the study of specimens taken from cancer patients. The pathologist can test the specimen to determine where the cancer originated, and to look for biomarkers which could indicate susceptibility to specific cancer treatments. For example, a breast cancer which is estrogen sensitive will be treated differently than a breast cancer which is not. Using molecular pathology, an oncologist can develop a treatment approach which is tailored to the patient.

Key techniques used in molecular pathology to identify relationships between gene alterations and disease include cell isolation and cell culture. Immunohistochemistry is not considered a molecular technique but it is based on the antigen-antibody affinity, it has emerged as a powerful investigative tool that can provide supplemental information to the routine morphological assessment of tissues. The antibody is usually linked to other molecules to aid visualization [(fluorophore, reporter enzyme, etc), FISH (A cytogenetic method of detecting and localizing specific DNA sequences on chromosomes)] and laboratory molecular biology techniques (identification of gene mutations, expression profiling, protein analysis, blotting, microarrays).

It is thought that the development of malignant disease progresses through defined stages such as hyperplasia, dysplasia, carcinoma in situ, primary carcinoma, invasive carcinoma and metastases, each of which may be linked to mutations and alterations in the expression of subsets of genes. Laser microdissection is useful for isolating particular cells, or populations of cells, from tissue (frozen sections, fixed sections and in cell culture monolayers) for genetic analysis allowing direct comparison of nucleic acid from cells in different stages of disease progression.

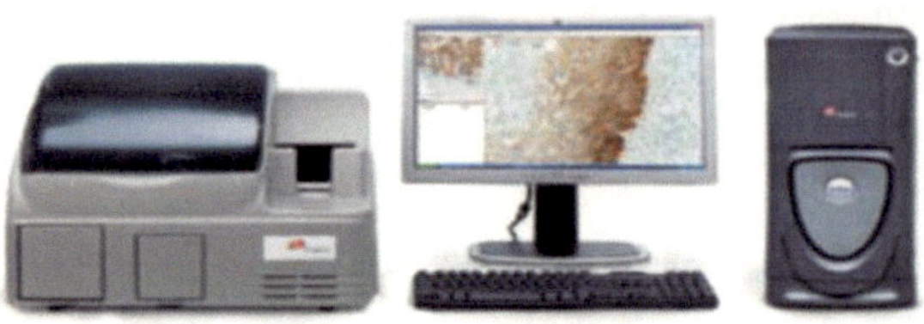

Figure 1. Automated Cellular Imaging System (ACISR III), an example of an image acquisition and image analysis instrument.

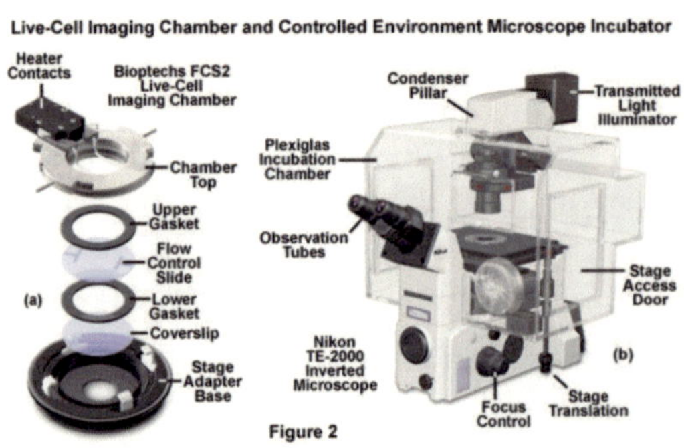

Figure 2.

The impact of gene alterations on protein function and disease can be investigated using a variety of imaging techniques (Figs.1 and 2). Of particular importance is the imaging of protein-protein interactions using time-lapse imaging, TIRF microscopy and confocal fluorescence microscopy techniques such as 3-D rendering, FRET/BRET. These enable spatial and temporal analysis of dynamic events involving, for example, receptor interactions and other signaling events (Fig.3).

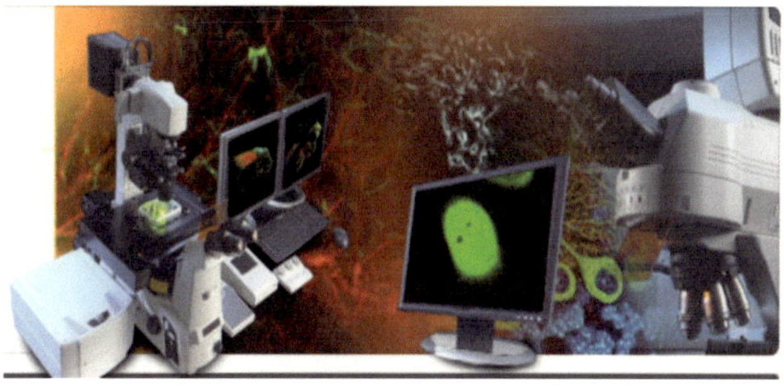

Figure 3. Nikon's powerful fully-automated confocal imaging system, capable of capturing high-quality confocal images of cells and molecular events.

1.1. Immune system (tumor immunology)

Another important role of the immune system (Fig.4) is to identify and eliminate tumors. The *transformed cells* of tumors express antigens that are not found on normal cells. To the immune system, these antigens appear foreign, and their presence causes immune cells to attack the transformed tumor cells. The antigens expressed by tumors have several sources [1] some are derived from oncogenic viruses like human papillomavirus, which causes cervical cancer,[2] while others are the organism's own proteins that occur at low levels in normal cells but reach high levels in tumor cells. One example is an enzyme called tyrosinase that, when expressed at high levels, transforms certain skin cells (e.g. melanocytes) into tumors called melanomas [3, 4]. A third possible source of tumor antigens are proteins normally important for regulating cell growth and survival, that commonly mutate into cancer inducing molecules called oncogenes [1,5,6].

The main response of the immune system to tumors is to destroy the abnormal cells using killer T cells, sometimes with the assistance of helper T cells [4, 7]. Tumor antigens are presented on MHC class I molecules in a similar way to viral antigens. This allows killer T cells to recognize the tumor cell as abnormal [8] NK cells also kill tumorous cells in a similar way, especially if the tumor cells have fewer MHC class I molecules on their surface than normal; this is a common phenomenon with tumors [9] .Sometimes antibodies are generated against tumor cells allowing for their destruction by the complement system [5].

Clearly, some tumors evade the immune system and go on to become cancers [10]. Tumor cells often have a reduced number of MHC class I molecules on their surface, thus avoiding detection by killer T cells [8]. Some tumor cells also release products that inhibit the immune response; for example by secreting the cytokine TGF-β, which suppresses the activity of macrophages and lymphocytes [11]. In addition, immunological tolerance may develop against tumor antigens, so the immune system no longer attacks the tumor cells [10].

Paradoxically, macrophages can promote tumor growth [12] when tumor cells send out cytokines that attract macrophages, which then generate cytokines and growth factors that nurture tumor development. In addition, a combination of hypoxia in the tumor and a cytokine produced by macrophages induces tumor cells to decrease production of a protein that blocks metastasis and thereby assists spread of cancer cells.

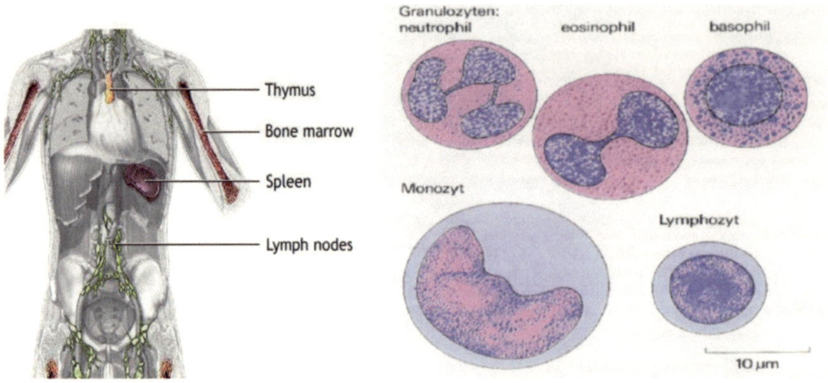

Figure 4. The immune system protects the body from potentially harmful substances. The inflammatory response (inflammation) is part of innate immunity. It occurs when tissues are injured by bacteria, trauma, toxins, heat or any other cause.

1.2. Genetic diseases (genetic disorders)

A genetic disorder is an illness caused by abnormalities in genes or chromosomes, especially a condition that is present from before birth. Most genetic disorders are quite rare and affect one person in every several thousands or millions.

A genetic disorder may or may not be a heritable disorder. Some genetic disorders are passed down from the parents' genes, but others are always or almost always caused by new mutations or changes to the DNA. In other cases, the same disease, such as some forms of cancer, may be caused by an inherited genetic condition in some people, by new mutations in other people, and by non-genetic causes in still other people.

2. Methods in molecular pathology

Nucleic acid–based testing is becoming a crucial diagnostic tool not only in the setting of inherited genetic disease (e.g., cystic fibrosis and hemochromatosis) but also in a wide variety of hemato-oncologic, solid neoplastic and infectious conditions. Molecular diagnostics provides the necessary underpinnings for any successful application of gene therapy or biologic response modifiers. It offers a great tool for assessing therapy response and detecting minimal residual disease. Currently, it is estimated that more than 5% of all laboratory testing is based on DNA or RNA analysis.

2.1. Tissue microdissection methods

Microdissection can be performed in a variety of ways, all of which have different advantages and disadvantages. These methods range from the simple and inexpensive manual methods to laser-capture microdissection (LCM) methods that require expensive and complex equipment. These methods are reviewed here, with particular emphasis on manual microdissection, which can be performed easily with common equipment in the pathology laboratory (Fig. 5).

One of the major benefits of microdissection is the production of relatively pure samples of morphologically confirmed cellular populations [13]. This relative purity may be essential for assessing a genetic change or for quantification of genetic changes. For example, in assessing possible loss of heterozygosity of tumor suppressor genes, normal contaminating cells will artifactually equalize the allelic balance, and it may appear that the tumor cells contain normal DNA. In molecular identity testing for tissue floaters (tissue carryover artifacts), microdissection is essential for separating the fragments of the suspected floater from the rest of the tissue sample [14, 15] . When examining expression of some gene targets in tumor cells at the mRNA level, results may be confounded by the expression found in normal contaminating stromal and lymphoid cells. In some diseases it may be important to measure events in rare single neoplastic cells [16-18] . Perhaps the most notable example is in Hodgkin lymphoma, where molecular experiments require detailed microdissection to isolate the Reed-Sternberg cells from the surrounding lymphoid infiltrates.

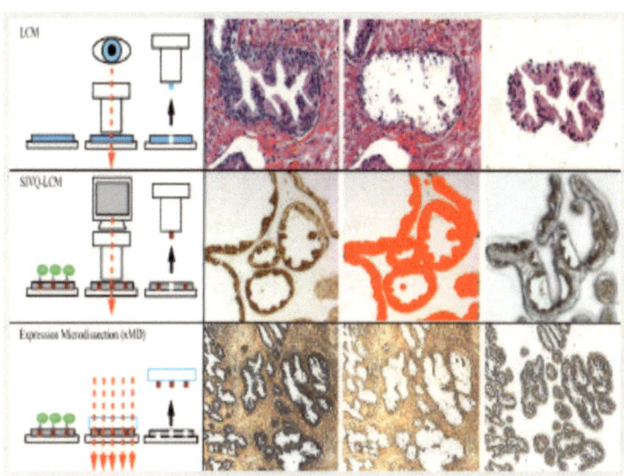

Figure 5. This method "microdissection", can be performed easily with common equipment in the pathology laboratory.

2.2. Amplification methods

The polymerase chain reaction (PCR) is a laboratory technique for "amplifying" a specific DNA sequence (Fig.6). PCR is extremely efficient and sensitive; it can make millions or billions of copies of any specific sequence of DNA, even when the sequence is in a complex mixture. Because of this power, researchers can use it to amplify sequences even if they only have a minute amount of DNA. A single hair root, or a microscopic blood stain left at a crime scene, for example, contains ample DNA for PCR.

PCR is based on the way cells replicate their DNA. During DNA replication, the two strands of each DNA molecule separate, and DNA polymerase, an enzyme, assembles nucleotides to form two new partner strands for each of the original strands. The original strands serve as templates for the new strands. The new strands are assembled such that each nucleotide in the new strand is determined by the corresponding nucleotide in the template strand. The nucleotides adenine (A) and thymine (T) always lie opposite each other, as do cytosine (C) and guanine (G). Because of this base-pairing specificity, each newly synthesized partner strand has the same sequence as the original partner strand, and replication produces two identical copies of the original double-stranded DNA molecule.

In PCR, a DNA sequence that a researcher wants to amplify, called the "target" sequence, undergoes about thirty rounds of replication in a small reaction tube. During each replication cycle, the number of molecules of the target sequence doubles, because the products and templates of one round of replication all become the templates for the next round. After n rounds of replication, 2^n copies of the target sequence are theoretically produced. After thirty cycles, PCR can produce 2^{30} or more than ten billion copies of a single target DNA sequence. This is called a polymerase chain reaction because DNA polymerase catalyzes a chain reaction of replication.

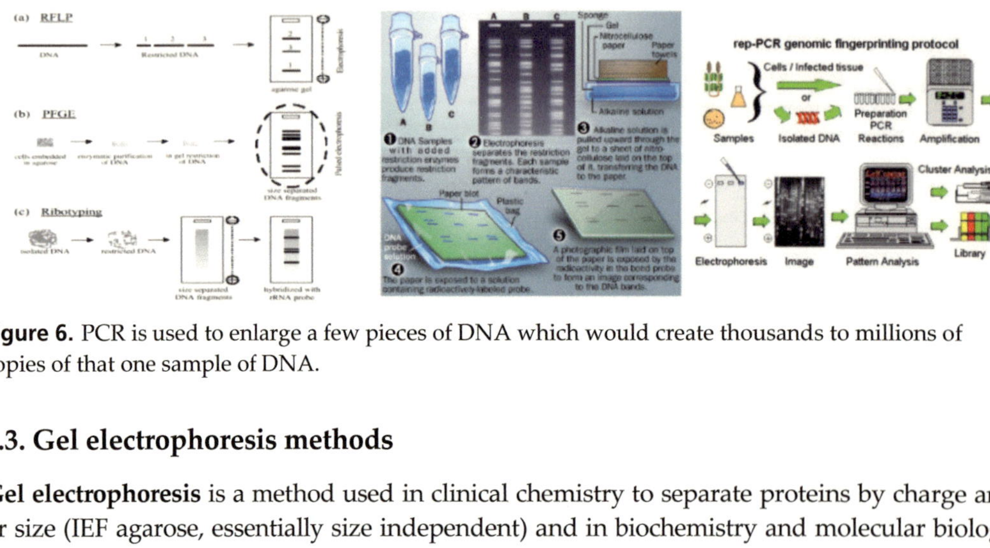

Figure 6. PCR is used to enlarge a few pieces of DNA which would create thousands to millions of copies of that one sample of DNA.

2.3. Gel electrophoresis methods

Gel electrophoresis is a method used in clinical chemistry to separate proteins by charge and or size (IEF agarose, essentially size independent) and in biochemistry and molecular biology to separate a mixed population of DNA and RNA fragments by length, to estimate the size of DNA and RNA fragments or to separate proteins by charge [19]. Nucleic acid molecules are separated by applying an electric field [20] to move the negatively charged molecules through an agarose matrix. Shorter molecules move faster and migrate farther than longer ones because shorter molecules migrate more easily through the pores of the gel. This phenomenon is called sieving. Proteins are separated by charge in agarose because the pores of the gel are too large to sieve proteins. Gel electrophoresis can also be used for separation of nanoparticles.

Gel electrophoresis uses a gel as an anticonvective medium and or sieving medium during electrophoresis, the movement of a charged particle in an electrical field. Gels suppress the thermal convection caused by application of the electric field, and can also act as a sieving medium, retarding the passage of molecules; gels can also simply serve to maintain the finished separation, so that a post electrophoresis stain can be applied [21].DNA Gel electrophoresis is usually performed for analytical purposes, often after amplification of DNA via PCR, but may be used as a preparative technique prior to use of other methods such as mass spectrometry (Fig.7), RFLP, PCR, cloning, DNA sequencing, or Southern blotting [22] for further characterization.

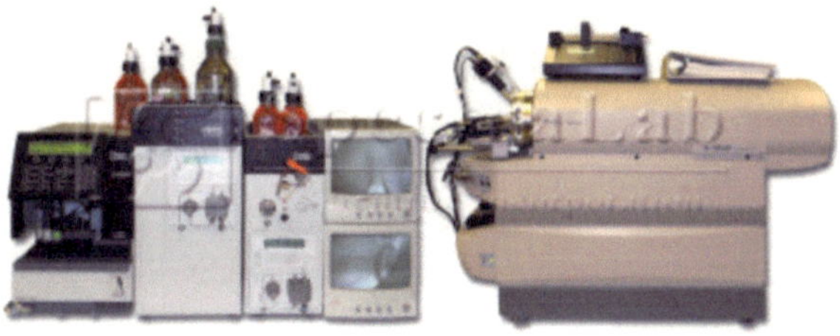

Figure 7. Mass spectrometry

2.4. Hybridization methods

In situ hybridization is a technique used to detect specific DNA and RNA sequences in a biological sample. Deoxyribonucleic acid (DNA) and ribonucleic acid (RNA) are macromolecules made up of different sequences of four nucleotide bases (adenine, guanine, uracil, cytosine, and thymidine). *In situ* hybridization takes advantage of the fact that each nucleotide base binds with a complementary nucleotide base. For instance, adenine binds with thymidine (in DNA) or uracil (in RNA) using hydrogen bonding. Similarly, guanine binds with cytosine.

In a specialized molecular biology laboratory, researchers can make a sequence of nucleotide bases that is complementary to a target sequence that occurs naturally in a cell (in a gene, for example). When this complementary sequence is exposed to the cell, it will bind with that naturally occuring target DNA or RNA in that cell, thus forming what is known as a hybrid. The complementary sequence thus can be used as a "probe" for cellular RNA or DNA.

Thus, the term "hybridization" refers to the chemical reaction between the probe and the DNA or RNA to be detected. If hybridization is performed on actual tissue sections, cells, or isolated chromosomes in order to detect the site where the DNA or RNA is located, it is said to be done "*in situ*." By contrast, "in vitro" hybridization takes place in a test tube or other apparatus, and is used to isolate DNA or RNA, or to determine sequence similarity of two nucleotide segments.

Application of the Probe for DNA or RNA to Tissues or Cells: *In situ* hybridization allows us to learn more about the geographical location of, for example, the messenger RNA (mRNA) in a cell or tissue. It can also tell us where a gene is located on a chromosome. Obviously, a detection system must be built into the technique to allow the cytochemist to visualize and map the geography of these molecules in the cells in question.

When *in situ* hybridization was first introduced, it was applied to isolated cell nuclei to detect specific DNA sequences. Early users applied the techniques to isolated chromosomal preparations in order to map the location of genes in those chromosomes. The technique has also been used to detect viral DNA in an infected cell. *In situ* hybridization of RNA has also been used to show that RNA synthesis (transcription) occurs in the nucleus, while protein synthesis (translation) occurs in the cytoplasm.

2.5. Nucleic acid sequencing

A process by which the sequence of nucleotides along a strand of DNA is determined. Originally a difficult process to carry out, DNA sequencing can now be done routinely by machines. The completion of the Human Genome Project in 2000 produced the largest DNA sequence ever assembled. To carry out the sequencing of the human genome, scientists cut the DNA up into short fragments, sequenced these fragments simultaneously, and then assembled the entire genome by using sophisticated computer techniques to match the fragments to each other.

2.5.1. DNA microarrays

Gene expression profiling using DNA microarrays holds great promise for the future of molecular diagnostics. This technology allows, in one assay, for simultaneous assessment of the expression rate of thousands of genes in a particular sample. The 2 types of DNA microarrays that are widely used are cDNA microarrays and oligonucleotide/ DNA chips.

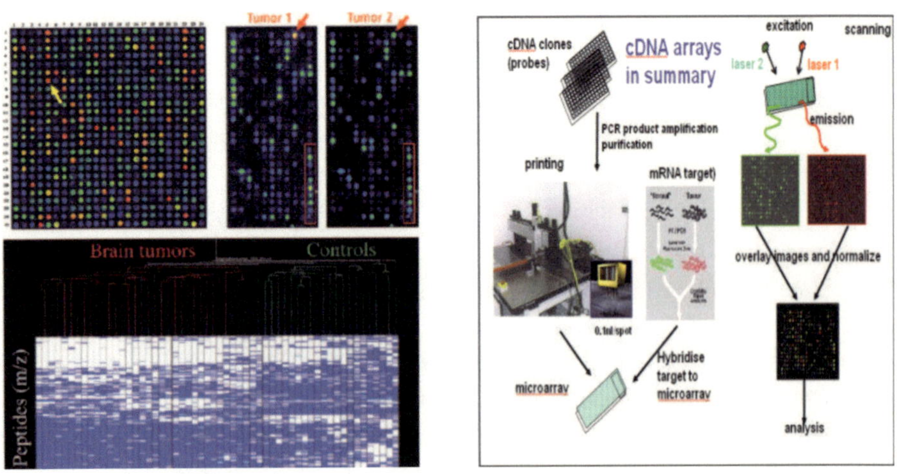

Figure 8. A lung primary tumor, for example, has a different fingerprint than an ovarian or colonic primary. This feature can be exploited in the setting of tumors of unknown primary, in which DNA microarrays have been shown to predict the correct primary site with an amazing accuracy rate of 99%.

In cDNA microarrays, DNA sequences complementary to a library of mRNA from thousands of genes are mechanically placed on a single glass slide. The immobilized cDNA sequences serve as anchoring probes to which mRNA extracted from the tested sample will specifically attach during hybridization. If the tested mRNA is first tagged with a fluorescent dye, the intensity of fluorescence at each anchoring probe location will be proportional to the amount of mRNA (degree of expression) of the gene at that location. A microarray reader displays the intensity of fluorescence at each cDNA location as a colored dot per gene location on a grid.

The applications of these technologies are limitless. By analyzing and comparing hundreds of tumor samples, databases of gene expression "fingerprints" are being built and specific patterns of expression linked to both prognosis and outcome of therapy.11–16 Patterns of gene expression in tumors are also linked to the primary site of origin (Fig.8).

2.5.2. Proteomics

The term *proteomics* indicates a large-scale characterization of the entire protein complement of a cell type, tissue, or organism. Two-dimensional gel electrophoresis has been, and remains, a widely used technique that offers a high-resolution capacity to separate and characterize proteins in complex mixtures. More recently, 2-dimensional electrophoresis (Fig.9) has been coupled with mass spectrometry analysis as a means to characterize complex milieus under study [23, 24]. Several mass spectrometry platforms are commercially available. We will focus our discussion on surface-enhanced laser desorption/ionization technology [25, 26].

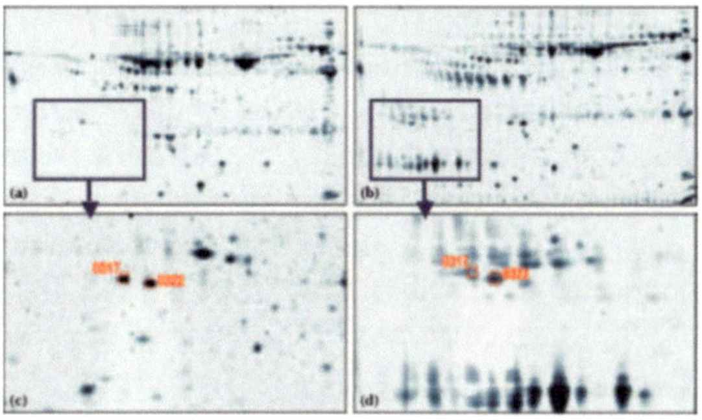

Figure 9. Proteomic analysis of nipple aspirate fluids using 2-dimensional gel electrophoresis. Spots in the bottom panel (enlarged from the top panel) indicate proteins expressed solely by nipple aspirate fluids from breasts containing tumor and not by the contralateral control breast. Copyright 2002 American Cancer Society. Reprinted with permission of Wiley-Liss, Inc, a subsidiary of John Wiley & Sons, Inc. [27].

These technology uses matrix-assisted lasers desorption and time-of-flight analysis to allow fully automated separation of even minute amounts of protein components. The assay exploits variations in mass and electric charge of different protein components in a given sample (e.g., serum). It is the variation in time of flight—based on the mass/charge ratio of each peptide—that allows for separation of the different protein components. With the aid of computer analyses, results are displayed as peaks representing the different peptide components of a given sample. By characterizing proteomic "fingerprints" associated with a particular type of tumor, it is possible to identify an unknown sample that matches a previously defined fingerprint. This can be done on the basis of the ''peaks'' pattern without knowing which protein each peak represents. Appropriate integration of genomic and proteomic data is crucial to elucidate protein functions as they relate to pathogenesis. This integration will help highlight potential pathogenically important epigenetic deviations at the protein level.18 Integration of genomics and proteomics will no doubt facilitate discovery of novel drug target proteins and biomarkers of diseases.

3. Molecular pathological diagnostics

Molecular diagnostics can be widely defined as the measurement of deoxyribonucleic acid (DNA), ribonucleic acid (RNA), proteins, or other metabolites to detect certain genotypes, mutations, or biochemical changes that may be associated with certain states of health or disease, main applications of molecular genetic testing … [28]. The emergence of molecular diagnostics is due to advances in biology that have resulted in an understanding of the mechanisms of normal and disease processes at the molecular level. Prior to this understanding, many disease states were diagnosed from morphologic observations.

The first widely used molecular tests were for infectious diseases, such as for hepatitis B and C or human papillomavirus (HPV), and this continues to be the largest molecular diagnostics market. Certain other fields, such as molecular tests for oncology, inherited conditions, cardiovascular disease, neurological disorders, and forensic testing, are rapidly growing areas of interest. Additionally, molecular diagnostics can be used to monitor a patient's response to a particular drug treatment.

Many different biological techniques fall under the "molecular diagnostics" umbrella. One of the most common techniques is the polymerase chain reaction (PCR), a method of producing large amounts of specifically defined DNA or RNA fragments that can then be used for multiple purposes, including pathogen identification and detection of aberrant gene expression associated with certain diseases. PCR fragments may also be sequenced to detect gene mutations connected to certain disease states, such as the detection of mutations in the BRCA1 and BRCA2 genes that are often associated with an increased risk of hereditary breast cancer and ovarian cancer.

3.1. Molecular genetic testing

Examples of main genetic testing….. [29].

- **Bone Marrow Transplant Engraftment** [Short tandem repeat (STR) polymorphic DNA markers used to distinguish patient from donor].

3.1.1. Indications for molecular testing

Allogeneic, HLA-matched hematopoietic stem cell transplantation (BMT) related or non-related donor. Donor and recipient specific DNA fragment patterns are utilized to distinguish the origins of each cell population.

3.2. Testing methodology

Applied Biosystems AmpFLSTR Profiler Plus Kit utilizes short tandem repeat (STR) polymorphic DNA markers to distinguish patient and donor cells. Fluorescent multiplex polymerase chain reaction (PCR) is used to amplify the markers.

3.2.1. Interpretation of DNA analysis

DNA isolated from the WCB's (lymphoid or myeloid cells) of the patient and donor is characterized with 10 polymorphic DNA markers prior to the bone marrow transplantation. The patterns are compared and one marker is selected to distinguish donor and patient as uniquely different from one another.

This will be subsequently used to assess the status of donor cell engraftment. In related family members one or more of these markers may demonstrate high incidence of non-identity in the BMT setting. The alleles range in size and heterozygosity.

In the general population, only identical twins have identical DNA profiles at all of these STR loci.When more than one of the ten STR markers has an informative (not identical) pattern between patient and donor, the one that demonstrates the most clearly distinguished differences in size or mobility is selected to follow engraftment status post-transplant. Amelogenin distinguishes X and Y chromosomes and may be used when the patient and donor are not of the same gender. Enriched subpopulations of hematopoietic cells (E.g. T lymphocytes and myeloid cells) may also be assayed

Specimen Requirements: Peripheral Blood--1 lavender-top (EDTA) tube. Invert several times to mix blood. Bone Marrow--Place 1-2 mL of anticoagulated bone marrow in a lavender-top (EDTA) tube. Invert several times to mix bone marrow. Do not freeze, forward promptly at ambient temperature. Buccal swab, cord blood, blood spots, and frozen tissue.

- BRCA Ashkenazi Jewish Mutations

BRCA1 and BRCA2 are human genes that belong to a class of genes known as tumor suppressors. Mutation of these genes has been linked to hereditary breast and ovarian cancer.

A woman's risk of developing breast and/or ovarian cancer is greatly increased if she inherits a deleterious (harmful) BRCA1 or BRCA2 mutation. Men with these mutations also have an increased risk of breast cancer. Both men and women who have harmful BRCA1 or BRCA2 mutations may be at increased risk of other cancers.

Genetic tests are available to check for BRCA1 and BRCA2 mutations (Fig.10). A blood sample is required for these tests, and genetic counseling is recommended before and after the tests. If a harmful BRCA1 or BRCA2 mutation is found, several options are available to help a person manage their cancer risk.

Several methods are available to test for *BRCA1* and *BRCA2* mutations. Most of these methods look for changes in *BRCA1* and *BRCA2* DNA. At least one method looks for changes in the proteins [(PROH-teen) A] molecule made up of amino acids that are needed for the body to function properly. Proteins are the basis of body structures such as skin and hair and of substances such as enzymes, cytokines, and antibodies] produced by these genes. Frequently, a combination of methods is used.

A blood sample is needed for these tests. The blood is drawn in a laboratory, doctor's office, hospital, or clinic and then sent to a laboratory that specializes in the tests. It usually takes several weeks or longer to get the test results. Individuals who decide to get tested should check with their health care provider to find out when their test results might be available.

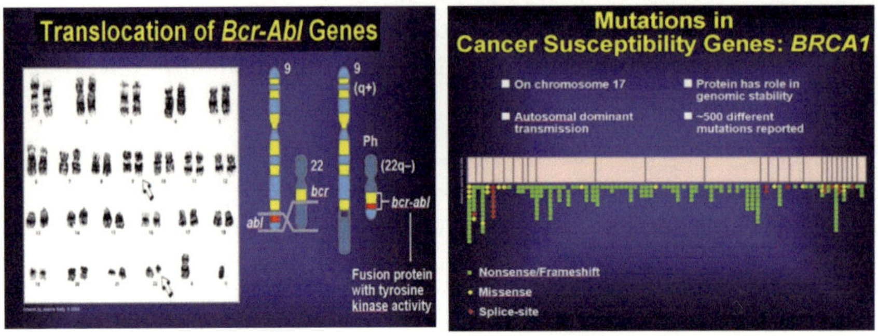

Figure 10. Genetic tests are to check for BRCA1 and BRCA2 mutations

- Cystic Fibrosis Mutation Analysis

Cystic fibrosis (CF) occurs at increased frequency in Caucasians and individuals of Ashkenazi Jewish descent, but can occur in any ethnic group (Fig.11). It is a disorder of mucus production, primarily affecting the pulmonary, gastrointestinal and reproductive systems. Although there is some variability of clinical expression, most individuals with CF require lifelong medical care and experience reduced life expectancy.

Molecular Testing: The preferred sample type is ACD or EDTA anticoagulated blood (pale yellow top or lavender top, 3ml), which may be refrigerated up to 48 hours before analysis. A mutation panel is tested by PCR followed by oligonucleotide ligation assay using commercial analyte specific reagents (ASRs) available through Abbott diagnostics that were validated in laboratory. In diagnostic (as opposed to screening) tests, three polymorphisms that have the potential to confound mutation analysis are also evaluated along with analysis of the intron 8 polypyrimidine tract polymorphism (5T, 7T and 9T). Intron 8 analysis is also done as a reflex test when an R117H mutation is detected because 5T in cis with R117H is a disease-related allele. Individuals of Ashkenazi Jewish descent are tested for D1152H in addition to the routine panel of mutations. Testing for D1152H is performed by the Third Wave InPlexTM CF Assay. Results are reported as either consistent with a diagnosis of CF (two mutations found); at least carrier status (one mutation identified); or no detectable mutation (which reduces the probability of CF or carrier status). We recommend that screening (carrier testing) of the partner of a carrier be sent to an outside laboratory where more extensive mutation testing is possible. When screening is simultaneously requested on both partners, testing is done in-house.

- DNA Fingerprinting

The process begins with a sample of an individual's DNA (typically called a "reference sample"). The most desirable method of collecting a reference sample is the use of a buccal swab, as this reduces the possibility of contamination. When this is not available (e.g. because a court order may be needed and not obtainable) other methods may need to be used to collect a sample of blood, saliva, semen, or other appropriate fluid or tissue from personal items (e.g. toothbrush, razor, etc.) or from stored samples (e.g. banked sperm or biopsy tissue). Samples obtained from blood relatives (biological relative) can provide an indication of an individual's profile, as could human remains which had been previously profiled.

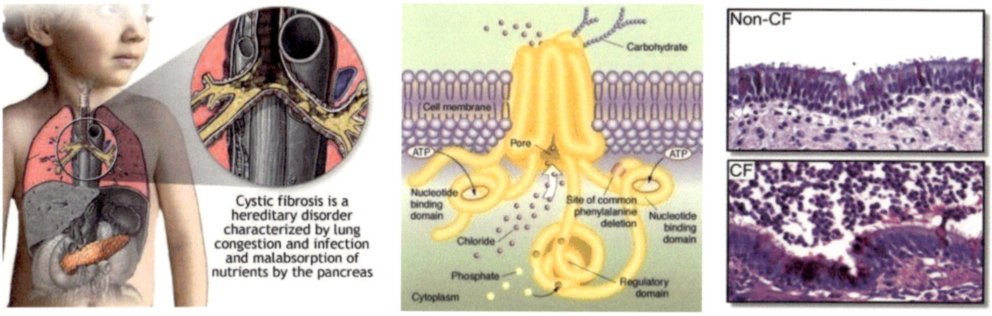

Figure 11. Cystic fibrosis (CF)

A reference sample is then analyzed to create the individual's DNA profile using one of a number of techniques, discussed below. The DNA profile is then compared against another sample to determine whether there is a genetic match.

Another technique, AmpFLP, or amplified fragment length polymorphism was also put into practice during the early 1990s. This technique was also faster than RFLP analysis and used PCR to amplify DNA samples. It relied on variable number tandem repeat (VNTR) polymorphisms to distinguish various alleles, which were separated on a polyacrylamide gel using an allelic ladder (as opposed to a molecular weight ladder). Bands could be visualized by silver staining the gel. One popular locus for fingerprinting was the D1S80 locus. As with all PCR based methods, highly degraded DNA or very small amounts of DNA may cause allelic dropout (causing a mistake in thinking a heterozygote is a homozygote) or other stochastic effects. In addition, because the analysis is done on a gel, very high number repeats may bunch together at the top of the gel, making it difficult to resolve. AmpFLP analysis can be highly automated, and allows for easy creation of phylogenetic trees based on comparing individual samples of DNA. Due to its relatively low cost and ease of set-up and operation, AmpFLP remains popular in lower income countries.

- Factor V Mutation Analysis

Factor V Leiden (F5) point mutation G1691A (Formerly FVL) (Fig.12).

Indications for Molecular Testing. Family history of venous thrombosis- Unprovoked thrombotic event at <45 years of age- Women with multiple stillbirths or spontaneous abortions - Confirmation of diagnosis of F5 by non-molecular means

Testing Methodology. Screening utilizes polymerase chain reaction (PCR) and restriction fragment length polymorphism (RFLP) techniques to detect the Factor V Leiden point mutation (G1691A). The base pair change results in the loss of a recognition site for the restriction enzyme MnlI. (PCR is utilized pursuant to a license agreement with Roche Molecular Systems, Inc.)

Interpretation of DNA analysis. Factor V Leiden, a point mutation (G1691A) in the gene coding for coagulation Factor V, has been associated with an increased risk of venous thrombosis due to increased resistance to degradation of factor V by activated Protein C. For individuals presenting with venous thrombosis, FVL occurs in 11 – 20% of those in all age groups and 50% of individuals under 50 years of age. Heterozygosity for this mutation produces a 7 – fold increase relative risk of venous thrombosis. Approximately 5% of Caucasians are heterozygous for this mutation. The homozygous occurrence of this mutation has been associated with an 80 – fold increased risk for venous thrombosis.

Specimen Requirements [Peripheral blood--1 lavender-top (EDTA) tube. Invert several times to mix blood].

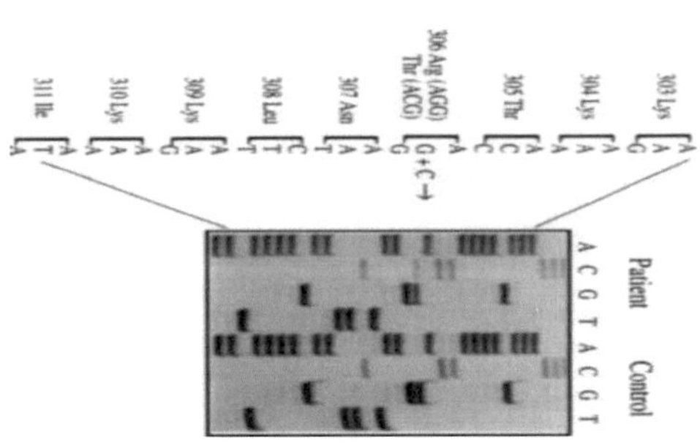

Figure 12. Factor V Leiden (F5) point mutation G1691A (Formerly FVL)

- Familial Mediterranean Fever Mutation

The MEFV gene (Fig.13) provides instructions for making a protein called pyrin (also known as marenostrin). Although pyrin's function is not fully understood, it likely assists in keeping the inflammation process under control. Inflammation occurs when the immune system sends signaling molecules and white blood cells to a site of injury or disease to fight microbial invaders and facilitate tissue repair. When this has been accomplished, the body stops the inflammatory response to prevent damage to its own cells and tissues.

Pyrin is produced in certain white blood cells (neutrophils, eosinophils, and monocytes) that play a role in inflammation and in fighting infection. Pyrin may direct the migration of white blood cells to sites of inflammation and stop or slow the inflammatory response when it is no longer needed. Pyrin also interacts with other molecules involved in fighting infection and in the inflammatory response. Research indicates that pyrin helps regulate inflammation by interacting with the cytoskeleton, the structural framework that helps to define the shape, size, and movement of a cell.

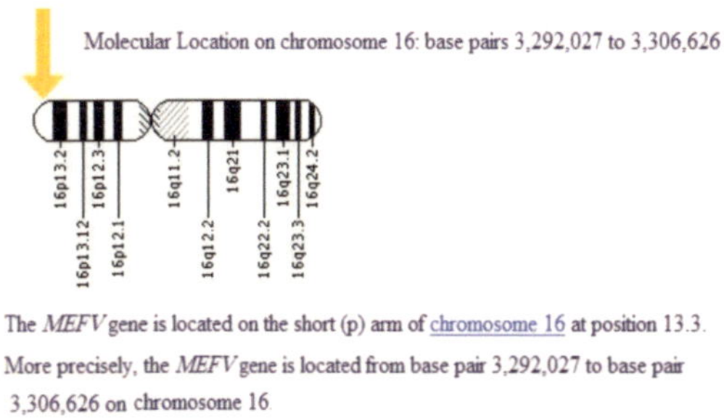

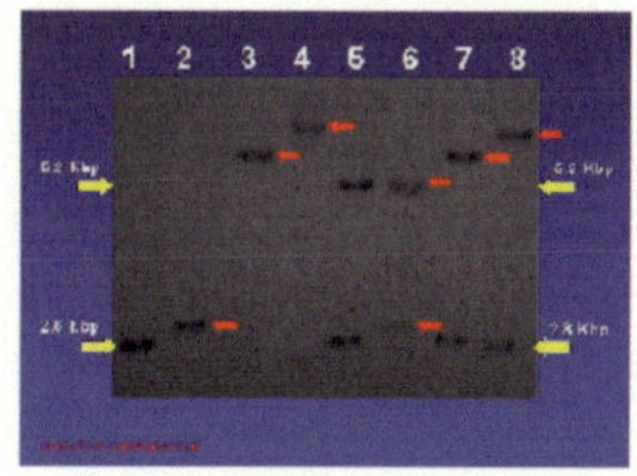

Figure 13. Familial Mediterranean Fever Mutation & Fig.14: Fragile X syndrome (FXS), Martin–Bell syndrome.

- Fragile X Mutation Analysis

Fragile X syndrome (FXS), Martin–Bell syndrome, or Escalante's syndrome (more commonly used in South American countries,Fig.14), is a genetic syndrome that is the most common known single-gene cause of autism and the most common inherited cause of mental retardation among boys. It results in a spectrum of intellectual disability ranging from mild to severe as well as physical characteristics such as an elongated face, large or protruding ears, and larger testes (macroorchidism), behavioral characteristics such as stereotypical movements (e.g. hand-flapping), and social anxiety.

Fragile X syndrome is associated with the expansion of the CGG trinucleotide repeat affecting the *Fragile X mental retardation 1* (*FMR1*) gene on the X chromosome, resulting in a failure to express the fragile X mental retardation protein (FMRP), which is required for normal neural development. Depending on the length of the CGG repeat, an allele may be classified as normal (unaffected by the syndrome), a premutation (at risk of fragile X associated disorders), or full mutation (usually affected by the syndrome). A definitive diagnosis of fragile X syndrome is made through genetic testing to determine the number of CGG repeats. Testing for premutation carriers can also be carried out to allow for genetic counseling.

This molecular test detects the DNA expansion observed in approximately 99% of Fragile X Syndrome carriers or affected individuals. Normal individuals have between about 6 and 50 FMR1 CGG repeats. The FMR1 CGG repeats tend to undergo expansion when repeat numbers exceed about 50. Premutation carrier females and normal transmitting males have between about 50 and 200 repeats. Affected males typically have many more than 200 repeats. Females with an X chromosome having greater than 200 FMR1 CGG repeats may or may not be affected depending on X chromosome inactivation patterns. FMR1 CGG repeats of about 50 to 200 show a dynamic instability directly related to their length, to the sex of the transmitting individual, and to subtle DNA sequence variation within the repeat itself. Premutation alleles tend to be unstable when transmitted by females and stable when transmitted by males (stability in males may be a consequence of selection against expanded FMR1 CGG alleles during spermatogenesis). Repeats greater than about 90-100 repeats have nearly a 100% risk of expansion into the affected range when transmitted by a female. The FMR1 CGG repeat demonstrates significant somatic instability when repeat sizes enter the premutation range. Premutation and larger sized CGG repeats determined from peripheral blood DNA may not reflect FMR1 CGG repeat sizes in other tissues.

- Friedreich's Ataxia Mutation Analysis

Friedreich's ataxia is an inherited disease that causes progressive damage to the nervous system, resulting in symptoms ranging from gait disturbance to speech problems; it can also lead to heart disease and diabetes (Fig.15).

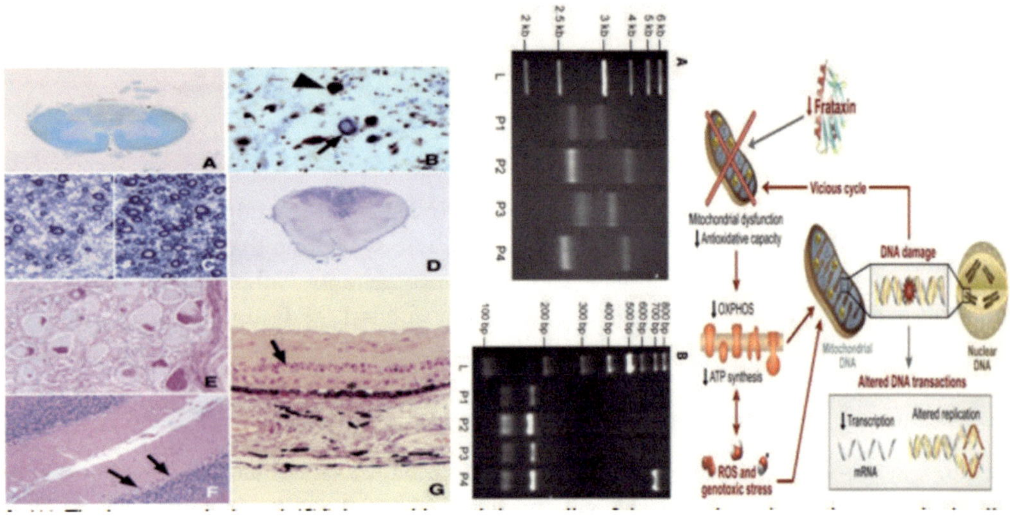

Figure 14. (A) The lower cervical cord (C6) is atrophic, and the myelin of the posterior column shows marked pallor (Klüver-Barrera stains originally×6.0). (B) Numerous axonal spheroids immunostained by antineurofilament antibody, SMI-31 (brown, arrow head) and corpora amylacea by antibiquitin antibody (purple, arrow) in the posterior column nucleus (originally×514). (C) The gracile fasciculi of the upper cervical cord (C3, left) and lower lumbar cord (L2, right) (toluidine blue stain×514), show decreased axon density and thin myelin. These changes are more marked in C3 than those in L2. (D) Lower medulla (Holzer stain originally×4.4). Marked gliosis is present in the gracile and cuneate nuclei. (E) The dorsal root ganglion of right C7 (periodic acid-Shiff originally×210). Ganglion cells are well preserved and Nageotte's nodules are very rare. (F) Cerebellar hemisphere (haematoxylin and eosin originally×64). There is focal loss of Purkinje cells. Purkinje cells have almost disappeared in the upper folium, but are relatively preserved in the lower folium (arrow). (G) Retina (haematoxylin and eosin originally×257). The outer segment layer of photoreceptor cells has disappeared (asterisk) and the outer nuclear layer is not obvious. The inner layers of the retina are thin and atrophic (arrow). Journal of Neurology, Neurosurgery & Psychiatryjnnp.bmj.com- *J Neurol Neurosurg Psychiatry 2000;68:521-525 doi:10.1136/jnnp.68.4.521. Analysis of the GAA trinucleotide repeats expansion in the FXN gene of individuals with Friedreich ataxia. (A) The length of the GAA repeat region in each allele of the FXN gene was determined by long-range PCR and agarose gel electrophoresis. Patient 1, 770 and 870 repeats; Patient 2, 760 and 1170 repeats; Patient 3, 790 and 940 repeats; Patient 4, 650 and 1140 repeats; L: DNA size ladder. (B) PCR products following digestion with MboII. Complete digestion of pure GAA repeat sequences leaves flanking regions of 157 bp and 125 bp. The occurrence of an additional band of ~680 bp in lane P4 indicates the presence of non-GAA sequence within the GAA trinucleotide repeat expansion region [31].*

The ataxia of Friedreich's ataxia results from the degeneration of nerve tissue in the spinal cord, in particular sensory neurons essential (through connections with the cerebellum) for directing muscle movement of the arms and legs. The spinal cord becomes thinner and nerve cells lose some of their myelin sheath (the insulating covering on some nerve cells that helps conduct nerve impulses).

The condition is named after the German physician Nikolaus Friedreich, who first described it in the 1860s [30].

- Hereditary Hemochromatosis

Hemochromatosis gene (HFE) testing is a blood test used to check for hereditary hemochromatosis, an inherited disorder that causes the body to absorb too much iron. The iron then builds up in the blood, liver, heart, pancreas, joints, skin, and other organs (Fig.16).

In its early stages, hemochromatosis can cause joint and belly pain, weakness, lack of energy, and weight loss. It can also cause scarring of the liver (cirrhosis), darkening of the skin, diabetes, infertility, heart failure, irregular heartbeats (arrhythmia), and arthritis. But many people do not have symptoms in the early stages.

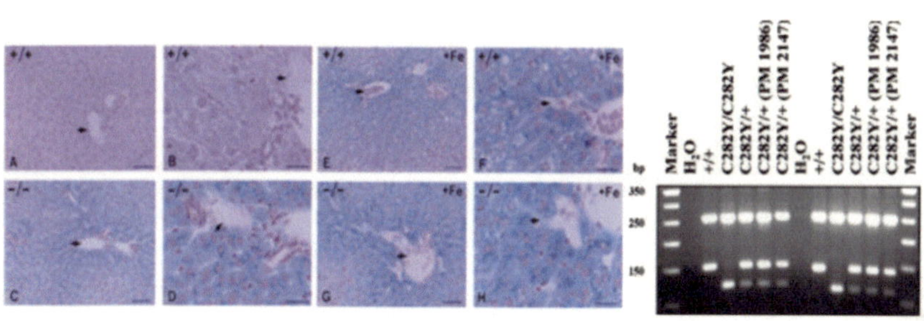

Figure 15. Perls' Prussian blue staining of liver sections from $HFE^{+/+}$ and $HFE^{-/-}$ mice fed control diet (*A–D*) or control diet supplemented with 2% (wt/wt) carbonyl iron (*E–H*). Shown are low-power views (*A, C, E,* and *G*) and high-power views (*B, D, F,* and *H*) of sections. *A* and *B* show the absence of stainable iron in the +/– mouse liver fed the control diet. *C* and *D* show prominent stainable iron in hepatocytes with periportal predominance in liver from $HFE^{-/-}$ mice fed the control diet. *E* and *F* show iron accumulation in $HFE^{+/+}$ mouse liver in response to iron loading. *G* and *H* show the stainable iron in the $HFE^{-/-}$ mice after 2 weeks of feeding with the iron-supplemented diet. The arrows indicate the location of branches of the portal vein. (Bars: *A, C, E,* and *G* = 50 μm in the low-power views; *B, D, F,* and *H* = 20 μm in the high-power views.)

In men, hereditary hemochromatosis is usually found between the ages of 40 and 60. In women, it is not usually found until after menopause because, until that time, women regularly lose blood and iron during their monthly periods. Genetic testing for hemochromatosis involves a simple blood test. DNA from the blood is extracted and the HFE gene is tested for two specific mutations in the gene known to cause the disease in most people. There are two laboratory techniques typically used to detect the two mutations: allele-specific oligonucleotide hybridization (ASO) and restriction fragment length polymorphism (RFLP) analyses. Both of these tests are designed to detect whether a specific mutation is present or absent in a DNA sample. These tests will also determine if an individual is a carrier of either mutation. The two mutations typically tested for are most commonly called C282Y and H63D. The mutations are named based on their location within the HFE gene and the change that they cause in the gene's instructions. The two mutations differ in how frequently they are found in the population, and in how severe your hemochromatosis is if you have them. There are other rare mutations that may predispose individuals towards abnormal iron storage. However they are not yet part of most laboratories testing panels for hemochromatosis.

- Huntington Disease

Huntington's disease (HD) is a neurodegenerative genetic disorder that affects muscle coordination and leads to cognitive decline and psychiatric problems (Fig.17). It typically becomes noticeable in mid-adult life. HD is the most common genetic cause of abnormal involuntary writhing movements called chorea, and indeed the disease used to be called Huntington's chorea.

Because HD follows an autosomal dominant pattern of inheritance, there is a strong motivation for individuals who are at risk of inheriting it to seek a diagnosis. The genetic test for HD consists of a blood test which counts the numbers of CAG repeats in each of the *HTT* alleles [32]. A positive result is not considered a diagnosis, since it may be obtained decades before the symptoms begin. However, a negative test means that the individual does not carry the expanded copy of the gene and will not develop HD [33].

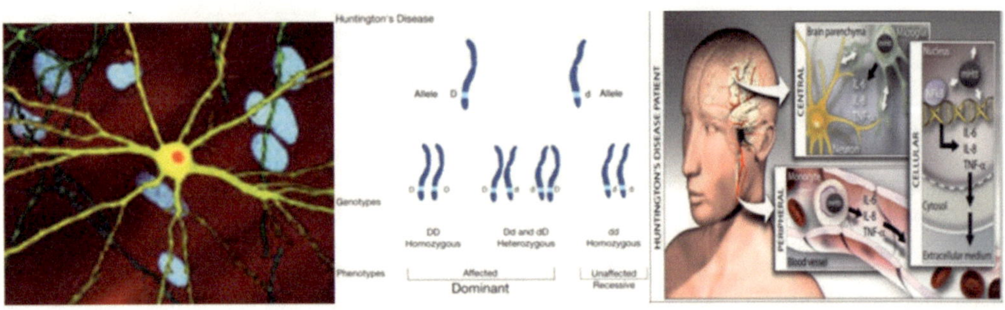

Figure 16. Huntington's disease (HD) is a neurodegenerative genetic disorder that affects muscle coordination and leads to cognitive decline and psychiatric problems. Neuron with inclusion (stained orange) caused by HD, image width 250 μm.

A pre-symptomatic test is a life-changing event and a very personal decision [33]. The main reason given for choosing testing for HD is to aid in career and family decisions [33]. Over 95% of individuals at risk of inheriting HD do not proceed with testing, mostly because there is no treatment.[38] A key issue is the anxiety an individual experiences about not knowing whether they will eventually develop HD, compared to the impact of a positive result [33] . Irrespective of the result, stress levels have been found to be lower two years after being tested, but the risk of suicide is increased after a positive test result [33] . Individuals found to have not inherited the disorder may experience survivor guilt with regard to family members who are affected [12]. Other factors taken into account when considering testing include the possibility of discrimination and the implications of a positive result, which usually means a parent has an affected gene and that the individual's siblings will be at risk of inheriting it. Genetic counseling in HD can provide information, advice and support for initial decision-making, and then, if chosen, throughout all stages of the testing process.[39] Counseling and guidelines on the use of genetic testing for HD have become models for other genetic disorders, such as autosomal dominant cerebellar ataxias [38]. Presymptomatic testing for HD has also influenced testing for other illnesses with genetic variants such as polycystic kidney disease, familial Alzheimer's disease and breast cancer [34].

4. Molecular oncology testing

- B-Cell Gene Rearrangement

The B- and T-cell rearrangement test [35] can detect a monoclonal population of B- and T-cells, strongly indicative of neoplasia. This is accomplished through the use of DNA probes. The presence of a unique band on the Southern blot (Fig.18) signifies a monoclonal gene rearrangement, which can make or confirm a diagnosis of a lymphoproliferative disorder and classify the lineage as B- or T-cell. T-cell neoplasms generally behave more aggressively than B-cell neoplasms, which can have important implications for prognosis and therapy. The unique gene rearrangement "signature" can be followed during and after therapy to document remission or recurrence. The most commonly examined samples are from the blood, bone marrow, and lymph nodes, but any tissue or fluid suspected of harboring a lymphoid neoplasm can be examined.

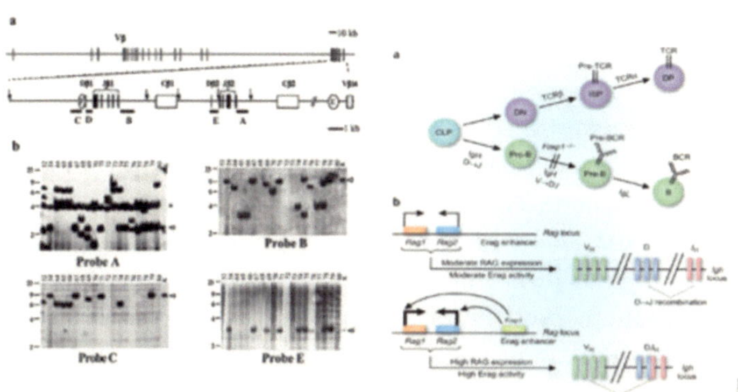

Figure 17. B-Lymphocyte Immunoglobulin; Heavy Chain Gene Rearrangement. Detection of monoclonal B-cell populations in B-lymph proliferative disorders.

This test is indicated for the accurate differentiation of malignant vs. benign lymphoproliferative disorders and for establishing T tumor cell lineage. Clonal proliferations of T lymphocytes can be detected by the identification of specific DNA rearrangements in the T-cell gamma chain antigen receptor gene. The majority of lymphocytic leukemias and non-Hodgkin's lymphomas arise from a clonal proliferation of a single lymphoid cell that has become aberrant. T cells normally differentiate from stem (precursor) cells in a highly specific and sequential manner. The malignant transformation may take place at any stage in the maturation process and when it occurs, the resulting malignant clone bears the characteristics of the originally transformed cell and is called monoclonal. Some of the early events in the maturation process of lymphoid cells involve specific nucleic acid rearrangements within the gamma chain antigen receptor gene in T-cells.

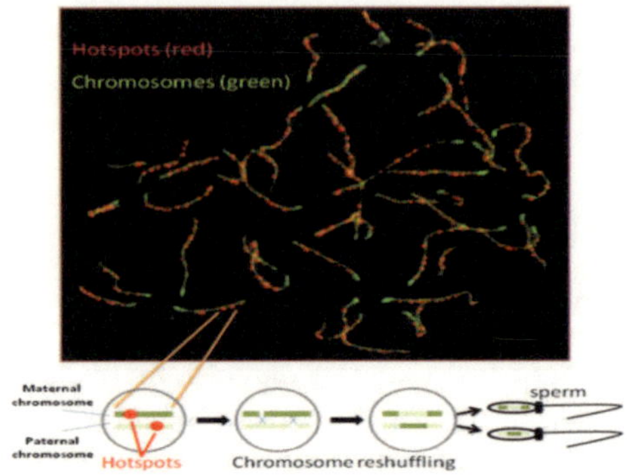

Figure 18. In this image, hundredfold magnification of a single sperm precursor cell shows the chromosomes – in green – and the places where these chromosomes are most likely to break apart and re-form, called genetic recombination hotspots – in red. Genetic rearrangements at these hotspots have the potential to shuffle maternal and paternal chromosomes, the end results of which ensure that the genetic information in every sperm cell is unique. Source: Fatima Smagulova, Ph.D., USU, and Kevin Brick, Ph.D., NIDDK, NIH.

This test is indicated for the accurate differentiation of malignant vs. benign lymphoproliferative disorders and for establishing B tumor cell lineage. Clonal proliferations of B-lymphocytes can be detected by the identification of specific DNA rearrangements in the immunoglobulin gene. The majority of lymphocytic leukemias and non-Hodgkin's lymphomas arise from a clonal proliferation of a single lymphoid cell that has become aberrant. B cells normally differentiate from stem (precursor) cells in a highly specific and sequential manner. The malignant transformation may take place at any stage in the maturation process and when it occurs the resulting malignant clone bears the characteristics of the originally transformed cell and is called monoclonal. Some of the early events in the maturation process of lymphoid cells involve specific nucleic acid rearrangements within the immunoglobulin genes in B cells. To detect B cell gene rearrangements using PCR, primers are constructed to amplify the DNA between the conserved framework (FR) and joining (J) regions. These conserved regions lie on either side of an area within the V-J region where programmed genetic rearrangements occur during maturation. In the germline configuration found in somatic cells, these areas are widely separated (by more than 70KB) making PCR amplification across the area impossible. The sequence alteration brought about by gene rearrangement brings these regions into close proximity, making the area of amplifiable length. Each B cell has a single productive V-J rearrangement that is unique in both length and sequence. The template-free incorporation of nucleotides (N-regions) between the spliced V, D, and J gene segments also adds uniqueness to the PCR product. Therefore, when this region is amplified using DNA primers that flank this region, a clonal population of cells yields one or two prominent amplified products (amplicons) within the expected size ranges. Two products are produced in cases when the initial rearrangement was non-productive and was followed by rearrangement of the other homologous chromosome. In contrast, DNA from a normal or polyclonal population produces a bell-shaped curve (or Gaussian distribution) of amplicon products that reflects the heterogeneous population of V-J region rearrangements. *Specimen:* Whole blood, bone marrow or tissue(10 mL blood; 4 mL bone marrow; 0.2 g or more of tissue)

- BCL-2 Gene Rearrangement

Gene Rearrangement *bcl-2*; Major Breakpoint Region (MBR); minor cluster region (mcr); t(14:18) Translocation. Applies to Follicular B-Cell Lymphomas. A translocation between immunoglobulin genes (heavy chain or light chain genes) and *bcl-2* results in the over expression of *bcl-2* protein and thus the expansion of B cells due to inhibition of cell death. This type of translocation is found in 100% at small cleaved type, 76% to 85% at mixed cell and 59% to 75% at large cell types of Bcell lymphoma. It is found in some cases of chronic lymphocytic leukemia, acute lymphoblastic leukemia, and small noncleaved cell lymphoma as well as some cases of Hodgkin's lymphoma and myeloid neoplasms. The t(14;18) is rarely detected in monocytoid B-cell lymphoma and MALT lymphomas. *bcl-2* rearrangement is not pathognomonic for lymphomas. It is found in 10% of reactive lymph nodes, and in some normal cells (eg, lymphoid and myeloid precursors, medullary thymocytes, T cells, nongerminal center B cells, and plasma cells). It is not expressed in centers.

- BCR-ABL Gene Rearrangement

Translocation *bcr/abl*; Gene Rearrangement *bcr*; Philadelphia Chromosome; t (9:22) Applies to Acute Myelogenous Leukemia (ALL); Chronic Myelogenous Leukemia (CML)

- BRAF Gene Mutation Detection

BRAF is downstream of KRAS in a signaling pathway involved in cell cycling. Both KRAS and BRAF are prone to mutations in sporadic colorectal carcinomas (CRC).

This assay is capable of detecting the V600E mutation in exon 15 of BRAF. The much rarer V600A or V600G mutations would also be detectable. Detection includes PCR amplification and a single-base extension reaction that generates allele-specific fluorescently labeled probes, detectable by capillary electrophoresis.

Several studies have demonstrated that mutations in KRAS lead to constitutive activation of this pathway, which may lead to cancer progression, and this activation results in a failure to respond to anti-EGFR therapy. Recent published results indicate that mutations in the KRAS gene are present in approximately 40% of patients with metastatic colorectal adenocarcinoma, and the presence of a K-ras mutation isassociated with resistance to cetuximab and panitumumab. BRAF mutations are responsible for an additional 12-15% of patients who fail to respond to anti-EGFR treatment. This finding suggests that testing for the BRAF V600E mutation can compliment KRAS mutation analysis and may be as important as KRAS testing for treatment decisions.

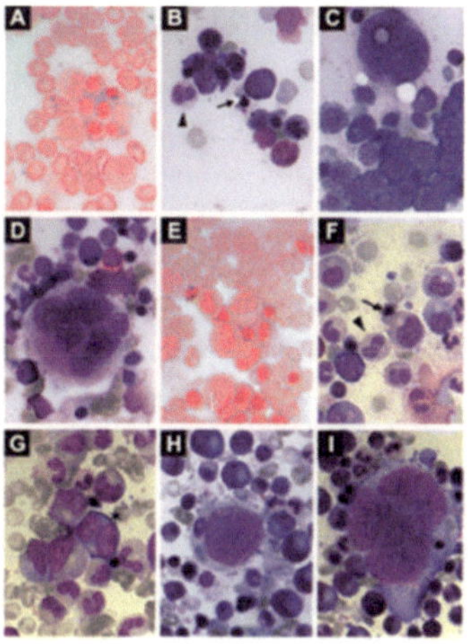

Figure 20. Bone marrow morphology demonstrating both dysplastic and proliferative features in a *JAK* V617F negative patient (n. 511; A-D) and a patient with the mutation (n. 510; E-I). Ringed sideroblastosis (A,E) associated with immaturity, megaloblastoid changes and abnormal nuclear budding (arrows) and binuclearity (asterix) of erythroblasts (B,C,F,G). Dysgranulopoiesis with numerous hypogranular (arrowheads) myeloid cells (B,F,G; Pappenheim's stain). Evidence of both small megakaryocytes with round nuclei and mature cytoplasm (C,H) and large multinucleated forms (D, I). A, E, Perls' stain; B-D, F-I, Pappenheim's stain; × 1000.

- KRAS Gene Mutation Detection

Mutations in the KRAS oncogene are highly prevalent in human tumors, and they most commonly occur in codons 12, 13, and 61. K-ras mutations have been detected in pancreatic, colorectal, lung, endometrial, gallbladder, and thyroid cancer at variable frequency. Accumulating evidence indicates that these mutations may play a role in prognosis and drug response. Specifically, recent published results indicate that mutations in the KRAS gene are present in approximately 40% of patients with metastatic colorectal adenocarcinoma, and the presence of a K-ras mutation is associated with resistance to cetuximab and panitumumab.

The ViennaLab K-ras StripAssay kit will detect 10 KRAS gene mutations in codons 12 and 13: G12V, G12D, G12L, G12S, G12A, G12I, G12C, G12R, G13C and G13D.

Specimen Formalin-fixed paraffin-embedded (FFPE) tissue, 10 precut, unstained slides from paraffin block in 10 μm (10-micron) sections or formalin-fixed paraffin-embedded tissue block containing ≥50% tumor. Either option needs to be accompanied by an H&E reference slide. Detection includes PCR amplification using biotinylated primers, reverse hybridization of PCR products to test strips containing specific mutant oligonucleotide probes, and visualization of bound products with streptavidin-alkaline phosphatase and color substrates.

- Microsatellite Instability

Microsatellites, also known as **Simple Sequence Repeats** (SSRs) or **short tandem repeats** (STRs), are repeating sequences of 2-6 base pairs of DNA.

Microsatellites are typically co-dominant. They are used as molecular markers in genetics, for kinship, population and other studies. They can also be used to study gene duplication or deletion. Microsatellites are also known to be causative agents in human disease, especially neurodegenerative disorders and cancer.

In cells with mutations in DNA repair genes, however, some of these sequences accumulate errors and become longer or shorter. The appearance of abnormally long or short microsatellites in an individual's DNA is referred to as microsatellite instability. **Microsatellite instability** (**MSI**) is a condition manifested by damaged DNA due to defects in the normal DNA repair process. Sections of DNA called microsatellites, which consist of a sequence of repeating units of 1-6 base pairs in length, become unstable and can shorten or lengthen. Microsatellites are also known as simple sequence repeats (SSRs). *Specimen*,1 normal tissue and 1 tumor tissue. Normal tissue may be substituted by a sample blood Each tissue sample must be ≥25 mg.. Amplification by Polymerase Chain Reaction (PCR) of 5 microsatellite short tandem repeats and detection of these alleles by electrophoresis and sizing on an automated fluorescence detector.

Muir Torre syndrome [MTS] is a rare autosomal dominant inherited genodermatosis with malignant potential. It consists of at least one sebaceous gland tumor such as sebaceous adenoma, epithelioma, or carcinoma, with at least one visceral malignancy [40].

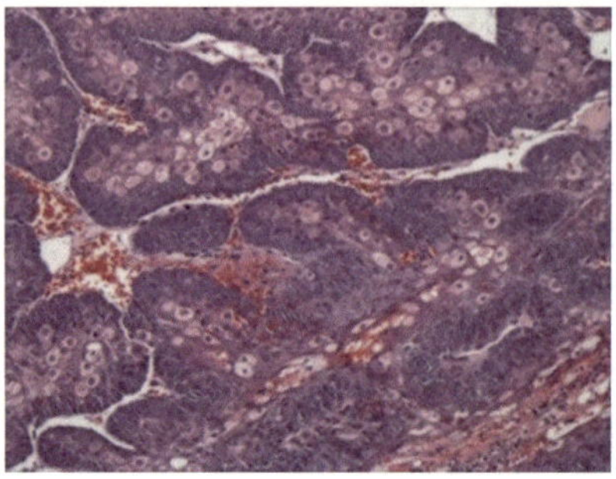

Figure 21. Components of Muir-Torre Syndrome. a). Sebaceous adenoma (100X) b). Colonic mucinous adenocarcinoma (100X).

Genetic mutations have been identified as the cause of inherited cancer risk in some colon cancer-prone families. The most common clinical syndromes associated with these mutations include familial adenomatous polyposis (FAP) and hereditary non-polyposis colorectal cancer (HNPCC). The former is associated with mutations of the APC gene, and the latter with mutations of MLH1, MSH2, MSH6, and PMS2 genes [41]. These inherited syndromes are estimated to account for only 2% to 6% of colorectal cancer cases overall. Turcot syndrome is a clinically defined, inherited syndrome associated with both colorectal cancer and a primary brain tumor.

- PMLRAR Alpha t(15;17) Translocation

AMLs (Acute Myeloid Leukemias, Fig.23) [42] are characterized with chromosomal translocations resulting in the formation of fusion proteins. Understanding PML (Acute

Promyelocytic Leukemia Inducer) function has become an area of intense research because of its involvement in the pathogenesis of APL (Acute Promyelocytic Leukemia), a distinct subtype of Myeloid Leukemia. In the vast majority of APL case studies, the PML gene (on Chromosome-15) fuses to the RAR-Alpha gene (Retinoic Acid Receptor-Alpha) (on Chromosome-17) as a consequence of reciprocal and balanced chromosomal translocations. In the t(15;17) chromosomal translocation, which is specific for APL, PML is found in a reciprocal translocation with the RAR-Alpha resulting in the formation of PML-RAR-Alpha and RAR-Alpha-PML fusion proteins . In a normal cell Vitamin-A (all-*trans*-Retinol) from dietary sources is converted to all-*trans*-Retinoic Acid in the liver through Retinol Metabolism and all-*trans*-Retinoic Acid is translocated to tissues by CRABP (Cellular Retinoic Acid Binding Protein) where it regulates target genes by binding with RARs (Retinoic Acid Receptors). Retinoic Acid is the only metabolite of Vitamin-A which regulates gene expression and all-*trans*-Retinoic Acid, the Carboxylic Acid form of Vitamin-A is of biological significance since it has high circulating levels than other isomers of Retinoic Acid. Biologically active ligands for the RARs include all-*trans*-Retinoic Acid, 9-*cis*-Retinoic Acid among others. 13-*cis*-Retinoic Acid is not a ligand for the RARs, but, it is readily converted into a RAR ligand by intracellular reciprocal isomerization. Less is understood about the fate of intracellular all-*trans*-Retinoic Acid is its isomerization to 9-*cis*-Retinoic Acid and 13-*cis*-Retinoic Acid. The RARs have a conserved modular structure consisting of six regions from A-F, viz., AF-1 or A/B (Amino-Terminal Activating Factor-1 Transcriptional Activation) Domain; a zinc-finger DBD or C (DNA-Binding Domain); a CoR or D (Hinge/Corepressor Binding) Domain; a LBD or AF-2 or E (Ligand-Binding/Transcriptional Activation) Domain; and a variable F (Carboxyl-Terminal) Domain. In RAR the DBD binds to the RARE (Retinoic Acid Response Element) region in the DNA. The RAREs consists of DRs (Direct Repeats) of AGG/TTCA motif with a spacer region of (n)25. Upon Retinoic Acid binding, RAR-Alpha regulates Retinoic Acid mediated gene expression and transactivates PML target genes critical for the induction of Myeloid Hemopoietic Cells' terminal differentiation.

In this assay, extracted RNA is subjected to 2 separate quantitative real-time reverse transcription-polymerase chain reaction (RT-PCR) procedures to detect the 2 types of PML/RARA fusion transcripts (long and short isoforms). An additional amplification for the abl gene is performed as a control for sample RNA quality and as a reference for relative quantification. The results are reported as positive or negative; the ratio of target (PML/RARA) to control (ABL) mRNA is reported for positive specimens. The isoform (short or long) is also reported. If available, a previously stored sample will be tested alongside the current specimen to assess quantitative changes with time (trend). The analytical sensitivity of this test is 1 tumor cell in 100,000 normal cells.

In APL cells due to t(15;17) chromosomal translocation the fusion protein PML-RAR-Alpha retains both DBD and LBD of RAR-Alpha, compete with normal RAR-Alpha for ligand binding and inhibits its transcriptional function through aberrant recruitment of HDACs (Histone Deacetylases). Recruitment of HDACs to PML also leads to inhibition of p53 activity and Sumolation. HDACs therefore, represent an ideal candidate for blocking the action of the fusion proteins. PML-RAR-Alpha and RAR-Alpha-PML fusion protein expression disrupts formation of NBs and paralyzes Tumor Suppression, Cellular Senescence, Mature PML degradation and normal Cell Growth and Survival. Co-expression of RAR-Alpha-PML with PML-RAR-Alpha thus results in an increase of Leukemia incidence and makes a cell more prone to pathogen invasions. All-trans-Retinoic Acid is a standard therapy for the management of APL. However, 13-*cis*-Retinoic Acid and 9-*cis*-Retinoic Acid implication reduce the incidence of secondary head and neck tumors and APL, respectively. It is apparent that PML is essential for critical tumor suppressive pathways that are deregulated in APL and therapies such as induction of Retinoic Acid and As2O3 can be helpful in restoring normal PML function in APL cells that can cause the reappearance of NBs, and the reversal of T-Cell Gene Rearrangement.

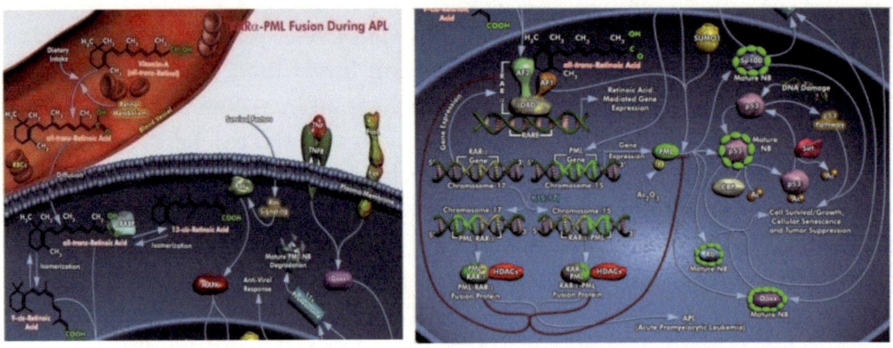

Figure 22. Under normal conditions PML is a potential Tumor Suppressor and is involved in Cellular Senescence, a process that controls Oncogenic Signaling leading to normal Cell Growth and Survival. PML is the organizer of nuclear matrix domains, NBs (Nuclear Bodies), with a proposed role in Apoptosis control. PML being a member of the RBCC (RING-B-Box-Coiled-Coil) Protein Family, contains three Zinc Finger-Like domains (a RING Finger and two B-Boxes) and a Coiled-Coil Dimerization domain. PML organizes NBs by targeting proteins such as Sp100 (Nuclear Antigen-Sp100), p53, Rb (Retinoblastoma) or Daxx onto these domains. These domains are also known as PODs (PML Oncogenic Domain/Promyelocytic Oncogenic Domains). PML levels increase during both Ras-induced Senescence, leading to a dramatic increase in the size and number of PODs. Survival factors/Ras signaling induce Cellular Senescence by up-regulating PML gene expression though MAPK (Mitogen-Activated Protein Kinase) activation. PML is covalently modified and conjugated to SUMO1 (Small Ubiquitin Related Modifier-1). This enables PML to form NBs and enhances their interaction with other proteins. A specific dephosphorylation event triggered by As2O3 (Arsenic Trioxide) targets PML to the nuclear matrix to form Primary PML bodies. Sumolation then induces the maturation to Secondary PML bodies. In mature PML-NBs (or Secondary PML bodies), PML forms the outer shell and many proteins (Sp100, Rb, p53, Daxx, etc) are found within its electron clear core. DNA damage induced activation of p53-dependent Apoptosis requires PML. PML acts as a coactivator for p53 and increases acetylation of p53 by the transcriptional coactivator CBP (CREB-Binding Protein). This acetylation of p53 is reversed by Sirt (Sirtuin (Silent Mating Type Information Regulation-2 Homolog)) releasing p53 into p53 Pathway. PML associates with Daxx-mediated Apoptosis induced by Fas/FasL (Fas Ligand) and TNF (Tumor Necrosis Factor)/TNFR (Tumor Necrosis Factor Receptor) and regulates the transcriptional repressor activity of Daxx. PML acts with Rb and p53 to promote Ras-induced Senescence. PML-Sp100 NBs act against viral invasions. Mature PML-NBs are finally degraded by the 11S Proteasome Complex.

- Immunohistochemistry Stains

Immunohistochemistry is not considered a molecular technique but it is based on the antigen-antibody affinity, it has emerged as a powerful investigative tool that can provide supplemental information to the routine morphological assessment of tissues. The use of immunohistochemistry to study cellular markers that define specific phenotypes has provided important diagnostic, prognostic, and predictive information relative to disease status and biology. The application of antibodies to the molecular study of tissue pathology (Fig.24) has required adaptation and refinement of immunohistochemical techniques, particularly for use in fixed tissues. In contrast to solution-based immunoassays that detect relatively abundant native proteins, in fixed tissues the preservation of antigen is variable and unpredictable. Thus, the history of immunohistochemistry has been a constant effort to improve sensitivity for detection of rare surviving antigenic targets with the ultimate goal of integrating tissue-based analysis with proteomic information.

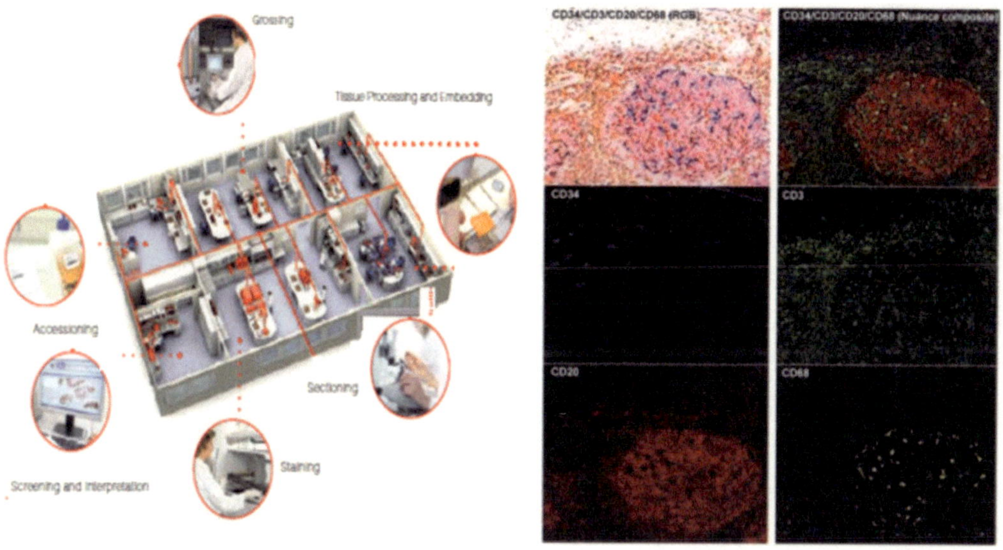

Figure 23. Immunohistochemistry Staining Stages.

- Nanotechnology in clinical laboratory diagnostics

Nanotechnologies enable diagnosis at the single-cell and molecule levels, and some can be incorporated in current molecular diagnostic methods, such as biochips. Nanoparticles, such as gold nanoparticles and quantum dots, are the most widely used, but various other nanotechnological devices for manipulation at the nanoscale as well as nanobiosensors are also promising for potential clinical applications, main applications of nanotechnology [43] .

Nanotechnologies will extend the limits of current molecular diagnostics and enable point-of-care diagnostics, integration of diagnostics with therapeutics, and development of personalized medicine. Although the potential diagnostic applications are unlimited, the most important current applications are foreseen in the areas of biomarker discovery, cancer diagnosis, and detection of infectious microorganisms. Safety studies are needed for in vivo use. Because of its close interrelationships with other technologies, nanobiotechnology in clinical diagnosis will play an important role in the development of nanomedicine in the future.

Author details

Hussein A. Kaoud
Department of Hygiene and Environmental Pollution, Faculty of Veterinary Medicine, Cairo University, Giza, Egypt.

5. References

[1] Andersen MH, Schrama D, Thor Straten P, Becker JC. "Cytotoxic T cells". The Journal of Investigative Dermatology 2006; 126 (1): 32–41.
[2] Boon T, van der Bruggen P. "Human tumor antigens recognized by T lymphocytes". The Journal of Experimental Medicine 1996;183 (3): 725–9.
[3] Castelli C, Rivoltini L, Andreola G, Carrabba M, Renkvist N, Parmiani G . "T-cell recognition of melanoma-associated antigens". Journal of Cellular Physiology 2000;182 (3): 323–31.
[4] Romero P, Cerottini JC, Speiser DE. "The human T cell response to melanoma antigens". Advances in Immunology. Advances in Immunology 2006;92: 187–224
[5] Guevara-Patiño JA, Turk MJ, Wolchok JD, Houghton AN (2003). "Immunity to cancer through immune recognition of altered self: studies with melanoma". Advances in Cancer Research. Advances in Cancer Research 90: 157–77.
[6] Renkvist N, Castelli C, Robbins PF, Parmiani G. "A listing of human tumor antigens recognized by T cells". Cancer Immunology, Immunotherapy 2001;50 (1): 3–15.
[7] Gerloni M, Zanetti M. "CD4 T cells in tumor immunity". Springer Seminars in Immunopathology 21005; 27 (1): 37–48.
[8] Seliger B, Ritz U, Ferrone S. "Molecular mechanisms of HLA class I antigen abnormalities following viral infection and transformation". International Journal of Cancer 2006;118 (1): 129–38.
[9] Hayakawa Y, Smyth MJ. "Innate immune recognition and suppression of tumors". Advances in Cancer Research 2006;95: 293–322.
[10] Seliger B . "Strategies of tumor immune evasion". BioDrugs 2005; 19 (6): 347–54.
[11] Frumento G, Piazza T, Di Carlo E, Ferrini S. "Targeting tumor-related immunosuppression for cancer immunotherapy". Endocrine, Metabolic & Immune Disorders Drug Targets 2006; 6 (3): 233–7.
[12] Stix, Gary. "A Malignant Flame" (PDF). Scientific American 2007;297 (1): 60–67.
[13] Erickson HS, Gillespie JW, Emmert-Buck MR. Tissue microdissection. Methods Mol Biol. 2008;424:433-48.
[14] Pagedar NA, Wang W, Chen DH, Davis RR, Lopez I, Wright CG, Alagramam KN. Gene expression analysis of distinct populations of cells isolated from mouse and human

inner ear FFPE tissue using laser capture microdissection--a technical report based on preliminary findings. Brain Res.2006;1091(1):289-99.
[15] Huang Q, Sacks PG, Mo J, McCormick SA, Iacob CE, Guo L, Schaefer S, Schantz SP. A simple method for fixation and microdissection of frozen fresh tissue sections for molecular cytogenetic analysis of cancers. Biotech Histochem 2005; 80(3-4):147-56.
[16] Shibutani M, Uneyama C. Methacarn fixation for genomic DNA analysis in microdissected cells. Methods Mol Biol 2005; 293:11-25.
[17] Erickson HS, Gillespie JW, Emmert-Buck MR. Tissue microdissection. Methods Mol Biol 2008;424:433-48.
[18] Kryndushkin DS, Alexandrov IM, Ter-Avanesyan MD, Kushnirov VV. "Yeast [PSI+] prion aggregates are formed by small Sup35 polymers fragmented by Hsp104". Journal of Biological Chemistry 2003;278 (49): 49636–43.
[19] Sambrook J, Russel DW. Molecular Cloning: A Laboratory Manual 3rd Ed. Cold Spring Harbor Laboratory Press 2001. Cold Spring Harbor, NY.
[20] Berg JM, Tymoczko JL Stryer L. Biochemistry (5th ed.) 2002. WH Freeman.
[21] http://www.answers.com/topic/gel-electrophoresis#ixzz1viquzJx9
[22] Liotta L, Kohn EC, Petricoin EF. Clinical proteomics: personalized molecular medicine. JAMA.2001;286:2211–2214.
[23] Lau AT, He QY, Chiu JF. Proteomic technology and its biomedical applications. (Shanghai) 2003;35: 965–975.
[24] Paweletz CP, Trock B, Pennanen M, et al. Proteomic patterns of nipple aspirate fluids obtained by SELDI-TOF: potential for new biomarkers to aid in the diagnosis of breast cancer. Dis Markers 2001;17:301–307.
[25] Issaq HJ, Veenstra TD, Conrads TP, Felschow D. The SELDI-TOF MS approach to proteomics: protein profiling and biomarker identification. Biochem Biophys Res Commun 2002;292:587–592.
[26] Copyright 2002 American Cancer Society. Reprinted with permission of Wiley-Liss, Inc, a subsidiary of John Wiley & Sons, Inc.
[27] http://www.wisegeek.com/what-is-oncology.htm
[28] UCLA diagnostic molecular pathology laboratory, Department of Pathology and Laboratory Medicine, David Geffen School of Medicine.
[29] J Neurol Neurosurg Psychiatry (2000);68:521-525 doi:10.1136/jnnp.68.4.521
[30] BioTechniques, Vol. 50, No. 3, March 2011, pp. 182–186
[31] Myers RH. "Huntington's Disease Genetics". NeuroRx 2004;1 (2): 255–62.
[32] Walker FO. "Huntington's disease". Lancet 2007;369 (9557): 218–28.
[33] Hayden MR. "Predictive testing for Huntington's disease: a universal model?". Lancet Neurol 2003; 2 (3): 141–2.
[34] Fatima Smagulova, Ph.D., USU, and Kevin Brick, Ph.D., NIDDK, NIH.
[35] Leukemia 26, 708-715 (April 2012) | doi:10.1038/leu.2011.255
[36] haematol January 1, 2008 vol. 93 no. 1 34-40
[37] Scott LM, Tong W, Levine RL, Scott MA, Beer PA, Stratton MR, Futreal PA, Erber WN, McMullin MF, Harrison CN, Warren AJ, Gilliland DG, Lodish HF, Green ARJAK2 exon

12 mutations in polycythemia vera and idiopathic erythrocytosis. N Engl J Med. 2007;356(5):459-68.

[38] Oki, E.; Oda, S.; Maehara, Y.; Sugimachi, K. "Mutated gene-specific phenotypes of dinucleotide repeat instability in human colorectal carcinoma cell lines deficient in DNA mismatch repair". Oncogene 1999; 18 (12): 2143–2147.

[39] https://www.pathnet.medsch.ucla.eud/referral/ODTCenter

[40] Torre D. Multiple sebaceous tumors. Arch Dermatol. 1968;98 (5):549-51.

[41] Heavey PM, McKenna D, Rowland IR. Colorectal Cancer and the Relationship Between Genes and the Environment. Nutr Cancer. 2004;48(2):124-141.

[42] https://www.qiagen.com/geneglobe/pathwayview.aspx?pathwayID=381&ID=NM_000964,NM_016152,NM_000966

[43] Kewal K. Jain. Nanotechnology in clinicallaboratorydiagnostics. Clinica Chimica Acta 2005;Volume 358, Issues 1–2, Pages 37–54

- c-kit Mutation Detection for Systemic Mastocytosis

Nucleotide substitutions at and adjacent to codon 816 in the catalytic domain of c-kit are common in SM. Detection of a codon 816 c-kit mutation is included as a minor diagnostic criterion in the WHO's diagnostic criteria for SM. Determining mutational status of the c-kit gene also has pharmacogenetic implications in patients considered for investigational mast cell cytoreductive therapies and targeted small-molecule tyrosine kinase inhibitors Sequencing analysis. Polymerase Chain Reaction (PCR) is performed for DNA amplification. Primers are designed specifically for exon 17 of the c-kit gene. PCR products are sequenced and analyzed on the ABI 3130xl Genetic Analyzer.

- JAK2 Mutation Analysis

The *JAK2* V617F substitution, located in the pseudokinase domain of JAK2, relieves the autoinhibition of its kinase activity; the resulting constitutively active kinase augments downstream JAK2-STAT signaling pathways. Other *JAK2* mutations in humans include translocations, point mutations, deletions, and insertions [36, 37]. However, the most frequent mutations are those seen in patients with *JAK2 V617F*-negative polycythemia vera or idiopathic erythrocytosis (Fig.20 and 21), the exon 12 mutations. Documented high-frequency *JAK2* exon 12 mutations include in-frame deletions, missense, and tandem point mutations such as del/F537-K539ins/L, del/N542-E543, K539L, and H538QK539L [38]. Whereas *JAK2 V617F* mutations are typically homozygous (by mitotic recombination), exon 12 mutations are often heterozygous in patients with polycythemia vera. In addition, exon 12 mutations can induce cytokine-independent hypersensitive proliferation in erythropoietin-expressing cell lines and are sufficient for the development of a polycythemia vera-like phenotype in a murine model.

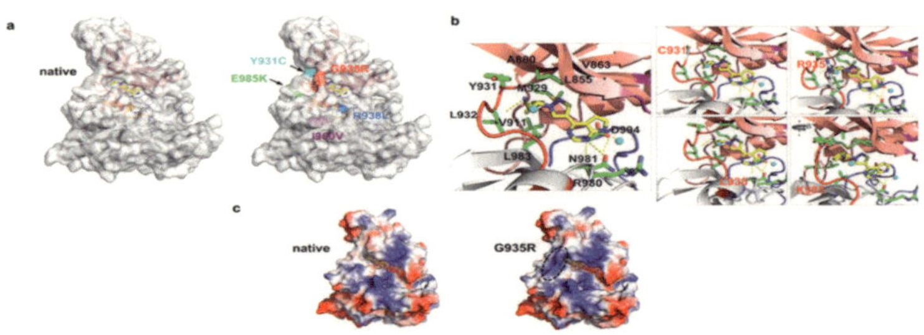

Figure 19. Structural analysis of JAK2V617F kinase domain mutations. (**a**) Cartoon and transparent surface representation of ruxolitinib-docked JAK2 kinase domain (**a**, **b**) (left) and JAK2 with location of point mutations that lead to drug resistance (right). N-terminal lobe (salmon), C-terminal lobe (gray), glycine loop (purple), activation loop (blue) and hinge region (red) form the boundaries for the binding site of ruxolitinib (stick representation in yellow (carbon) and blue (nitrogen)). The I960V side chain (purple) is buried within the protein interior. (**b**) Enlarged ruxolitinib-binding pocket with secondary structure elements (cartoon) and the interactions of the side chains (labeled sticks) with the inhibitor. Hydrogen bonds between the inhibitor and the protein are indicated as dotted yellow lines (one hydrogen bond between backbone of Y931 and L932; and two hydrogen bonds with R980 and N981 and pyrrolopyrimidine ring of the inhibitor; additional hydrogen bonds are with water molecules (cyan spheres) . Mutated amino acids are labeled red (right panels). (**c**) Surface electrostatic potential representation of the native (left) and G935R (right) containing JAK2 JH1 domain with ruxolitinib. Charged surfaces are displayed in shades of blue (positive), red (negative) and white (non-polar) [39].